BIOMEDICAL
COMMUNICATIONS

• • • • • • • • •

Purposes, Audiences, and Strategies

BIOMEDICAL
COMMUNICATIONS

· · · · · · · · · · · · · · · · ·

Purposes, Audiences, and Strategies

Jon D. Miller
Linda G. Kimmel

Center for Biomedical Communications
Northwestern University Medical School
Chicago, Illinois

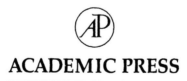

ACADEMIC PRESS
A Harcourt Science and Technology Company

San Diego   San Francisco   New York   Boston   London   Sydney   Tokyo

Contents

· · · · · · · · · ·

PART II
• • • • • • •

COMMUNICATIONS TO INFORM CONSUMERS

PART III
•••••••

COMMUNICATIONS TO INFLUENCE PUBLIC POLICY

PART IV
• • • • • •

BIOMEDICAL COMMUNICATION POLICIES
FOR THE 21st CENTURY

12. POLICIES TO IMPROVE BIOMEDICAL COMMUNICATIONS   287

APPENDIX A. QUESTIONNAIRES   309

Acknowledgments

Biomedical Communications is a data-based analysis of communications. It is built on a set of national surveys, some of which were designed and conducted by the authors of this book and some of which were conducted by other organizations.

To a large extent, the intellectual roots of this project grew from the 1993 Biomedical Literacy Study, sponsored by the National Institutes of Health through a joint agreement with the National Science Foundation. David Chananie was an ideal project officer, providing constructive guidance and keeping us on schedule and on task. Joan Bailey (NIH) provided important technical assistance in launching the project, and Don Dillman (Washington State University), Willie Pearson Jr. (Wake Forest University), Peter Rossi (University of Massachusetts), Antonio Rigual (Our Lady of the Lake University, San Antonio), and Alan Levy (University of Illinois) provided invaluable substantive and statistical advice for the project.

The data from the Science and Engineering Indicators studies, sponsored by the National Science Foundation, provided important change measures over time. Jennifer Bond (NSF) was an exemplary program officer, sharing a basic commitment to the importance of good time series measures and an understanding of the importance of scholarly inquiry as a part of this process. Throughout the past two decades, the members of the National Science Board have been unwavering supporters of the measurement of public understanding and attitudes, and we are grateful for that commitment in good budget years and in not-so-good budget years.

The 1998 Social and Behavioral Indicators Study provided useful insights into the process of information acquisition and use. Norman Anderson (then at NIH, now at Harvard), Virginia Cain (NIH), and Margaret Huyck (then at NIH, now at the Illinois Institute of Technology) provided invaluable leadership in conceptualizing and launching the project. Tom Smith, Director of the General Social Survey (National Opinion Research Center), provided both administrative leadership and substantive insights into the development and conduct of the study.

The 1997–1998 U.S. Biotechnology Study was designed to provide a parallel survey to the work of the Eurobarometer and provided additional insights into the biomedical communications process. Funded by the NSF, we are grateful for the support of Jennifer Bond, without whose commitment to cross-national studies this work would not have taken place, and to our colleague and co-investigator Tom Hoban (North Carolina State University) for his extensive understanding of consumer information and attitudes toward biotechnology.

Equally important, we are grateful to the approximately 16,000 adults who took the time to talk with an interviewer and share some information about their lives and activities. Survey research depends on a broad public commitment to openness in our public discourse, and we are most grateful to those adults who have withstood the abuses of telemarketers and continued to be willing to participate in responsible telephone surveys.

We are grateful to Graham Lees from Academic Press for his original interest in this project and for his advice and encouragement in shaping this book. The conversion of a manuscript into a book requires extraordinary efforts by a wide array of talented people. We are indebted to Noelle Gracy from Academic Press for her encouragement and patience and for her occasional haiku. Brian Rose provided a good technical editing of the book, Kathy Nida provided production management, and Liz Miller provided invaluable proofreading and editing help.

Despite the kind and generous help from all of those listed above, we are sure that some errors have escaped our notice and we urge our readers to share their observations, findings, and suggestions with us at j-miller8@northwestern.edu or l-kimmel@northwestern.edu.

Jon D. Miller
Linda G. Kimmel

A BASIC FRAMEWORK

1

....

USING RESEARCH TO IMPROVE BIOMEDICAL COMMUNICATIONS

....

The challenge of communicating biomedical information to the broader public is as old as medical research itself. From the early struggles of Joseph Lister to persuade the public, as well as his fellow physicians, of the existence of germs and the importance of sterilization to more recent struggles to educate the public about the transmission of the AIDS virus, the task is challenging because it often means changes in traditional beliefs and behaviors in response to new biomedical knowledge that is poorly understood by the vast majority of adults at any point in time. With the invention of radio, television, personal computers, optical fibers, satellite telecommunications, high-speed printing presses, and relatively cheap paper manufacture, the twentieth century has experienced a revolution in the speed and reach of communications. With the extraordinary growth of satellite communications and the Internet in recent years, we have become a global village in a manner that even McLuhan did not foresee in the 1970s.

In fact, the problem for most Americans has become how to filter, evaluate, organize, store, and manage the vast array of communications that they receive daily. Most Americans have available on a daily basis numerous television channels, dozens of radio stations, at least one daily newspaper with national and international wire services, hundreds of magazines, thousands of videotapes, and thousands of books. A 1999 national study (NSB, 2000) found that, on average, Americans watch 1017 hours of television each year, including 431 hours of television news and 42 hours of science television shows. Seventy-eight percent of Americans—approximately 155 million individuals—live in a household serviced by a television cable or a television satellite system. It is clear that these new technologies make a difference in information acquisition patterns: Americans living in households served by cable watched an average of 48 hours of science television shows compared to 20 hours for persons living in households without cable or satellite services.

The first broadcast medium—the radio—is still a major source of information and entertainment. The average American adult reported listening to 918 hours of radio broadcasts in 1999, including 228 hours of radio news. For individuals who spend a large number of hours in a vehicle or in a work setting in which they can listen, but not watch, radio remains an important communications channel.

Print-based communications remain an important source of information for a significant segment of the public. In 1999, the typical American reported reading 178 newspapers each year, visiting a public library 9 times, and borrowing 11 books from a public library (NSB, 1998). Magazines are an important source of information for many Americans, becoming increasingly specialized in their audience definition and editorial content. In 1999, three of five American adults—about 144 million individuals—claimed to have bought one or more books during the previous year, and 33 percent of adults indicated that they have purchased one or more scientific or technical books (including computer books) in the preceding 12 months.

The new era of electronic computer-based communications is already here for most Americans. A majority—65 percent—of American adults reported that they used a computer at home, work, or both in 1999. Forty-two percent of American adults use a computer in their work and 54 percent reported having a computer at home. Thirty-one percent of adults used a computer at work and at home. Nearly half of Americans live in a household that includes a computer with a modem. In 1999, the average American used a computer 421 hours at work and 153 hours at home. It is important to recognize that most of the information presently transmitted through computer-based systems is still in a text format, requiring reading and information management skills similar to those needed to utilize a traditional library.

THE STUDY OF HUMAN ATTITUDES AND BEHAVIORS

Since the 1950s, social scientists have documented and studied the transformation of the United States and other major industrial nations into information-oriented societies. In broad strokes, this literature may be classified as (1) primarily descriptive studies with some reference to theory, (2) experimental and quasi-experimental studies focused on specific messages or information campaigns, or (3) multivariate analyses designed to use data to test models of development and change in human attitudes and behaviors. Throughout the following chapters, the relevant literature will be discussed in conjunction with each analysis rather than as a separate freestanding review. It is important, however, to introduce at this point the major analytic ideas that are the intellectual foundation of this book.

The fundamental objective of all social science and communications research is to identify those factors that are responsible for the development, maintenance, and change of human knowledge, attitudes, and behaviors. Parallel to the categorization of the biomedical communications literature proposed above, scholars have utilized observation and description, experimentation, and model building as strategies or techniques for seeking to understand and explain human learning, attitudes, and behaviors. It is important to understand the role, value, applicability, and limitations of each of these techniques.

Most science and social science began with observation and description, and these remain necessary and useful tools in understanding human learning, attitudes, and behaviors. Indeed, observation and description should be viewed as the original empirical method, enhanced over the centuries by improvements in writing, printing, photography, and audio and visual recording devices. Inherently, description must precede explanation or understanding.

Although observation and description are necessary, they are rarely sufficient for understanding human learning, attitudes, or behaviors. There are several fundamental limitations to observation. First, there are numerous factors or variables that operate simultaneously in human events, and it is difficult to sort out the influence of each factor or variable by simple observation. For example, if you wanted to know whether a particular brochure was effective in communicating information about a set of early warning signs for a certain kind of cancer, you might go to a local shopping mall and ask several people to read the brochure and rate its clarity and effectiveness. After several hours, you may have talked to five men and five women. Three of the women and two of the men were able to describe the early warning signals correctly after reading the brochure. Two of the women who were able to correctly identify the early warning signs were college graduates, as was one of the men. One of the three women who was able to describe the early warning signs correctly was of Hispanic descent, as was one of the women who could not recall the information after reading the brochure. One of the two men who was able to describe the early warning signs was an African-American. From these conversations, what might we conclude about the effectiveness of the brochure in communicating the early warning signs for a particular kind of cancer? Not much. The process of observation may provide some rich and suggestive details about individual cases, but a more rigorous analytic technique is required to sort out the relative effectiveness of the brochure among different age groups, among men and women, and among individuals with differing levels of education.

Second, the observation procedure described above did not check to see how much information each person held prior to reading the brochure, thus it is impossible to determine whether the ability to list the early warning signs was the result of the brochure or of prior education or from reading other materials elsewhere. When we ask about the impact of a brochure on the level of understanding, we are asking about a potential change in human learning or knowledge.

Third, the selection of a convenience sample in a shopping mall is not a representative sample of the population of the community, the city, the state, or the nation. Sometimes, this informal selection approach is formalized into a focus group format, but focus groups are nearly always composed of volunteers rather than randomly selected respondents, thus most focus groups should be viewed as a slightly more formal observation and description approach.

One of the major social science inventions of the twentieth century was the work of Fisher in developing the concept of randomized assignment of subjects (plants in Fisher's case) to control and treatment groups and the development of statistical procedures for the analysis of the results. Although the randomized experimental model controls for all possible background variables and isolates the impact of the treatment variable, it does not control for the selection of the original pool of cases or respondents. Nonetheless, it is a powerful tool for understanding the impact of definable interventions, such as the example of a brochure about early warning signs discussed above. Returning to this example, a rigorous test of the impact of this brochure might select a random sample of adults in a community and ask each person selected to answer some question about early warning signs. A randomly selected half of this pool of respondents would be asked to read the brochure and then answer the same questions about early warning signs that they were asked some days earlier. The other half of the original sample—the control group—would not be given the brochure, but would be asked the same questions a second time. As a result of this procedure, it would be possible to isolate the impact of the brochure from general background information available in the media and from other sources and to eliminate all other variables as explanatory factors for any changes in the level of awareness or understanding of the early warning signs.

Unfortunately, the range of applications of a rigorous experimental model in biomedical communications is limited. If, for example, we want to understand the impact of children in the home on an adult's level of understanding of biomedical science concepts, we cannot randomly assign children or families to adults. Families are preexisting groups, and we cannot randomly modify the education, age, or gender of the family members. For problems of this kind, the development of models provides a useful tool for seeking to identify the relative impact of factors such as age, gender, and education that are related to each other and may be independently related to a knowledge, attitudinal, or behavioral outcome of analytic interest. This book will make extensive use of models of knowledge, attitudes, and behaviors, thus it is important to discuss some of the basic premises of models as a preface to the chapters that follow.

Models may be thought of as empirical tests of theories about human learning, attitudes, or behaviors, or various combinations of those outcomes. By carefully selecting variables thought to be influential on a selected outcome and by collecting systematic information about a relatively large and representative sample of respondents, it is possible to specify the relationships that we would expect among these factors and to determine how accurately measures of these independent factors can predict the outcome variable of interest. In more concrete terms, to estimate the importance of formal education in the development of a positive attitude toward biomedical research, we might interview a national sample of adults and collect information about each individual's educational background, their attitude toward biomedical research, and other variables that we might think relevant to the formation of this attitude. If we were able to use the measures of age, gender, and education to predict each individual's attitude toward biomedical research with a high degree of accuracy, we would think that these factors were important influences on the development of an individual's attitude toward biomedical research.

It is important to recognize that a high level of prediction does not prove the existence of a relationship or a set of relationships. It is always possible that several of the variables included in the model were caused by another variable that was omitted from the model and that the relationships found are spurious. The likelihood of a completely spurious model decreases markedly with the inclusion of more variables in a model and, when possible, with repeated measures over a period of time. In the spirit of Karl Popper's work, however, the absence of a high level of prediction would tend to discount, or falsify, the plausibility of the expected relationships. A low level of prediction may mean that other important variables have been left out of the model, or it might mean that the outcome measure includes a high level of noise and is not related to any other variable or measure.

In the chapters that follow, a series of models will be presented that will seek to predict the level of biomedical literacy, interest in health information, attitudes toward biomedical and biotechnology policies, and other outcome variables. In this usage, prediction is a measure of the degree of fit between what our model projects to be the outcome—given the variables included in the analysis—and the actual data collected in national surveys. When the level of fit is relatively high, we should have more confidence that the relationships specified in the model are realistic, and we should have correspondingly less confidence in the results of poorly fitting models. The use and interpretation of models will be revisited in the chapters and analyses that follow. The use of models is an important tool in understanding human behavior, and we hope that readers will become sufficiently comfortable with the concept to eventually take ownership and use it in their own thinking.

TWO PURPOSES FOR BIOMEDICAL COMMUNICATION

It is important to distinguish between two basic, but different, purposes that biomedical communications are designed to serve. First, most biomedical communications are designed to convey health and medical information to individuals to assist them in making nutritional, medical, and behavioral decisions, or to help them identify conditions or symptoms that merit examination by a health professional. Ranging from news releases provided by the *New England Journal of Medicine* to recipes distributed by the American Heart Association, a large and growing volume of messages are provided for media and public consumption on a continuing basis.

Second, some biomedical communications are designed to stimulate citizens to become aware of and concerned about a particular problem and to join in the policy formulation debate. For example, numerous health organizations and facilities may become concerned about the level of governmental support for biomedical research generally, or for a specific disease or problem, and urge citizens to pressure their legislators to support higher appropriations for this purpose. Other organizations or institutions may develop communications to encourage citizens to intervene in the public policy process to allow or prohibit a specific biomedical procedure. The analyses included in this book will examine the structure of policy preferences in the public, identify segments of the public mostly likely to participate in a biomedical policy dispute, and outline strategies to improve the effectiveness of this kind of communication.

Although this differentiation of purposes may seem obvious, it is often ignored or misunderstood in practice.

A FRAMEWORK FOR THINKING ABOUT BIOMEDICAL COMMUNICATION

In four parts, organized into 12 chapters, this book seeks to provide a general introduction to the current levels of biomedical literacy in the United States, examine the communication of messages to inform consumers and potential patients about specific health issues or problems, examine the communication of messages designed to influence public policy, and to set these processes in the general context of the political and communications systems of modern American society. Using data from recent national studies, the analysis will describe present patterns of knowledge, attitude, and information acquisition; discuss some of the implications for communicators and communications programs; and outline strategies to enhance the effectiveness of biomedical communication.

In this initial section, Chapter 2 will introduce the concept of biomedical literacy and provide some national estimates, using studies from 1988 to 1999. Although a part of these discussions will inevitably involve some technical terminology, all readers—with and without statistical training—should be able to follow the basic line of argument and the implications for biomedical communications. Additional technical information for interested analysts is provided in footnotes and appendices.

Part II focuses on the communication of health and medical information to consumers and potential patients. Chapter 3 will examine the level of interest in health information, and Chapter 4 will describe current patterns of health and medical information acquisition by consumers, linking these patterns to basic population segments. Chapter 5 will explore in greater depth the dominant information acquisition patterns for several populations that are often the targets of biomedical communications: senior citizens, parents of young children, adult men, adult women, adolescents and young adults, African-Americans, and Hispanic-Americans. Part II will conclude, in Chapter 6, with a general model of health and medical communications for consumers and the presentation of specific strategies to improve this kind of communications.

Communications designed to inform citizens about biomedical and biotechnology policy issues are the focus of Part III. Chapter 7 will describe the process of biomedical and biotechnology policy formulation in the American political system and introduce the concepts of political specialization and issue attentiveness, which will provide a useful framework for understanding the evolving role of interest groups in American politics. The acquisition of biomedical and biotechnology policy information will be examined in Chapter 8. The concept of attitudinal schema—general organizing units that filter, organize, and interpret biomedical news and events—will be introduced in Chapter 9, along with a comprehensive analysis of the development of specific biomedical policy attitudes. Chapter 10 will present a parallel analysis of the development of public awareness of and attitudes toward biotechnology policy in the United States. Part III will conclude in Chapter 11 with a general model of biomedical/biotechnology policy communications and the presentation of specific communication strategies to influence public policy.

Part IV of this book, consisting of Chapter 12, will place the preceding analyses in the more general context of American educational, communications, and political systems. To a large extent, the baseline for biomedical and biotechnology communications must reflect the predominant knowledge level of high school graduates, thus the role of formal educational systems in transmitting basic health and scientific information will be the focus of the first section of Chapter 12. This analysis will describe the present range of baseline knowledge held by precollegiate students and discuss specific strategies for intervention in this system. The second section of Chapter 12 will review the present patterns of adult information acquisition and examine the resources available for enhancing adult understanding of health, biomedical, and biotechnology issues. The third section of Chapter 12 will discuss the formulation of biomedical and biotechnology policy, including the role of the attentive public in the resolution of disputes unresolved by policy leaders and decision-makers. Chapter 12 will conclude with a discussion of an agenda for biomedical communications research.

THE NEED FOR FEEDBACK

This is the first edition of this book. Like all works based on current data, it will age over the next few years. If this approach and this material prove to be useful for communicators, subsequent editions should reflect the experiences of practicing communicators and program managers. Your comments, corrections, and suggestions are encouraged and welcomed. The most efficient means of sharing your ideas, comments, and suggestions is through e-mail at j-miller8@northwestern.edu. Ordinary mail may be directed to the authors at the Center for Biomedical Communications, Ward 18-142, Northwestern University Medical School, 303 East Chicago Avenue, Chicago, Illinois 60611.

2

•••••••••

THE PUBLIC UNDERSTANDING OF BIOMEDICAL SCIENCE

•••••••••••••••••

In the course of everyday life, individuals encounter a wide array of biomedical terms and concepts. The evening television news may report that medical researchers have identified the gene or set of genes responsible for a particular disease. A magazine advertisement may promote a food product as being low in cholesterol and infer that it will reduce the likelihood of heart disease. A newspaper story may discuss the safety and effectiveness of a particular pharmaceutical product, basing the discussion on the results of an experiment involving several hundred patients. A movie or television drama may involve the unintentional release of a genetically modified virus into the atmosphere. The scope and depth of understanding of biomedical terms and concepts will differ among individuals, ranging from virtually no recognition of any of these terms to a comprehensive understanding of all of the concepts.

The very nature of communication assumes a language. The preceding list of examples illustrates the breadth and diversity of biomedical concepts and terms that might occur in only a limited list of possible news stories. As a foundation for communicating with individuals and groups of individuals about biomedical concepts, it is essential to have a summary measure of the scope and depth of individual understanding of a core set of biomedical terms and concepts. Although it is often interesting to look at the percentage of individuals able to identify selected terms and concepts correctly, the results of single items are inherently too narrow to serve as an indicator of understanding that is helpful for communicating health and biomedical information to individuals or groups of individuals.

How much biology or biomedical science does the public need to know? How would a citizen use this information? These are basic and important questions concerning the public understanding of science and technology generally, and they are particularly important in regard to the biomedical sciences. As noted in the previous chapter, the two major purposes of biomedical communications are to inform consumers and patients about personal and public health matters and to inform citizens about public policy issues involving biomedical science. Although the kind of biomedical information needed for each of these purposes may differ to some degree, there is a core of terms and concepts that are essential for either of these purposes.

Building on previous work by Miller (1983a, 1987a, 1989, 1995, 1998) defining civic scientific literacy, the public understanding of biomedical science is conceptualized as having two dimensions—one that reflects a vocabulary of basic terms and concepts and a second that reflects an understanding of the nature of scientific inquiry. A basic vocabulary of biomedical terms and concepts is needed to be able to read a newspaper report on a new medical discovery or to judge the relative merits of contrasting arguments about government policy in regard to funding for biomedical research. A citizen who does not understand the role of DNA in living systems is likely to have a great deal of difficulty in understanding a news story about the identification of a gene related to a particular disease or disorder and the implications of this finding for his personal health in the years ahead. Similarly, a citizen who does not understand the difference between a bacterial infection and a viral infection may not be able to understand a news report about the growth of bacteria resistant to a particular antibiotic and relate that report to the reluctance of her physician to prescribe an antibiotic for her cold. At the policy level, a citizen who does not understand the genetic basis of many diseases may be unable to reconcile substantial government expenditures for the study of molecular biology with a commitment to cure cancer.

At the same time, it is important for consumers, patients, and citizens to understand the nature of scientific inquiry, which is the foundation of virtually all biomedical and biotechnology research. The nineteenth century saw a period of popularity for medical tonics and elixirs that their salesmen claimed would cure a wide range of diseases and conditions and produce happiness. In the postwar decades in the United States, there have been major disputes over substances such as Krebiozen and Laetrile, whose advocates claimed would cure cancer, but for which there was no accepted empirical data. At least once a week, major U.S. newspapers and television newscasts report the results of one or more medical studies, often including a brief mention of the nature of the study and the number of subjects included. This pattern of reporting will undoubtedly increase in the years ahead, and it is important that consumers and citizens understand the empirical nature of scientific investigation and the general structure of experimental methods. It is also important that informed adults learn that nonempirical approaches such as astrology provide no information comparable in reliability to the cumulative results of scientific investigation.

THE MEASUREMENT
OF BIOMEDICAL LITERACY

Fortunately, several major studies conducted in the United States in recent years included a broad set of knowledge questions that allow an estimation of the number of Americans who understand a sufficient set of biomedical terms, concepts, and methods to make informed health and medical decisions for themselves and their families and to follow and participate in public discourse about biomedical policy issues. The National Science Board's *Science and Engineering Indicators* studies have included a sufficient set of biomedical vocabulary and process measures to allow the estimation of a biomedical literacy score in 1988, 1990, 1995, 1997, and 1999. The 1993 Biomedical Literacy Study asked a national sample of adults a wide range of knowledge, behavior, and attitude questions about health and biomedical matters, and this National Institutes of Health (NIH)-sponsored study was designed to disproportionately sample African-Americans, Hispanic-Americans, and Other Americans[1]—including educational oversampling—to allow reliable racial and ethnic comparisons. The 1998 U.S. Biotechnology Study included a broad set of biomedical and agricultural biotechnology knowledge items with sufficient overlap with the preceding U.S. studies to provide another measurement of biomedical literacy as well as a link to a 19-nation study that included Canada, Norway, Switzerland, and the 15 member states of the European Union (Table 2-1).

Although previous studies of civic scientific literacy—including the physical sciences, earth sciences, and biological sciences—have found two separate, but closely related, measures of (1) a vocabulary of terms and constructs and (2) an understanding of the nature of scientific inquiry, these two dimensions merge into a single measure when applied to biomedical literacy. Using standard confirmatory factor analysis procedures, it is possible to identify a set of items that measure biomedical vocabulary and a set of items that measure an understanding of scientific inquiry, but the two measures

[1]Other Americans is a Census Bureau category that includes all individuals who are not classified as African-Americans or Hispanic-Americans. In the present analysis, Other Americans refers to all adults aged 18 and over who are not African-American or Hispanic-American.

Table 2-1 Knowledge and Process Questions Used in Index of Biomedical Literacy

				Percent correct			
	SEI[a] 1988	SEI 1990	NIH[b] 1993	SEI 1995	SEI 1997	Biotek 1998	SEI 1999
Open-ended definition of scientific study	17	18	22	16	23	29	21
Open-ended explanation of experiment	—[c]	—	22	27	39	37	35
Multipart question on probability (1-in-4)	57	52	55	54	53	50	55
Open-ended definition of DNA	22	24	19	21	22	—	29
Open-ended definition of molecule	—	—	—	—	11	15	13
Open-ended definition of radiation	—	—	—	11	11	—	—
Open-ended definition of bacteria	—	—	9	—	—	—	—
Agree that "The oxygen we breathe comes from plants"	81	85	84	85	84	—	85
Disagree that "Antibiotics kill viruses as well as bacteria"	26	30	—	40	43	48	45
Agree that "It is the father's gene that decides whether the baby is a boy or a girl"	—	—	—	64	62	—	66

Disagree that "The earliest humans lived at the same time as the dinosaurs"	37	47	—	48	51	—	51
Open-ended explanation of acid rain	10	15	—	7	—	—	—
Open-ended explanation of the health effects of the thinning of the ozone layer	—	29	32	—	—	—	—
Disagree that "All bacteria are harmful to humans"	—	—	82	—	—	86	—
Disagree that "Senility is inevitable as the brain ages and loses tissue"	—	—	46	—	—	49	—
Disagree that "Ordinary tomatoes do not contain genes while genetically modified tomatoes do"	—	—	—	—	—	43	—
Disagree that "Human beings can survive on almost any combination of foods, provided the total diet includes enough calories"	—	—	42	—	—	39	—
Number of respondents	2041	2033	1628	2066	2000	1076	1882

[a]SEI = *Science and Engineering Indicators.*

[b]NIH = National Institutes of Health.

[c]— = Not asked.

15

are correlated at .95 or higher in each of the 7 years for which reliable data are available, indicating that individuals who score high (or low) on a measure of biomedical vocabulary score equally high (or low) on a measure of understanding scientific inquiry. Given the virtually identical nature of these two measures, it is appropriate to combine these items into a single Index of Biomedical Literacy, which will provide a more statistically reliable measure than two smaller separate measures.

The 1988, 1990, 1995, 1997, and 1999 *Science and Engineering Indicators* studies; the 1993 Biomedical Literacy Study; and the 1998 Biotechnology Study all included sets of questions to measure each respondent's understanding of basic biomedical concepts and the nature of scientific inquiry. Because each of these studies was developed for somewhat different purposes, the terms and concepts included in each study differed slightly, but there were numerous questions that appeared in two or more studies (Table 2-1). Because each question provides some additional information about each respondent's level of biomedical understanding, it is important to include as many of these items as possible in our analysis. Fortunately, modern testing and measurement methods provide a good statistical technology for placing all of these separate questions on a single metric, producing a comparable total score for biomedical literacy. Known as item response theory (IRT), this technique—often used in major tests such as the Graduate Record Examination—allows the development of a common metric under overlapping sets of items or the same set of items given to different groups at different times (Bock and Aitkin, 1981; Bock and Zimowski, 1997; Zimowski *et al.*, 1996).

Because the Index of Biomedical Literacy will be used extensively in subsequent chapters, it is important to examine the items included in this measurement. Although the measures of vocabulary and process understanding merged into a single index statistically, it is useful to discuss the selection of the items and the rationale for their inclusion in terms of the two dimensions. We recognize that some readers may find this extended discussion of measure to be tedious, but communicators are increasingly expected to be involved in the measurement and evaluation of information programs and campaigns, and it is important to understand some of the logic and rationale for the development of a measure such as the Index of Biomedical Literacy.

A Vocabulary of Biomedical Terms and Concepts

A vocabulary of basic biomedical terms and concepts is an essential component of biomedical literacy. Whereas a sound biomedical vocabulary might include several hundred words or concepts, it is obviously impossible to measure any individual's full vocabulary in the context of a personal or telephone interview. It is possible, however, to identify a set of words, terms, and concepts that is sufficiently central to an understanding of biomedical science to serve as a reasonable estimator of an individual's full biomedical vocabulary. In the studies used in this analysis, the basic objective was to identify sets of words, terms, and constructs that would be necessary to read an article or report in a popular publication such as the Tuesday science section of the *New York Times.*

The simplest approach would be to write several questions about health or medicine and then sum the number of correct responses. This approach is often seen in a health or medical information quiz in a newspaper or magazine. There are, however, important limitations to this approach. In terms of elementary test theory, the items that are summed into a total score ought to correlate positively with each other. Decades of research on test construction have demonstrated that there is a structure to virtually any set of test items, but that some structures provide more accurate and reliable test results than other structures.

Looking at the substantive items included in the seven studies included in this analysis, a significant number of items were asked in an open-ended format. This approach effectively eliminates the guessing component of responses to multichoice questions, and requires each respondent to demonstrate both understanding and vocabulary in providing a response. Because respondents in telephone surveys always have the option of hanging up and terminating the interview, it is important to provide an escape option for individuals who have no idea about a particular item. This objective is achieved by asking a two-part question:

> *In articles and on television shows, the term DNA has been used. When you hear the term DNA, do you have a clear understanding of what it means, a general sense of what it means, or little understanding of what it means?*

Respondents who reported having a clear understanding or a general sense of the term were then asked:

> *Please tell me, in your own words, what is DNA?*

The interviewer entered each respondent's response into a computer, and the responses were later read and coded independently by graduate-student coders. Individuals who reported that they had little understanding of the term were not asked to provide an open-ended explanation.

Similar open-ended questions were asked about the meaning of molecule, radiation, and bacteria in various studies during the 1990s. Other open-ended questions were asked about the sources and consequences of acid rain and about the possible health consequences of a thinning of the ozone layer around the earth. These items are good indicators of the level of biomedical literacy and generally had the highest loadings on the factor analyses for each of the seven studies included in this analysis.

To gain additional information about the level of respondent understanding of biomedical science, a series of closed-ended questions were included in all seven of the studies used in this analysis. The standard format for these questions is reflected in the following introduction to a series of closed-ended knowledge questions:

> *Now, I would like to ask you a few short quiz-type questions such as you might see on a television game show. For each statement that I read, please tell me if it is true or false. If you don't know or aren't sure, just tell me and we will skip to the next question. Remember, true, false, or don't know.*

For the construction of the Index of Biomedical Literacy, the following items from these series were used:

The oxygen we breathe comes from plants.

Antibiotics kill viruses as well as bacteria.

It is the father's gene that decides whether the baby is a boy or a girl.

The earliest human beings lived at the same time as the dinosaurs.

All bacteria are harmful to humans.

Senility is inevitable as the brain ages and loses tissue.

Ordinary tomatoes do not contain genes while genetically modified tomatoes do.

Human beings can survive on almost any combination of foods, provided the total diet includes enough calories.

As noted above, some of these items were asked in some years, but not in other years (Table 2-1). The equating and calibrating techniques in IRT-based measurement allow the construction of a set of difficulty coefficients for each item that act as relative weights. A more difficult item would have a higher weight, and a less difficult item would have a lower weight. If a respondent answered an item correctly, he or she would get the full value of the item. If a respondent answered an item incorrectly, he or she would get no value for their response. Using this approach, it is possible to compute a score for each individual on a common metric even though some individuals took one set of items and other individuals took a partially different—but partially overlapping—set of items.

An Understanding of Scientific Inquiry

The second essential component of biomedical literacy is an understanding of the nature of scientific inquiry. It is important for citizens to be able to distinguish between scientific investigation and nonscientific or pseudoscientific approaches, especially in media reports of biomedical research and claims. Looking back on the public debates on issues such as the fluoridation of water and the efficacy of Laetrile, those citizens who understood the need for empirical testing and the logic of experimentation had a much better chance of comprehending and evaluating the competing claims offered in the media by scientists and pseudoscientists.

The primary difficulty in measuring the public understanding of scientific inquiry is that science does not utilize a single uniform procedure. Whereas the biomedical sciences rely heavily on experimental procedures, some sciences, such as astronomy, depend primarily on observation, measurement, and model building and testing. Other sciences, such as paleontology, depend on fossil discovery, classification, and the construction or integration of possible developmental sequences, in the context of our growing understanding of molecular biology and the broader knowledge of biological systems. Under the broad umbrella of scientific endeavor covered by the biomedical sciences, virtually all of these approaches are utilized to some degree.

What is central to all scientific endeavor, however, is the effort to build theories or models to enhance our understanding of nature and the materials and processes found in nature. Parallel to the theory building process is a commitment that all theories must be subject to logical or empirical falsification. Some individuals are able to conceptualize scientific inquiry at this level and utilize this conceptualization in reading and thinking about news reports concerning biomedical research.

At a slightly less sophisticated level, some individuals think of scientific inquiry primarily in terms of experimental investigation. In some cases, this may reflect a basic understanding of scientific ideas as being subject to testing. Popper's concept of falsification is not widely understood by nonscientists, and most people think that scientists prove their theories or ideas, much as a mathematician might prove a theorem. In this context, then, a second important level of public understanding of scientific inquiry involves a view of science as the conduct of experimentation.

Below these theory and experimentation levels, some people hold a simpler view of science, thinking of it as a combination of rigorous comparison and precise measurement. This view is largely devoid of any notion of theory building. Most often, this view of science lacks any understanding of experimentation as the use of random assignment and control groups, or any appreciation of the purposes for those procedures. This view does see science as being empirical in character and precise in its measurements, often resulting in a view of science as "testing" against some known standard. It is not a very sophisticated view, but most individuals holding this view would have greater confidence in a product that was "tested scientifically" than one that was not so tested.

To measure each individual's understanding of the nature of scientific inquiry, the Index of Biomedical Literacy includes three question sets. Some questions necessarily involve a set or sequence of questions rather than a single inquiry.

Scientific Study

Each respondent was asked an initial screening question and then an open-ended question concerning the meaning of a scientific study:

When you read news stories, you see certain sets of words and terms. We are interested in how many people recognize certain kinds of terms and I would like to ask you a few brief questions in that regard. First, some articles refer to the results of a scientific study. When you read or hear the term scientific study, do you have a clear understanding of what it means, a general sense of what it means, or little understanding of what it means?

IF CLEAR UNDERSTANDING OR GENERAL SENSE: In your own words, could you tell me what it means to study something scientifically?

The resulting open-ended response is coded by a set of independent coders into a multilevel classification reflecting the levels of understanding described above. Respondents who provided an answer that included theory building, experimentation, or comparative measurement were coded as correct.

Experiment

Beginning in the 1993 Biomedical Literacy Study, each respondent was asked a two-part open-ended question concerning the rationale for an experiment:

Now, please think of this situation. Two scientists want to know if a certain drug is effective against high blood pressure. The first scientist wants to give the drug to 1000 people with high blood pressure and see how many experience lower blood pressure levels. The second scientist wants to give the drug to 500 people with high blood pressure, and not give the drug to another 500 people with high blood pressure, and see how many in both groups experience lower blood pressure levels. Which is the better way to test this drug? Why it is better to test the drug this way?

All respondents were asked the follow-up probe, regardless of which group they selected. This decision proved to be essential to assessing these responses. Among the 76 percent of individuals who selected the two-group design in the 1993 study, the open-ended probe found substantial misunderstanding of the rationale for experimental design. A substantial portion of this group—representing approximately 32 percent of the total population—indicated that they selected the two-group design so that if the drug "killed a lot of people," it would claim fewer victims since it would have been administered to fewer subjects. This is not the understanding of experimental logic that one would infer from the selection of the two-group design and illustrates one of the hazards of closed-ended questions. In the 1993 study, approximately 22 percent of American adults selected the two-group design and were able to explain the logic of control groups. An additional 20 percent of Americans interviewed selected the two-group design and provided a general rationale that included a "comparison" between the two groups, but lacked the language or logic of control groups. A similar pattern was found in the 1995, 1997, and 1999 *Science and Engineering Indicators* studies and in the 1998 Biotechnology Study.

Probability

Each respondent in all seven studies was told about a couple who wanted to have a baby, but were informed by their doctor that there was a one-in-four chance that a child of theirs would have an inherited illness. Each respondent was then offered four possible explanations of the meaning of this one-in-four probability and asked to agree or disagree with each of the four choices. The four queries were:

(a) *Does this mean that if their first three children are healthy, the fourth will have the illness?*

(b) *Does this mean that if their first child has the illness, the next three will not?*

(c) *Does this mean that each of the couple's children will have the same risk of suffering from the illness?*

(d) *Does this mean that if they have only three children, none will have the illness?*

Agreement with statement (c) and disagreement with the other three statements was coded as correct. Agreement with more than one statement was coded as incorrect even if it included agreement with statement (c).

An Estimate of Biomedical Literacy

Although it is useful to think of biomedical literacy as being composed of two separate dimensions, an empirical examination of the responses from more than 12,000 respondents in seven national studies since 1988 found that the two dimensions were so highly correlated that they are best represented by a single factor, and therefore, a single score. Using the IRT methods described above, the mean Index of Biomedical Literacy increased from 45.4 in 1988 to 51.2 in 1999 (see Figure 2-1). It is apparent that the mean level of biomedical literacy in the United States has been relatively stable during the 1990s.

A comparison of the mean score on the Index of Biomedical Literacy in 1988 and 1999 indicates that the growth in the public understanding of biomedical science has been relatively uniform across major educational and demographic classifications (see Figure 2-2). Biomedical literacy was strongly associated with formal education. Individuals who did not complete high

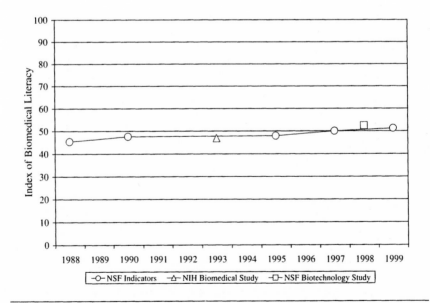

Figure 2-1   Mean biomedical literacy score, 1988 to 1999.

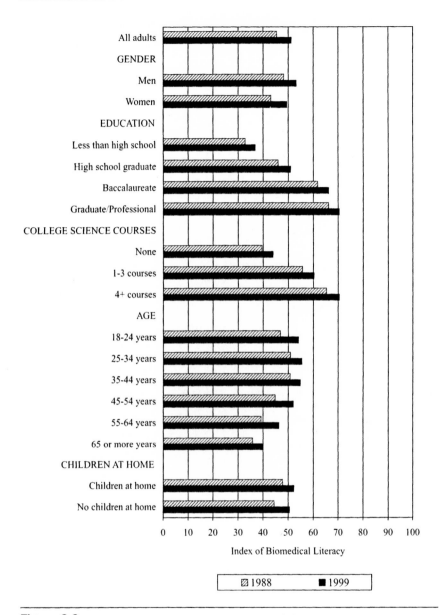

Figure 2-2   Mean biomedical literacy score, 1988, 1999.

school had a mean score of 32.8 in 1988 and a mean score of 36.8 in 1999, while graduate and professional degree holders had a mean score of 66.0 in 1988 and 70.4 in 1999. Clearly, adults with more years of formal education were more likely to be biomedically literate in both 1988 and 1999, and the difference between the two groups remained relatively the same. Men were slightly more likely to be biomedically literate than women in both 1988 and 1999.

What level of biomedical literacy is adequate? This is a difficult question and one that demands careful thought and discussion.

For managing one's personal and family health and for following biomedical policy issues, a higher level of knowledge and understanding is more desirable than a lower level. Although the selection of a single cut-point to describe biomedical literacy is inherently arbitrary, individuals with very low scores on the Index of Biomedical Literacy have an inadequate framework to understand or utilize a great deal of currently available information about personal health and wellness issues. Conversely, individuals with high scores on the Index of Biomedical Literacy are more likely to be able to read biomedical news stories in newspapers and magazines and use the information to make better decisions on both personal health matters and on public policy issues.

To estimate how many individuals are inadequately informed about biomedical matters and how many are sufficiently literate to be able to understand and utilize biomedical information, it is necessary to venture into

Table 2-2   Percent Correct on Biomedical Literacy Items, by Grouped Total Score, 1999

	Biomedical literacy score		
	0 thru 49	50 thru 69	70 or more
Open-ended definition of scientific study	3.2	25.8	63.7
Open-ended explanation of experiment	9.1	47.6	82.5
Multipart question on probability (1-in-4)	29.9	75.9	88.3
Open-ended definition of DNA	2.1	36.2	88.6
Open-ended definition of molecule	1.8	3.7	60.5
Agree that "The oxygen we breathe comes from plants"	77.8	93.5	92.1
Disagree that "Antibiotics kill viruses as well as bacteria"	20.3	65.2	79.3
Agree that "It is the father's gene that decides whether the baby is a boy or a girl"	53.3	77.7	80.1
Disagree that "The earliest humans lived at the same time as the dinosaurs"	42.5	51.4	75.1
Number of respondents	942	597	342

making cut-point decisions. Working from the general observation that individuals with low scores on the Index of Biomedical Literacy will have substantially more difficulty understanding and using biomedical information, it is useful to look at the percentages of individuals with low scores who were able to answer each of the knowledge questions correctly. Looking at all of the individuals with a score of less than 50 on the Index of Biomedical Literacy in 1999, fewer than 3 percent of these individuals were able to define the meaning of DNA or a molecule, and only 9 percent were able to describe the meaning of an experiment (see Table 2-2). Only 20 percent knew that antibiotics do not kill viruses, and only 30 percent could apply the meaning of a probability of one-in-four. We can be reasonably comfortable in saying that individuals with a score of less than 50 on the Index of Biomedical Literacy are inadequately informed about biomedical science.

At the other end of the distribution, an examination of the percentage of individuals with a score of 70 or more on the Index of Biomedical Literacy answering each of the knowledge items correctly suggests that virtually all of these individuals have a sufficient level of understanding of basic biomedical concepts to be able to read a biomedical story in the Tuesday *New York Times* or to follow a *Nova* show on a biomedical subject (see Table 2-2). Nearly 90 percent of this group was able to provide a correct definition of DNA in response to an open-ended question in 1999, and the same proportion was able to apply the meaning of one-in-four chances to a concrete health issue.

It is important to note the difference in the performance of these three groupings on the three open-ended questions and on the multipart probability question. Although half of any group of respondents should be able to answer a true–false question by guessing alone, open-ended questions re-

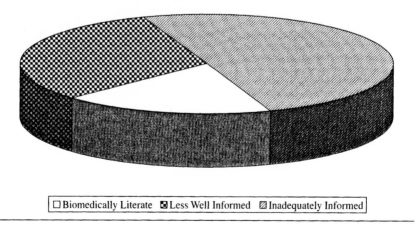

☐ Biomedically Literate   ☒ Less Well Informed   ▨ Inadequately Informed

Figure 2-3   **Proportion of American adults biomedically literate, 1999.**

quire a respondent to utilize their retained understanding of a concept to make a response. Thus, only 2 percent of individuals with a score of less than 50 were able to define the meaning of DNA, compared to 89 percent of individuals with a total score of 70 or more on the Index of Biomedical Literacy. Although open-ended knowledge questions are more difficult to collect and score, they are invaluable in estimating the level of retained understanding held by an individual or group of individuals.

Using these groupings, approximately half of American adults were inadequately informed about biomedical science in 1999 and 18 percent were well-informed, or biomedically literate (see Figure 2-3). The remaining 32 percent of adults displayed a level of biomedical understanding higher than the lowest group, but not sufficient to understand and use biomedical information proficiently for either personal health decisions or for public policy participation.

A Basic Learning Model for Biomedical Literacy

To develop sound communication strategies, it is necessary to go beyond the categorization of individuals by level of biomedical literacy and seek to understand the relative influence of major background, educational, and experiential factors on the level of biomedical literacy. As noted in Chapter 1, it is not feasible to design experiments to randomly assign education, for example, but it is possible to construct models that use these background variables as predictors of an outcome and then compare the predicted result to the actual result recorded for the same individuals. The basic technique that will be used in these analyses—structural equation modeling—has a mathematical basis. We will attempt to describe the use and results of this methodology without extensive statistical discussion. When possible, necessary statistical information will be provided in footnotes and appendices.

In thinking about the personal characteristics and factors that influence the likelihood that an individual will be biomedically literate, the most likely source of biomedical knowledge is formal education. It is reasonable to expect that individuals who have completed a baccalaureate and taken several college-level science courses, for example, would have a larger biomedical vocabulary and would be more likely to understand the nature of scientific inquiry than individuals without those educational experiences. Because this analysis will look closely at the impact of media use in later chapters, a simple measure of news reading (in newspapers, newsmagazines, science magazines, or health magazines) is included in the model to illustrate the relative placement and role of information acquisition, and it is reasonable to expect that individuals who read one or more news sources regularly would

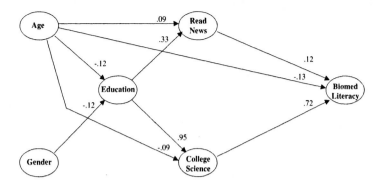

Figure 2-4 A path model to predict biomedical literacy, 1997.

be more likely to be biomedically literate than individuals who do not regularly read major news sources. It is a simple conceptualization, but one that is often ignored in the rush to explore the impact of a new brochure or public service message.

The basic design of the model is shown in a path diagram (see Figure 2-4). The model is structured so that all of the background variables are placed on the left side of the model, and influence is assumed to flow from left to right in the path diagram. In this basic learning model, each respondent's age and gender is placed on the left side of the model, because these characteristics are acquired at birth and cannot be influenced by subsequent variables, such as education. The level of formal education completed, however, may be influenced by an individual's age or gender or both. The number of college-level science courses taken is undoubtedly influenced by the level of formal education completed and could have been influenced by either age or gender. The likelihood that an individual will be a regular reader of newspapers, newsmagazines, and health or science magazines may be influenced by age, gender, and the level of formal education attained. Although it is possible that news reading might be influenced marginally by the number of college-level science courses taken, this model treats the number of college science courses taken and the frequency of news reading as two logically (but not necessarily chronologically) parallel activities that are both included by the level of educational attainment. All of these variables may have some influence on the likelihood that an individual is biomedically literate.

In a path model, a line—called a path—between two variables means that there is a significant relationship between those two variables and the direction of the arrow shows the expected direction of the influence. The number above, or close to, the path is called a path coefficient and is an in-

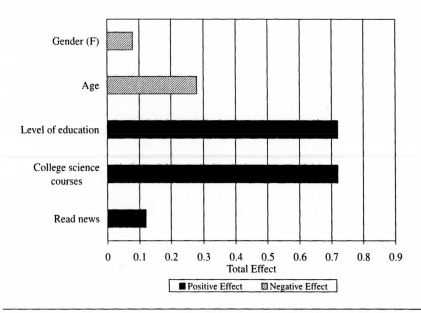

Figure 2-5   Total effects of selected factors on biomedical literacy, 1997.

dicator of the relative influence of the one variable on the other variable. An examination of the two paths from respondent age to education and to current news reading frequency in a 1997 national study may illustrate the nature of paths and path coefficients. The path from age to education has a coefficient of −.12, meaning that older persons are likely to have slightly less formal education than younger respondents. The path from age to news reading frequency has a coefficient of .09, which indicates that older respondents were likely to read slightly more newspapers, newsmagazines, and health and science magazines than younger respondents, holding constant the level of formal educational attainment and the gender of the respondents. The direct path from age to biomedical literacy means that, after all of the other variables in this model are taken into account, older adults are slightly less likely to be biomedically literate than younger adults.

It is possible to estimate the total influence of each of the variables in the model by multiplying all of the coefficients in each possible path to the outcome variable—biomedical literacy—and then summing all of the paths that go from that variable to the outcome variable. For example, age has five paths that reach biomedical literacy, illustrating the complex impact of what are often thought of as simple background variables. One path runs from age to education to college science courses to biomedical literacy. A second path runs from age to education to news reading to biomedical literacy. A third path runs from age to news reading to biomedical literacy. A fourth path runs from age to college science courses to biomedical literacy. And, a fifth path runs directly from age to biomedical literacy. When the coefficients in these paths are multiplied and summed, the total influence of age on biomedical literacy is $-.28$ (see Figure 2-5), meaning that younger persons are more likely to qualify as biomedically literate than older respondents.

Looking at the estimates of total effects, it is clear that formal education and the number of college science courses taken are the major predictors of biomedical literacy, each with an estimated total effect of .72. Regular reading of newspapers and magazines had a small positive total effect of .12, suggesting that keeping up with the news has some additive effect, but it is icing on the educational cake. The total effect of gender was $-.08$, indicating that men were slightly more likely to be biomedically literate than women, holding constant differences in age, education, college science courses, and news reading, but the magnitude of the difference is not substantively important when compared to educational effects and college science course effects higher than .70.

In the discussion of models in Chapter 1, the point was made that the degree of confidence that a reader might have in these relationships should reflect the fit of the predicted outcomes to the observed outcomes. There are several indicators of fit, but the multiple R^2 is the simplest. The R^2 for this model is .65, indicating that 65 percent of the total variance in the model is accounted for, or explained, by the variables in this basic learning model. All of the other fit indicators confirm that this is a good fitting model and that we should have a high level of confidence in the relationships described above.

Differences by Gender

In the preceding model, the results indicated that gender does not substantially influence the likelihood that an individual is biomedically literate. It is possible, however, that there are structural differences in the ways that men and women combine formal education, college-level science courses, and news reading to become or remain biomedically literate. Because structural differences could be important in thinking about biomedical communication strategies, the previous model was run with men and women treated as two separate groups, but using a common metric for comparison. The results found several interesting differences.

First, there is an important structure difference in the relationship between age and education for men and women (see Figures 2-6 and 2-7). Although the combined model showed a small negative relationship between age and education $(-.12)$, the separate models indicate that there is a substantial negative relationship between age and education for women $(-.20)$

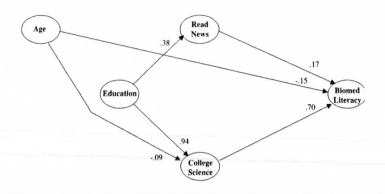

Figure 2-6   A path model to predict biomedical literacy among men, 1997.

and no relationship between age and educational attainment for men. This result reflects the impact of the veterans' educational benefits programs for men who served in the Second World War and in the Korean War. During those years, millions of young men were offered support for as much education as they could complete successfully, fostering a social revolution in American society. Since fewer women served in the armed forces and the social conventions associated with the beginning of the post-World War II baby boom, fewer young women in the 1940s and 1950s entered post-high school education. While this gap has now been closed and reversed—a higher percentage of female high school graduates enter and complete college than young men—the stronger negative path coefficient between age and educational attainment for women reflects the educational opportunity differ-

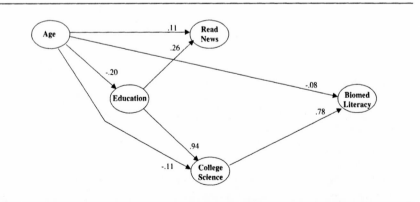

Figure 2-7   A path model to predict biomedical literacy among women, 1997.

Table 2-3   Total Effects of Selected Factors, by Gender, 1997

	Total effects	
	Men	*Women*
Age	−.21	−.31
Level of education	.72	.73
College science courses	.70	.78
Reads news	.17	.00
R^2	.67	.64

entials prior to the 1960s or 1970s. This difference is summarized in the total effects of age, with a total age effect of −.21 for men and −.31 for women (see Table 2-3).

Second, reading current news is related to biomedical literacy among men, but not among women (see Figures 2-6 and 2-7). This result suggests that women rely more on formal education for health and medical information and that their use of current news sources does not significantly improve their biomedical literacy score.

Without entering into a technical discussion of model building, these results demonstrate the error of taking simple two-variable tabulations—the common tables presented in most reports—at face value. The mean scores shown in Table 2-3 indicate that men, individuals with more years of formal education, and individuals with some college science courses tend to have higher biomedical literacy scores, but it masks important structural differences. Although the model for all adults suggested that gender had only a minor effect (−.08), the separate analyses of men and women indicated that the root cause was a significant difference in educational opportunity and experience and not something uniquely related to gender itself. The magnitude of the importance of education is shown more clearly from the model results than from the simple tables.

Differences by Race and Ethnicity

Following the same process used in the analysis of gender differences, the basic model was re-run using data from the 1993 NIH Biomedical Literacy Study and treating African-Americans, Hispanic-Americans, and Other Americans as three separate groups. In this case, the analysis found several interesting structural differences among the three groups (see Figure 2-8).

First, news reading had a significant effect on biomedical literacy among

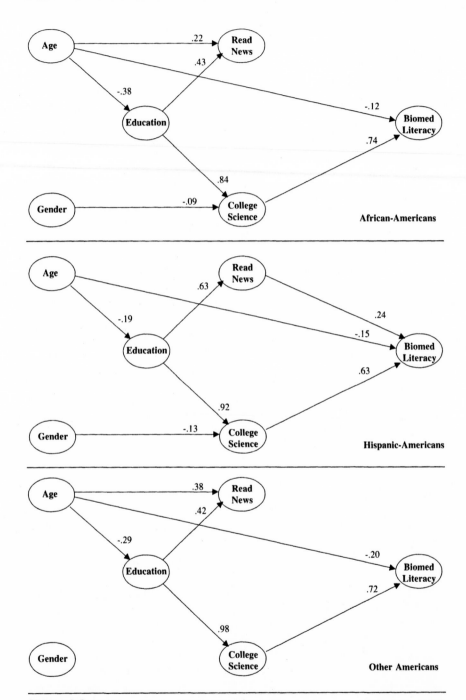

Figure 2-8 Path models to predict biomedical literacy, by race and ethnicity, 1993.

Table 2-4   Total Effects of Selected Factors, by Race and Ethnicity, 1993

	Total effects		
	African-Americans	Hispanic-Americans	Other Americans
Age	−.36	−.29	−.40
Gender (female)	−.07	−.08	.00
Level of education	.62	.73	.71
College science courses	.74	.63	.72
Reads news	.00	.24	.00
R^2	.62	.72	.63

Hispanic-Americans, but no relationship among African-Americans and Other Americans (see Table 2-4). This result means that for Hispanic-Americans reading current news and information about biomedical matters makes a contribution toward biomedical literacy above and beyond the influence of formal education or college-level science courses. To some degree, the greater influence of news and information reports by Hispanic-Americans may be a compensation for less formal instruction in science and mathematics and a need to learn or relearn some biomedical terms in English.

Second, age has a smaller effect among Hispanic-Americans and a larger effect among African-Americans and Other Americans (see Table 2-4). This difference is a reflection of the magnitude of educational growth or improvement among the three racial/ethnic groups during the last two generations. Reflecting the college opportunities afforded by the veterans educational programs associated with the Second World War and the Korean War, a relatively larger proportion of African-Americans and Other Americans were able to obtain baccalaureate, graduate, or professional training relative to Hispanic-Americans. The more recent growth of the Hispanic-American population in the United States largely eliminated the advantages of federal veterans educational programs and continuing language barriers may reduce access to and use of other educational scholarship and assistance programs.

For all three racial/ethnic groups, the importance of formal education and participation in college-level science courses were the primary predictors of biomedical literacy. This is consistent with the earlier discussion of the central role of education in building a foundation for adult biomedical literacy.

There was a small, but significant, gender difference among African-Americans and Hispanic-Americans, with men being slightly more likely to score higher on the Index of Biomedical Literacy than women. There was no gender difference among Other Americans. Some of the structural differences between men and women noted in the preceding section are masked in this analysis of racial and ethnic groups, but the size of the available samples does not allow the simultaneous analysis of racial, ethic, and gender differences as subgroups.

THE MARGINAL IMPACT OF SELECTED FACTORS

It is possible to use this basic learning model to assess the marginal impact of other factors on the level of biomedical literacy. For example, many health care communicators assume that adults with children at home develop a higher level of health and medical understanding from their experiences as parents. It is possible to test this hypothesis by adding to the previous model a new variable that indicates whether or not a respondent has a child under the age of 18 at home. In 1993, approximately 31 percent of adults included in the study reported that they had one or more children under the age of 18 living in their home. An examination of the biomedical literacy scores suggests that 21 percent of adults with minor children at home qualify as biomedically literate, compared to 13 percent of adults without minor children at home. The analytic question here is whether this difference reflects the presence or absence of children or some other combination of differences in age, education, and other characteristics, and we will shortly turn to an analytic model to answer this question.

It is also widely believed among health care providers that individuals with personal health problems are more likely to be knowledgeable about biomedical terms and concepts, often reflecting their own encounters with well-informed patients. To test this proposition, data from the 1993 Biomedical Literacy Study was used to construct a measure of their own health status, using responses from a question asking each respondent to rate his or her own health on a zero to 10 scale (with zero representing serious health problems and 10 reflecting perfect health) and a self-report about any chronic or continuing illnesses. Approximately 61 percent of adults in 1993 reported good health without any problems, while 39 percent reported moderate to serious personal health problems. In this case, the simple cross-tabulation does not support the expectation. Twenty percent of adults reporting good personal health qualified as biomedically literate, compared to only 9 percent of individuals with moderate to serious health problems. Although this simple tabulation appears to go in an unexpected direction, it is reasonable to speculate that individuals with health problems may be older and come from a generation with less formal education, thus it is possible that adults with a personal health problem may be marginally better informed about biomedical matters than similar individuals without those problems. Again, we will test this proposition shortly with an analytic model.

A parallel argument might suggest that an individual's experience of health problems within his or her family might influence the likelihood of biomedical literacy, with individuals whose family includes one or more other individuals with a serious health problem acquiring more biomedical information and understanding. There are numerous instances of a parent or spouse who has become extraordinarily well-informed about a specific health problem experienced by another member of their family. The movie *Lorenzo's Oil* documented the struggle of one set of parents in this situation. Using a similar set of 1993 questions about the health of one's spouse (if married) and children (if any), a measure of serious health problems in the family was developed. In 1993, approximately 5 percent of adults reported that another member of their family had a serious health condition. In this case, the percentage of adults who qualify as biomedically literate does not differ significantly by the presence or absence of a serious medical problem in the family. As noted above, however, we can assess the relative impact of this factor by including the variable in a general analytic model.

Building on the previous general learning model for biomedical literacy, the three variables described above were inserted into this model (see Figure 2-9). To examine their relative contribution to biomedical literacy, each of the three new variables were added to the model in the same relative position as college science courses and news reading. This placement in the

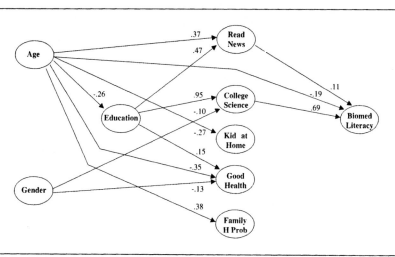

Figure 2-9   A path model to predict biomedical literacy, including selected family and health variables, 1993.

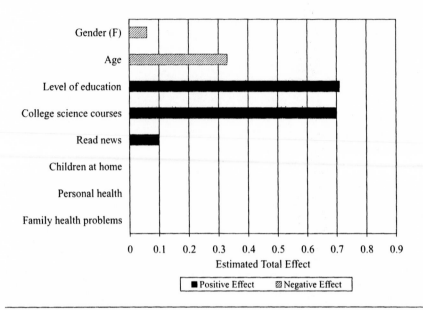

Figure 2-10   Total effects of selected factors on biomedical literacy, 1993.

model allows the possibility of influence from age, gender, and education, but does not attempt to examine any interactions among these potential intervening variables. The resulting analysis indicates that none of these additional variables were related to biomedical literacy (see Figure 2-10). The total effects of age, gender, education, college science courses, and news reading remained relatively unchanged.

This result is important because it illustrates one of the hazards of using simple tabulations of outcome variables by demographic category rather than looking at structured data sets. Given the statistically significant difference in the percentage of biomedically literate adults with and without minor children at home, it would have been easy to accept the conclusion that the experience of parenting a minor child or children produces a higher level of biomedical understanding. An analysis of the relative influence of this experience in the context of age, gender, educational attainment, exposure to college science courses, and other variables found, however, that the difference displayed in the tabulation was really the reflection of other variables and not the result of the parenting experience per se.

Because this chapter is the first introduction of the use of models to understand the relative impact of selected factors on an outcome variable (biomedical literacy, in this case), we are presenting more information about each of the models to illustrate the way that models can be used to define and test hypotheses about the sources or distribution of attitudes in the population generally or among various groups. In subsequent chapters, we will omit the details of models that confirm the absence of an effect, but note that the conclusion is based on an empirical model.

Differences by Gender

Although the preceding analysis looked at national samples of adults and included each respondent's gender as a variable, it is possible that there are structural differences between men and women in the ways that these additional factors included an individual's level of biomedical literacy. For example, minor children living at home might have a different influence on mothers and fathers. Following the same two-group procedure described in an earlier section of this chapter, a two-group analytic model was constructed. This procedure allows the computation of path coefficients and total effects estimates for men and women separately, but on a common metric that allows precise comparisons.

Compared to the general model described in the preceding section, the resulting two-group model found only minor variations between men and women in the factors associated with biomedical literacy (see Table 2-5). The level of educational attainment and the number of college-level science courses completed remain the major predictors of biomedical literacy for both men and women. Age is a slightly more important factor among women than men, and reading the news regularly is a more positive influence on biomedical literacy among men and women. Having minor children at home,

Table 2-5 Total Effects of Selected Factors, by Gender, 1993

	Total effects	
	Men	*Women*
Age	⎯.23	⎯.32
Level of education	.74	.73
College science courses	.62	.71
Reads news	.24	.16
Children at home	.00	.00
Personal health	.00	.00
Family health problems	.00	.00
R^2	.65	.69

Table 2-6   Total Effects of Selected Factors, by Race and Ethnicity, 1993

	Total effects		
	African-Americans	Hispanic-Americans	Other Americans
Age	−.37	−.26	−.42
Gender (female)	−.08	−.09	−.07
Level of education	.64	.73	.69
College science courses	.74	.64	.70
Reads news	.00	.22	.00
Children at home	.00	.00	.00
Personal health	.00	.00	0.00
Family health problems	.00	.00	.00
R^2	.61	.70	.63

having a personal health problem, or having someone else in an individual's family with a serious health problem were all unrelated to the likelihood of being biomedically literate for both men and women.

Differences by Race and Ethnicity

Following the same general logic and procedures, it is possible to examine the structure of biomedical literacy for American-Americans, Hispanic-Americans, and Other Americans using a three-group analytic model and a common metric. The results of this analysis found no significant differences among the three racial and ethnic groups in regard to the relatively influence of having minor children at home, personal health, and family health problems (see Table 2-6).

SUMMARY OF FINDINGS

This analysis indicates that there are substantial differences in the level of understanding of biomedical terms and concepts among American adults. In 1988, only 22 percent of American adults could define DNA as a part of the human that controls basic hereditary characteristics, and in 1999, 29 percent could provide a correct response. This is a disappointing level of understanding of one the central concepts of modern biology. Although the percentage of American adults who recognize that antibiotics do not kill viruses increased from 26 percent to 45 percent over the last decade, a majority of American adults still do not understand the scope of antibiotic impact. Just slightly more than half of American adults are able to apply the concept of a one-in-four probability to a practical heredity problem. For large segments of the adult public, communicators must assume a limited understanding of basic biomedical terms and concepts.

A simple Index of Biomedical Literacy was constructed to measure the level of individual understanding of a core set of biomedical terms and concepts, with a distribution of scores from zero to approximately 100. The mean score of American adults on this Index of Biomedical Literacy increased from 45.4 in 1988 to 51.2 in 1999, a modest pattern of growth at best. An examination of the patterns of growth in biomedical literacy scores over the last decades found that better educated adults were more likely to be biomedically literate (throughout the 1990s), and that the rate of change or growth had been relatively stable across major educational, gender, and age groups during the 1990s.

Looking at the level of understanding associated with various scores on the Index of Biomedical Literacy, it appears that individuals with scores of less than 50 on this scale would be likely to encounter substantial difficulty in trying to make sense of a television or newspaper story about the ineffectiveness of antibiotics for the common cold, the linkage between specific genes and diseases, or the impact of the thinning of the ozone layer on human health. Stories about antibiotic resistance or the advantages and disadvantages of genetically modified foods would be beyond the comprehension of large segments of adults with scores below 50 on this index. In 1999, approximately half of American adults had biomedical scores below 50.

At the other end of the scale, individuals with a score of 70 or higher might be expected to be able to read stories similar to those described above, and to understand the implications of these stories for their personal health and for relevant health policy issues. Although the exact level of comprehension of any story will depend in part on its content, a core set of biomedical terms and concepts runs through a great deal of current health and medical reporting, and those individuals able to bring a solid level of biomedical understanding to current news stories will be able to build their cumulative stock of knowledge and information. In 1999, only 18 percent of American adults—about 36 million individuals—were able to demonstrate a level of understanding sufficient to be characterized as being biomedically literate.

Looking for the factors that might account for this differential distribution of biomedical literacy, a series of basic analytic models suggests that the probability that any individual will be biomedically literate depends on his or her level of formal education, number of college-level science courses, and age. A pattern of reading about news and science regularly provides a small additional bonus. An individual's gender, personal health, family health status, or the presence of minor children in the household have virtually no influence on the likelihood of being biomedically literate.

IMPLICATIONS FOR BIOMEDICAL COMMUNICATORS

What are the major implications of this model for communicating biomedical information to the public generally or to targeted segments of the public? Three major points emerge from the preceding analyses.

First, the substantial differences in the level of biomedical understanding between the most and least educated Americans indicate that it is necessary for communicators to send multiple messages with differential levels of substantive sophistication to different segments of the public. The most knowledgeable segment of the adult population is able to use relatively advanced information that includes some discussion of the biomedical science involved in various health or disease issues. The least knowledgeable segment of the adult population has difficulty with some of the most basic biomedical terms and concepts and has little understanding of the nature of scientific inquiry. Messages to this less well educated portion of the population must explain basic concepts in simpler terms and recognize the limited reading and language ability characteristic of individuals with limited formal education. Given the large difference in levels of language and understanding, efforts to reach a middle level that will serve both audiences are unlikely to succeed.

Second, long-term change is driven primarily by formal schooling, including the study of science and mathematics. Too often, schools are dismissed as being hard to work with and largely ineffective, and primary reliance is placed on media campaigns. Although short-term crises may demand some major media campaigns, the models examined in this chapter indicate that real changes over the long term will require the integration of health and biomedical messages into formal education, including course curricula and persuasive information campaigns within the school environment. Most students who graduate from high school without an understanding of a molecule, DNA, or other basic biomedical concepts are unlikely to acquire that information during the remainder of their lifetime. Further, numerous studies have found that important life shaping health decisions are made by adolescents, including the use of tobacco, alcohol, and other drugs. There is equally strong evidence that many lifestyle decisions made during adolescence—diet, exercise, smoking, sexual behaviors—have a direct and continuing influence on adult lifestyle behaviors. It is essential that health and biomedical education and communications begin during the school years.

Third, the preceding analyses suggest that some growth in understanding biomedical concepts and processes can and does occur during the adult years. For example, the growth in the proportion of adults with a basic understanding of the function of DNA was larger than could be accounted for by formal educational experiences alone, indicating that some additional growth did occur during the adult years. This example is useful because it illustrates both the possibility of successful informal learning during adulthood and suggests the scope and magnitude of the effort needed. During the 1990s, the coverage of DNA-based biomedical research grew steadily in virtually all major media. In recent years, one might even speak of the gene of the week! The cumulative impact of this kind of print and broadcast coverage over a decade, combined with extensive use of DNA-based plots in television dramas and motion pictures and the prominent role of DNA in showcase trials, has produced a modest growth in the percentage of adults who are able to associate DNA with the transmission of traits and characteristics in humans. The parallel role of DNA in plants and animals and the commonality of all DNA is recognized by only a small portion of the population. It is essential to recognize that this modest growth in understanding was not achieved by a campaign of public service announcements and brochures, but reflects thousands of news stories, thousands of television and movie dramas, thousands of magazine articles, and several national showcase trials. For the best educated segment of the population, later analyses will suggest that the time required to communicate new information may be shorter, and the growing use of the new electronic media by the best educated adults may expedite the process even more. For most Americans, however, the process of informal adult education is slow and requires a long-term communications commitment.

COMMUNICATIONS TO INFORM CONSUMERS

3

· · · · · · · · · ·

PUBLIC INTEREST
IN HEALTH INFORMATION

· · · · · · · · · · · · · · · · ·

Most American adults report a high level of interest in health information. A 1998 survey of 3000 Americans conducted by the Pew Research Center asked individuals whether they followed various issues "very closely, somewhat closely, not very closely, or not at all closely" in the newspaper, radio, or television. Thirty-four percent of Americans said that they followed news about health very closely, second only to news about crime. This pervasive interest is expressed in the readership of health news and columns in newspapers, the purchase of health magazines, and the growing use of the Internet to search for health-related information. Despite the appearance of a pervasive level of interest, there are some variations in the level of reported interest and, as will be observed in later chapters, variation in the actual levels of information consumption and the retention of health-related information. An understanding of the structure of public interest in health information will provide an essential framework for a discussion of the communication of consumer health information to the public.

In the first chapter of this book, we suggested that there are two major purposes for biomedical communications—the dissemination of consumer health information and the transmission of biomedical policy information. This section will focus on the dissemination of consumer health information and outline a general model to identify the factors that lead some individuals to have a high level of interest in health matters and become regular consumers of biomedical information, while others acquire and retain little or no health-related information.

PATTERNS OF INTEREST
IN HEALTH INFORMATION

One of the key elements in the biomedical communication process is the salience of health and medical information to each individual. At one level, virtually everyone is interested in health information. If they are injured, become ill, or are diagnosed as having a serious disease, the salience of health information may increase sharply. On any given day, however, most people are not ill or injured and generally feel in good health, and it is the salience of health information to this group that governs, in part, short-term patterns of information acquisition and retention. Parrott (1995) suggests that exposure to a health message is not adequate; people are exposed to health messages on a regular basis. It is the level of involvement an individual has with a particular health topic that will influence how, if at all, the message is processed.

Several small studies have been conducted to examine the relationship between the salience of health information and health-related behaviors. Turk-Charles *et al.* (1997) found that cancer patients with a strong desire for more information were more likely to seek information about health from nonmedical establishment sources. Severin and Tankard (1992) conclude that:

> *It has become clear that information sometimes causes knowledge gaps to widen and sometimes causes them to narrow. One of the crucial variables in the process identified by several studies is interest or motivation. If there is sufficient interest, and particularly if it is evenly distributed throughout a community, then information can help to close a knowledge gap. (Severin and Tankard, 1992, p. 245)*

Although many health professionals and communicators presume that everyone is interested in health, the evidence suggests that many adults have moderate to low levels of interest in health information on a daily basis. It is important to understand the factors associated with higher and lower levels of interest and to look at the levels of reported interest for various segments of American society.

Previous studies have found that interest in or concern about health is not evenly distributed in the population. Cangelosi and Markham (1994) examined health-consciousness in seven southern counties. They created a Preventive Health Care Index composed of how well informed individuals felt about preventive health care methods, the degree to which they sought out preventive health care information, and the extent to which this information had changed their lives. They found that older adults, women, and those with higher levels of education had higher levels of concern about preventive health care.

Numerous studies have found that women are more interested in health than men (Hibbard and Pope, 1987). Hibbard and Pope (1987) suggest that there "are at least three potential factors influencing women's interest in health: biological exigencies, gender-related socialization, and gender specific role responsibilities" (Hibbard and Pope, 1987). They studied 1155 women who were members of a large health maintenance organization, and measured interest in health through an index that combined four factors: frequency of reading health columns in newspapers and magazines; having health or medical books in the home; frequency of consulting health and medical reference books; and how informed the respondent felt about their health. They found that "women who are younger, have higher educational status and better health status are apparently more interested in health." (p. 77). They also found that women with at least one child in the home were more likely to be interested in health than those without, and suggest that:

> *Women may also be more concerned with health and take more preventive actions than men because women's role obligations center more attention and responsibilities on family health. In addition to providing direct nursing care to family members, women are also the primary brokers or arrangers of health services for children and spouses. (Hibbard and Pope, 1987, p. 68)*

The simplest way to measure interest in various substantive areas is to ask individuals how interested they are. While direct inquiry has been shown to lead to socially desirable responses in some cases, there is ample evidence that individuals are willing to report their level of substantive interest when asked directly and that there is little or no distortion if the list of areas is sufficiently broad. In a 1993 national study of biomedical literacy in the United States, respondents were asked to report whether they were very interested, moderately interested, or not interested in each of several substantive areas. Six of ten Americans reported that they were very interested in information about health and an additional 34 percent said that they were moderately interested in health information. Only 3 percent of American adults claimed to have no interest in health information.

The proportion of Americans who expressed a high level of interest in health information exceeded the reported levels of interest for economic and business conditions, environmental pollution, and local school issues—all of which have traditionally been viewed as the core issues of American public opinion (see Figure 3-1). Other studies of public interest in selected issues and areas have found that this pattern is generally stable over time, but there

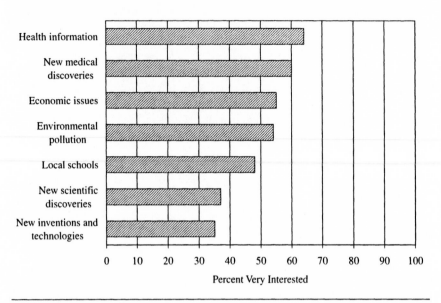

Figure 3-1 Public interest in selected topics, 1993.

may be temporary peaks of interest in response to unexpected events. The level of interest in foreign policy issues increased substantially in response to both the Vietnam War and the Persian Gulf War. In a similar manner, the level of interest in space exploration increased sharply immediately after the Challenger accident in 1986 (National Science Board, 1989, 1991, 1993, 1996, 1998).

A Sense of Being Well-Informed about Health Information

Although most Americans express a high level of interest in health information, most adults have substantially less confidence in their knowledge about health information. In the same 1993 survey, respondents were asked to indicate whether they were very well-informed, moderately well-informed, or poorly informed about information about health. Only 30 percent of Americans felt very well-informed about health information (see Figure 3-2). This is in sharp contrast to the 63 percent of Americans who reported being very interested in health information. An additional 60 percent of respondents felt moderately well-informed about health information, while only 10 percent felt that they were poorly informed.

Unfortunately, the level of self-reported knowledge about health information is only weakly related to the actual level of biomedical literacy re-

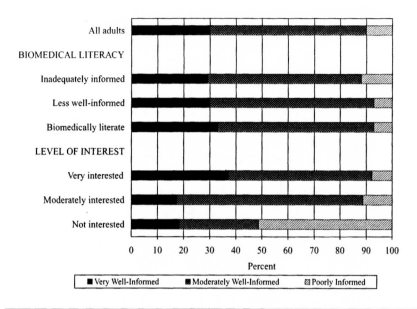

Figure 3-2 The public's perceived knowledge about health information, 1993.

ported in the previous chapter. This result can be seen by looking at the self-reported assessment of being well-informed about health information within each of the three levels of biomedical literacy described in the previous chapter (see Figure 3-2). The results show that 33 percent of adults classified as biomedically literate classified themselves as very well-informed about health information, compared to 30 percent of adults who were classified as partially biomedically literate and 29 percent of adults categorized as having a low level of biomedical literacy. The level of measured biomedical literacy accounts for only 9 percent of the variation in self-assessments of being informed about health information.

How can we explain this result? It appears that individuals may need some level of biomedical literacy to assess how much, or little, that they actually know about biomedical and health matters. The individuals with the lowest level of measured biomedical literacy may understand the basic information about nutrition and sanitation and have a general sense of the germ basis of illness and feel that they are very well-informed. If you do not know the difference between a bacteria and a virus, you may not think that your knowledge is inadequate. Conversely, those individuals with a better understanding of biomedical concepts such as DNA may recognize the complexity of the linkage between genetic findings and disease and classify themselves as being only moderately well-informed about health information.

The Relationship between Interest and Understanding

There is a strong, positive relationship between interest in and perceived knowledge about health information. Thirty-seven percent of adults who were very interested in health information also felt very well-informed about health information (see Figure 3-2). In contrast, fewer than 20 percent of those who were either moderately interested or not at all interested felt very well-informed. Whereas fewer than 10 percent of those who were very interested in health information felt that they were poorly informed, over half of those who were not at all interested in health information felt that they were poorly informed.

Does a low level of interest in health information lead to a low level of health knowledge (self perceived or measured), or does a low level of understanding of biomedical concepts reduce an individual's level of interest in health information? This is an important issue for communicators of health information, but our data provide limited insight into this important question. Since all of the variables in each of the surveys used in this analysis were collected at a single point in time, we cannot determine a causal order from the data alone. For example, our measures of the level of interest in health information and of self-assessed health knowledge were collected within 2 minutes of each other, and we cannot assert that interest caused a sense of being well-informed, or that a stronger sense of being well-informed caused a higher level of interest in health information.

Because the analysis in the preceding chapter found that the level of measured biomedical literacy is strongly related to formal schooling, we may reason that an individual's level of biomedical literacy was established some period of time prior to the interview, but that our measure of interest in health information is a reflection of interest at the time of the interview.[1] If the level of biomedical literacy influences the level of interest in health information, we would expect to see a moderate to strong positive relationship between our measures of biomedical literacy and interest. The data, however, show a weak negative relationship, casting doubt on the proposition that biomedical literacy leads to a higher level of interest in health information (see Figure 3-3). Because this result is based on only one simple cross-tabulation, we are not prepared to declare that this proposition is falsified, and we will return to this issue in our discussion of a formal model to test these relationships.

---

[1]This kind of assumption is commonly used in communications and social science research and we hope that our discussion of these assumptions will increase the general sensitivity of our readers to the logical structure of communications research found in reports and journals in this field.

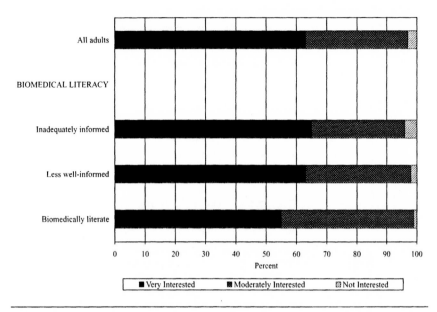

Figure 3-3   The public's interest in health information by biomedical literacy, 1993.

Some Factors Associated with Interest in Health Information

An examination of the levels of reported interest in health information by major educational and demographic groupings indicates that interest in health information in the United States is pervasive (see Figure 3-4). These simple cross-tabulations suggest that there is no clear relationship between overall educational attainment and college science courses and interest in health information. There is some relationship between gender and age and a high level of interest in health information, but when the very interested and moderately interested responses are combined, even this relationship appears to disappear.

Consistent with previous studies, women were significantly more likely to report a high level of interest in health information than were men within each age group. Among the youngest adults, those under age 25, 58 percent of women and only 45 percent of men reported being very interested in health information. The gender difference is greatest during the middle years. Nearly three-quarters of the women aged 35 through 44, but less than half of the men, reported that they were very interested in health information. The gender difference is smallest among adults 65 and older, when 81

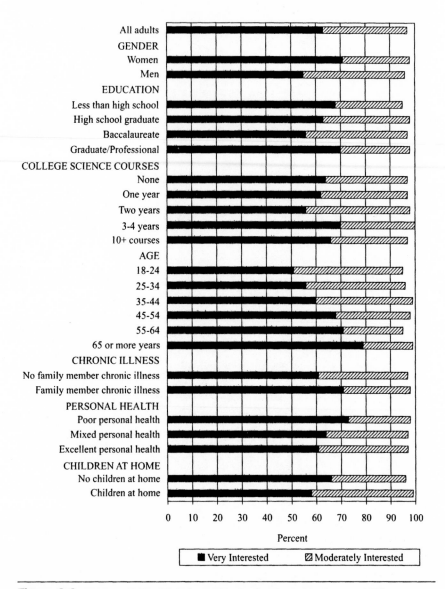

Figure 3-4 Interest in health information by demographic factors, 1993.

percent of women and 75 percent of men reported being very interested in health information (see Figure 3-5).

It is important to recognize, however, that each of these cross-tabulations fails to take into account differences in other variables. We know, for example, that educational attainment is negatively related to age, that is, old-

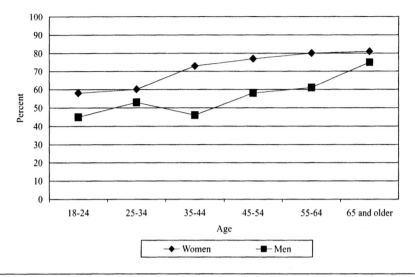

Figure 3-5 Interest in health information by age and gender, 1993.

er adults are likely to have less education than younger individuals in the United States. To provide a comprehensive assessment of the relative influence of each of several variables on the level of interest in health information, it is necessary to construct and examine a model that includes all of these measures at the same time.

A MODEL TO PREDICT INTEREST IN HEALTH INFORMATION

Using the same multivariate methods employed to examine the level of biomedical literacy in Chapter 2, it is possible to estimate the relative influence of each of several factors associated with a high level of interest in health and medical information. We begin with the same model used to predict biomedical literacy (see Figure 2-9), including both basic demographic factors as well as measures of personal health, family health problems, and the presence of children in the household. As noted in Chapter 2, age and gender are presumed to be prior to educational attainment, which is assumed to be prior to college science courses. All of these basic factors are assumed to contribute to differences in personal health, family health, and the composition of the family. All of the variables in the model are assumed to be potentially related to interest in health information.

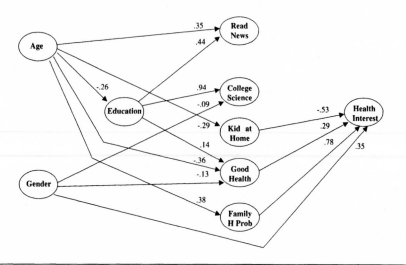

Figure 3-6   **Public interest in health information, 1993.**

This model[2] indicates that the strongest predictor (.78) of interest in health information is the presence of another family member with a chronic illness in the family, holding constant differences in age, gender, education, news reading, personal health, and the presence or absence of a child in the home (see Figures 3-6 and 3-7). This model also shows that individuals with good personal health are more likely to be interested in health information than individuals with personal health problems (.29). This set of results indicates that it is not personal illness, but rather the chronic illness of another family member, that stimulates a high level of interest in health information.

The second strongest predictor of interest in health information is the presence of minor children in the home (−.53), holding constant all of the other variables in the model. This result suggests that parents with children under the age of 18 living in the home may be busy with the demands of parenting, work, and other responsibilities and view health information as relatively less urgent than other matters. This result should not be interpreted to mean that the parent of a sick child would not be interested in information relevant to the illness or seek additional information, but rather that they might be less likely to report that they are very interested in health information than in other possible kinds of information. It should be noted that a chronically ill child would have been included in the previous measure of

[2]The model explains 76 percent of the total variance in interest in health information and has a good statistical fit, with 52.6 chi-squares with 29 degrees of freedom. The Root Mean Square Error of Approximation (RMSEA) is .023 (the upper limit of the 90 percent confidence interval of the RMSEA is .033).

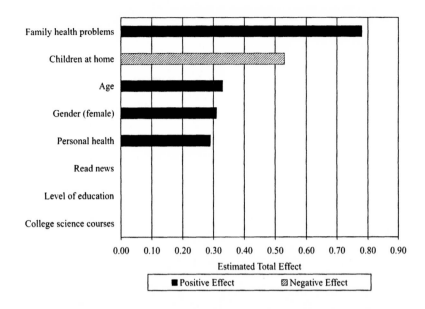

Figure 3-7   Total effects of selected factors on interest in health information, 1993.

other family members with a chronic illness, and that we might expect a parent of a chronically ill child to have and to report a high level of interest in health information.

Older adults are more likely to have a high level of interest in health information than younger adults (.33), holding constant the other variables in the model. This finding is consistent with a broad literature on health information acquisition and health services usage, and confirms our common sense understanding that adults become more sensitive to health issues as they grow older. The previously noted finding that individuals with good personal health are more likely to be interested in health information than adults with personal health problems, holding constant age and other variables, suggests that it is concern about potential illness that leads more senior citizens to have a high level of interest in health information rather than the actual presence of ill health.

Holding constant other factors, women are more likely to hold a high level of interest in health information than men (.31). We will return to a discussion of some of the reasons for a higher average level of interest in health information among women shortly.

The model also indicates that the level of educational attainment, the frequency of reading newspapers and magazines, and the number of college-level science courses do not influence the level of interest in health information (see Figures 3-6 and 3-7). This is an important finding for health communicators. Although education, college-level science courses, and news reading are positively related to biomedical literacy, the absence of significant relationships between these three variables and the level of interest in health information serves to reemphasize the relationships between life experience and patterns of interest in major topical areas.

The Hazards of Simple Cross-Tabulations

The results of this model provide a sharp contrast with the conclusions that we might have made on the basis of the simple cross-tabulations (expressed as bar charts) in Figure 3-4. Because the vast majority of health information is presented in this bivariate format, it is worthwhile to point to the level of misinformation often conveyed by simple bar charts.

The bar charts in Figure 3-4 indicate that approximately 72 percent of individuals with a family member with a chronic illness were very interested in health information in 1993, compared to 62 percent of respondents without a family member with a chronic illness. When the very interested and moderately interested responses are combined, it appears that the presence or absence of a chronic illness in one's family makes no difference in the level of that person's interest in health information. When differences in age, gender, education, personal health, and other variables in the model are held constant, however, a chronic illness by another family member becomes the best single predictor of the level of interest in health information, with a total effect of .78 (see Figure 3-7). If we had relied on only the bar charts, we would have missed an important finding that may be useful in thinking about health and biomedical communications.

Similarly, the bar charts in Figure 3-4 indicate that individuals with minor children in the home are slightly less likely to report that they are very interested in heath information than adults without children at home, but that they are slightly more likely to report that they are moderately interested in health information than adults without children at home. When the very interested and moderately interested responses are combined, parents with minor children at home are slightly more likely to be interested in health information than other adults. When viewed in the context of differences in age, gender, education, news reading, personal and family health, and other factors, however, the presence of minor children in the home has a significant negative effect on the level of interest in health information, with a total effect of −.53 (see Figure 3-7). Again, a literal interpretation of the bar charts would have led us to conclude that the presence or absence of minor children in the household had only a small influence in the level of interest in health information, but the analysis provided by the model found that was the second strongest predictor of interest in health information. We would have underestimated, if not totally missed, the influence of children in the home.

These two examples illustrate the danger of relying on simple cross-tabulations or bar charts in thinking about the factors involved in human behavior. Human behavior is complex. We are unlikely to obtain useful answers by using, or disseminating, simple frequency or cross-tabulated data.

Gender Differences

In the preceding model, the results indicated that women are more likely than men to be interested in information about health. It is possible that some of the relationships among the variables operate differently for men and for women. For example, it is often suggested that women serve as the primary caregivers in the family. As such, we might expect that the presence of children, or another family member with a chronic illness, might have a stronger effect on interest in health information for women than for men.

In order to test whether the relationships and effects discussed in the previous sections operate differently for men and women, a two-group model was run separately for men and women, but using a common metric so that differences in relationships or effects can be compared.[3] The results indicate that the effects of age and the presence of a chronic illness in the family remained essentially the same, but there were several importance differences between men and women in regard to the factors that influence the level of interest in health information among men and women.

Returning to our earlier hypothesis, having a family member with a chronic illness was the strongest predictor of interest in health information for both men and women, but the total effect of having a family member with a chronic illness was slightly stronger for women (.62) than for men (.56), holding constant all of the other variables in the model (see Table 3-1). This result indicates that women may bear a slightly greater sense of responsibility in families with a person (spouse, child, parent, or other relative living with the family) with a chronic illness, but that there is a substantial impact on both men and women in that situation.

The influence of age on the level of interest in health information was essentially the same for both men (.39) and women (.37), holding other variables in the model constant. The total effect of age was the second strongest

[3]The model to predict men's interest in health information accounted for 40 percent of the total variance in the outcome variable, whereas the model to predict women's interest in health information accounted for 69 percent of the variance in the outcome variable for women. The combined two-group model has a good statistical fit, with 145.7 chi-squares with 57 degrees of freedom and a Root Mean Square Error of Approximation (RMSEA) of .045 (the upper limit of the 90 percent confidence interval of the RMSEA is .054).

Table 3-1   Total Effects of Selected Factors on Interest in Health Information by Gender, 1993

	Women	Men
Age	.37	.39
Level of education	.21	.00
College science courses	.00	.00
Reading the news	.00	.34
Family health problems	.62	.56
Personal health	.21	.00
Children at home	.00	−.24
R^2 (proportion of total variance explained)	.69	.40

predictor of the level of interest in health information in the male and female model. The number of college-level science courses did not influence the level of interest in health information for either men or women, following the pattern in the aggregate model.

In contrast to these points of commonality, the two-group model found several interesting differences in the relative influence of other variables in the model. First, this two-group analysis found that the influence of minor children in the home on the level of interest in health information differed among men and women. Men who lived in a home with minor children were less likely to be interested in health information (−.24) than men in households without children, but the presence or absence of minor children in the home had no effect on women's interest in health information. Substantively, this result could support several different explanations. For example, this pattern is consistent with the view that there is a greater role differentiation in two-parent homes with minor children and that men are less likely to assume primary responsibility for the health of the children.

Second, the influence of reading newspapers and magazines on the level of interest in health information differed among men and women, holding constant the other variables in the model. Women who reported reading newspapers and magazines regularly were more likely to express a high level of interest in health information (.34) than women who reported less frequent news reading, but there was no relationship between the frequency of news reading and the level of interest in health information among men. This finding may point to the specialized nature of news reading. Our measure of news reading measures the regular reading of newspapers and magazines, but does not differentiate between the types of articles individuals read. This finding may suggest that the types of articles women read in magazines and newspapers enhance their interest in health information, while the types of articles men read have no effect on their interest in health.

Third, women with more years of formal education were more likely to report a high level of interest in health information than women with less education (.21), but the level of educational attainment was unrelated to the level of interest in health information among men. It will be recalled that there was a moderately strong positive relationship between the female gender and the level of interest in health information. In the context of path models, these additional paths provide an elaboration of the ways in which women develop or maintain a high level of interest in health information. The lower aggregate interest of men in health information did not demand—in statistical terms—an elaboration of the factors associated with the tendency of men to be less interested in health information.

Finally, women who reported having excellent personal health were more likely to be interested in health information (.21) than women with more health problems, but personal health status had no effect on the level of interest in health information among men. As noted above, this result is another elaboration of the total effect of being female on interest in health information. It suggests that women with good personal health are more likely to have a high level of interest in health information, reflecting both the traditional caregiver role of women and interest in preventive information to maintain their own health. The lower level of interest among men did not produce a differentiation sufficient to create a separate path in the male model.

Looking at the full pattern of differences in the two models, it appears that the level of interest in health information among men is driven by a few demographic or situational variables—age, a family member with a chronic illness, or children in the home—whereas the level of interest in health information among women is a more complex reflection of demographic, family, and behavioral variables. Numerous scholars and commentators have observed that many women live complex lives—balancing work, children, household management, health care coordination, and the coordination of social activities—and these results may simply mirror real differences in the life experiences of men and women at the beginning of the twenty-first century.

Racial and Ethnic Differences

The same multiple-group approach used above to examine structural differences in the level of interest in health information can also be utilized to look for structural differences among racial and ethnic groups. For this purpose, three groups were defined: African-Americans, Hispanic-Americans, and Other Americans. Three models reflecting the aggregate model defined above were run simultaneously, using a common metric to assure the comparability of effects and relationships across all three models.

It is important to note that the three-group analysis provided a much better explanation of Other Americans' interest in health information, explaining 83 percent of the total variance compared to 42 percent of the total variance for Hispanic-Americans and 35 percent of the total variance for African Americans.[4] The lower levels of prediction—the proportion of the total variance explained—means that some important variables were not included in the models for the prediction of interest in health information among African-Americans and Hispanic-Americans.

Consistent with the results of our original model for the total population, older adults were more likely to be interested in health information than younger adults in all three groups (see Table 3-2). However, the influence of age was greater for Other Americans (.38) and Hispanic-Americans (.25) than it was for African-Americans (.10). Enrollment in college sciences courses had no effect on interest in health information in our original model for the total population or in any of the three racial/ethnic groups.

The comparative three-group model found striking differences in the relative effect of the other variables in the model on interest in health information. In our aggregate adult model, having a family member with a chronic illness had the largest total effect on Americans' interest in health information (.78), it had a similar effect (.75) for Other Americans but no effect on African-Americans' or Hispanic-Americans' interest in health information. There are both methodological and substantive explanations of this result. Methodologically, it appears that a slightly lower proportion of African-Americans and Hispanic-Americans reported that another member of their family had a chronic illness. There is no evidence in the medical literature that there is a significantly lower incidence of chronic illness among African-Americans or Hispanic-Americans, thus we caution that there may be some difference in reporting, awareness, or understanding of chronic illness among these respondents. It is also possible that there is an underdiagnosis of chronic illnesses among these two minority groups. Substantively, this result could indicate that there is less of a linkage between the presence of a chronic illness in the family and the need for health information. This pattern could result from a cultural acceptance of illness as an uncontrollable fate, or stated conversely, from a lower sense of instrumental control over personal or family health conditions. Our data do not provide clear answers on this matter, but point to a need for more investigation of the factors involved in interest in health information.

---

[4]The combined model had a good statistical fit with 146.7 chi-squares with 84 degrees of freedom and a Root Mean Square Error of Approximation (RMSEA) of .048 (the upper limit of the 90 percent confidence interval of the RMSEA is .048).

Table 3-2   Total Effects of Selected Factors on Interest in Health Information by Race–Ethnicity

	African-American	Hispanic-American	Other American
Age	.10	.25	.38
Gender (female)	.19	.00	.35
Level of education	.21	.00	.00
College science courses	.00	.00	.00
Reading the news	.42	.00	.00
Family health problems	.00	.00	.75
Personal health	.00	−.68	.20
Children at home	−.36	.47	−.29
R^2 (proportion of total variance explained)	.35	.42	.83

Consistent with the aggregate model, Other American women and African-American women were more likely than men to be interested in health information, although the effects of gender were greater for Other Americans (.38) than African-Americans (.19). In contrast, Hispanic-American women and men were equally interested in health information, holding constant the other variables in the model. This is an interesting cultural difference, with implications for biomedical communicators. It suggests that African-American men and Other American men have relatively lower levels of interest in health information than other adults, and that communications targeted to these groups may require some attention to fostering interest as well as conveying information.

The relative effect of minor children in the home on interest in health information also differs among the three racial/ethnic groups. Consistent with the aggregate model, African-American (−.36) and Other American (−.29) adults with minor children in the home were less likely to report a high level of interest in health information than comparable adults without minor children in the home. In contrast, Hispanic-American adults with minor children at home were much more likely to be interested in health information (.47) than Hispanic-American adults without children at home. This result, in conjunction with the previous difference in regard to gender, suggests that in Hispanic-American families the presence of minor children in the home stimulates an increased interest in health information in both adults, diminishing the female role of health information monitoring found among African-Americans and Other Americans. These results should be taken as provisional and meriting more research and analysis with larger populations of all three groups.

Consistent with the aggregate model, neither regular news reading nor formal educational attainment had an effect on interest in health information for Hispanic-American adults or Other American adults, but African-American adults with more years of formal education (.21) and who read the news regularly (.42) were more likely to have a higher level of interest in health information than other African-Americans. For African-Americans, the factors associated with an interest in health information were similar to the factors related to biomedical literacy: formal educational attainment and regular news reading. For biomedical communicators, this result suggests that informal education is a potentially effective means for increasing the salience of health information among African-American adults.

Finally, the relative influence of personal health on the level of interest in health information varied greatly among the three racial and ethnic groups. Consistent with the aggregate model, Other American adults with good personal health (.20) were slightly more likely to be interested in health information than similar adults. In contrast, the opposite pattern was found among Hispanic-American adults, with those adults with good personal health being less likely to report a high level of interest in health information (−.68) than similar adults with personal health problems. Personal health status had no influence on the level of interest in health information among African-American adults. These results suggest that the social and cultural influence of personal health status varies among racial and ethnic groups and that health communicators need to think about these patterns in developing health information messages and campaigns.

Looking at the differences between the aggregate model and the three separate racial and ethnic models, it appears that Other American adults' interest in health information is driven primarily by a few situational and demographic factors—primarily having a family member with a chronic illness, being older, and being female. African-American adults' interest in health, in contrast, is strongly related to formal and informal education. Hispanic-American adults' interest in health is driven by two situational factors—suffering from poor health and having minor children—and being older.

THE IMPORTANCE OF SELECTED DISEASES

The preceding discussion and analysis have looked at health information broadly, including a full range of potential diseases and conditions. Some health communicators may wish to focus on a narrower range of diseases, and it is possible to provide some information about the interest in and attitudes toward specific diseases. A 1998 survey of American adults conducted by the National Opinion Research Center included a question asking Americans to rate the seriousness of selected diseases.[5] Respondents were told:

First, I'd like to ask you about health and social problems facing the country today. Please think of a scale from zero to ten where zero means that a problem is not at all serous and ten means that it is extremely serious. How serious a problem do you think _____ is?

Respondents were then read the names of seven different health problems and were asked to rate the seriousness of each one. Although American adults found all of the health problems to be relatively serious, cancer was rated the most serious health problem, with a mean rating of 8.3 on this index of seriousness (see Figure 3-8). Americans were least concerned about Alzheimer's disease, which received an average seriousness rating of 6.5.

Looking at simple bivariate tabulations, expressed as bar charts, there was a significant difference in the rating assigned to each of the seven conditions based on gender (see Figure 3-9). Women rated each of the seven conditions as being more serious than did men. The largest difference was on the perceived seriousness of mental illnesses such as depression. Women assigned an average seriousness rating of 7.1 to these illnesses, compared to an average seriousness rating of 6.1 by men.

Older adults rated heart disease, drug abuse, diabetes, and Alzheimer's disease as being more serious than did young adults. Young adults found AIDS to be a more serious problem than did older adults. There was no difference among age groups in the perceived rating of the seriousness of cancer, violence, or mental illnesses such as depression (see Table 3-3).

There was a significant difference regarding the relative seriousness of the seven conditions based on the level of educational attainment (see Table 3-4). Individuals who did not graduate from high school rated each of the seven conditions to be more serious than adults with more education. The largest difference was in the rating of the seriousness of drug abuse: adults who did not graduate from high school assigned a seriousness rating of 8.8 to drug abuse, while those adults who had graduated from college assigned

[5]The 1998 OBSSR/GSS survey was a telephone reinterview of households that participated in the 1998 General Social Survey (GSS), and was funded by the Office of Behavioral and Social Science Research (OBSSR) in the Office of the Director of the NIH. The GSS is a large omnibus survey that has been conducted annually for most of the last 27 years. The GSS includes a broad range of questions regarding education, family, and religious status, as well as the respondents' attitudes toward various social and religious topics. The OBSSR/GSS focused on the public's understanding of and attitudes about the causes and treatment of selected diseases.

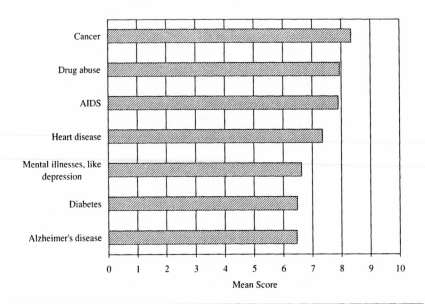

Figure 3-8 The public's assessment of the seriousness of selected health problems, 1998.

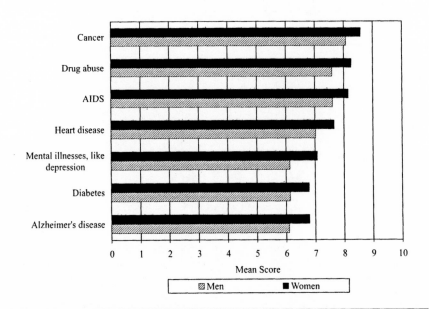

Figure 3-9 The public's assessment of the seriousness of selected health problems by gender, 1998.

Table 3-3 The Public's Assessment of the Seriousness of Selected Health Problems by Age, 1998[a]

	Cancer	Drug abuse	AIDS	Heart disease	Mental illnesses	Diabetes	Alzheimer's disease
All adults	8.3	7.9	7.9	7.4	6.6	6.5	6.5
Age							
18–24	8.3	7.7	8.3	6.7	6.6	6.0	5.7
25–34	8.2	7.9	8.2	7.2	6.6	6.2	6.2
35–44	8.3	7.8	7.8	7.2	6.5	6.4	6.2
45–54	8.4	8.0	7.8	7.7	6.8	6.7	6.8
55–64	8.6	8.1	7.7	7.7	6.7	6.8	6.7
65 or more years	8.4	8.2	7.5	7.6	6.6	6.8	7.2

[a]Cell entries are the mean score on an index of importance that ranges from zero to ten. Source: General Social Survey, 1998.

an average seriousness rating of 7.2 to drug abuse. This difference in perceived seriousness may reflect perceptions of the immediacy of the threat, the seriousness of the consequences, or fear of the unknown. A full exploration of the rationale that individuals use in assessing the seriousness of selected diseases is beyond the scope of this analysis, but these results are presented to demonstrate that many individuals do differentiate among different diseases in terms of perceived seriousness.

Table 3-4 The Public's Assessment of the Seriousness of Selected Health Problems by Education, 1998[a]

	Cancer	Drug abuse	AIDS	Heart disease	Mental illnesses	Diabetes	Alzheimer's disease
All adults	8.3	7.9	7.9	7.4	6.6	6.5	6.5
Less than high school	8.6	8.8	8.4	7.8	7.1	7.1	7.0
High school graduate	8.4	8.0	8.0	7.3	6.6	6.5	6.5
Baccalaureate or higher	8.1	7.2	7.2	7.3	6.4	6.0	6.1

[a]Cell entries are the mean score on an index of importance that ranges from zero to ten. Source: General Social Survey, 1998.

IMPLICATIONS FOR
BIOMEDICAL COMMUNICATORS

In summary, six of ten Americans have a high level of interest in health information, and an additional third report a moderate level of interest in health information. This level of interest is higher than comparable measures for economic policy, environmental issues, or local schools. It is substantially higher than the reported levels of interest in new scientific discoveries and the uses of new inventions and technologies.

A high level of interest in health information does not mean that an individual also has high levels of knowledge about biomedical information. In fact, many individuals who reported that they were very interested in health information also reported that they were only moderately well-informed about health and medical topics. As noted above, it may be necessary for an individual to understand some set of basic scientific and biomedical constructs to be able to recognize how much more there is to know about these subjects. Individuals who were very interested in health information had significantly lower levels of biomedical literacy than did those who reported being moderately, or not at all interested in health information.

On balance, the combination of a large number of American adults with a high level of interest in health information and a broader held sense of not being very well-informed on these matters indicates that there is a large and ready audience for health and medical information in the United States. In subsequent chapters, we will examine the efforts of American adults to find and understand health and biomedical information, but it is sufficient for now to simply note that there is a strong demand for timely and accurate health information.

Some adults have a higher level of interest in health information than others, and a series of multivariate models explored the factors most closely associated with higher levels of interest in health information. The results found that a chronic illness by another member of the family was the strongest predictor of a high level of interest in health information. A separate examination of the sources of interest in health information among men and women found significantly different patterns of influence. The factors associated with a high level of interest in health information among men reflected basic demographic and situational variables—age, a family member with a chronic illness, and the presence of minor children in the home. The factors associated with a high level of interest in health information among women were more diverse, reflecting a wider range of demographic, family, and behavioral experiences. It will be important for health and medical communicators to recognize these differences between men and women in designing and conducting information programs.

It is also important to recognize that biomedical literacy and interest in health information are largely unrelated. As demonstrated in the previous chapter, an individual's level of biomedical literacy is strongly related to formal education and to participation in college-level science courses. In sharp contrast, the level of educational attainment and the number of college sciences course taken were largely unrelated to interest in health information in the aggregate. The level of educational attainment was moderately related to interest in health information among women, and not at all related among men.

In this context, then, it is appropriate to turn to an examination in Chapter 4 of the sources of health and medical information used by various segments of the public.

4
• • • • • • • • •

PRIMARY SOURCES
OF BIOMEDICAL
INFORMATION

• • • • • • • • • • • • • • • • •

The traditional view of health care information dissemination was that "information circulated among medical professionals through a few, clearly defined channels—medical schools, professional journals, specialized conferences. From there it was dispensed to patients by doctors" (Bunn 1993, pp. 85–86).

> *Today, however, the doctor is no longer the only, or even necessarily the primary source of health information for the consumer. . . The system not only requires that the consumer have enough information to be able to make an informed choice of his or her physician. It also requires that the individual consumer possess health-related information on such a wide range of subjects—the effects of environmental pollutants, the merits of differing health plans, the health consequences of various lifestyles, etc.—that the information demand is beyond the capacity of a conversation between a physician and a patient. (Bunn, 1993 pp. 86)*

Americans have a long-standing interest in personal health and medical news. Adults in the United States are avid readers of newspaper and magazine stories about health-related issues and new medical discoveries. Atkin and Arkin (1990) report that "at least one-fourth of all articles in daily news-papers are in some way related to health." Virtually all major television stations now have at least one reporter assigned to health and medical news, and many major daily papers publish a weekly supplement devoted to health and medical news and features. By the end of the twentieth century, the Internet was home to more than 2000 e-health sites. The volume of health and medical information in the United States continues to grow rapidly, and the number of health information channels or outlets is growing exponentially.

Within this context of changing and expanding information sources, communicators need to understand current patterns of information exposure and retention. The use of information sources, and retention of health information is not evenly distributed throughout the population. Communications researchers speak of a knowledge gap, in which better educated segments of the population make more use of new information and new information sources, often widening the gap in knowledge, despite new communications campaigns (Donohue *et al.*, 1975, 1987; Severin and Tankard, 1992). Donohue *et al.* comment that:

> *A substantial body of research literature indicates that throwing more information into a system will not necessarily lead to an equalization of knowledge across social groups, any more than throwing more money at an unemployment problem will bring equity to income levels. While the general level of income or information per capita may increase, the relative gap in income or information may also increase. (Donohue et al., 1987, p. 87)*

As a result of differential use of information, public health campaigns may actually create a greater disparity in knowledge among the general public. Donohue *et al.* (1975) comment that,

> *As the flow of information into a social system increases, segments of the population with higher levels of education often tend to acquire this information at a faster rate than segments with lower levels of education. As a result, gaps in knowledge between these segments tend to increase rather than decrease. (Donohue et al., 1975, p. 4)*

Information seeking is generally considered to be one characteristic of individuals who will engage in preventive health behaviors (Rakowski *et al.*, 1990). Rakowski *et al.* (1990) surveyed a small sample of adults in one Rhode Island community and found that women were more likely than men to engage in health information-seeking activities. Additionally, Rakowski *et al.* (1990) found that individuals who engaged in information-seeking activities were more likely to have taken some new action to benefit their health. Cangelosi and Markham (1994) examined the acquisition of preventive health care information by residents of seven southern communities and found women, older adults, and better educated adults were more likely to seek out preventive health care information.

Lenz (1984), commenting on information-seeking behavior, notes that:

> Although active search for information is not prerequisite to information acquisition (information can be acquired passively), information-seeking patterns have potential to help explain discretionary health behavior because they affect the scope and nature of information acquired, the repertoire of alternative courses of action known to the searcher, and ultimately, the action taken. (Lenz, 1984, p. 60)

Lenz (1984) summarized the literature on health information searches, finding that women have been found to engage in more extensive health information searches than men, and those with higher socioeconomic status are also more likely to engage in health information searches. Hickey *et al.* (1988) examined gender differences in various health practices of a small sample of older adults. They found that women were more likely than men to read articles about health, to seek out television or radio programs about health, and to prepare in advance for health care appointments. There is some evidence that when faced with a threatening event, such as poor health, the information-seeking behavior of people varies along two main dimensions: the extent to which they seek out relevant information—or monitoring—and the extent to which they avoid relevant information—or blunting (Davey *et al.*, 1993).

This chapter will describe the current sources of health information for the American public and for selected segments of the public. The first section will describe the regular information consumption patterns of the adult population. A second section will examine the primary sources of information used by selected segments of the population. A final section will explore the levels of public trust in major health information sources, looking at both the full public and at selected segments of the public.

GENERAL PATTERNS OF MEDIA USE

Looking at trend data from the National Science Foundation's *Science and Engineering Indicators* studies since 1983, it appears that Americans utilize a variety of sources and institutions for scientific and technical information, but that television and the newspaper remain primary sources.

Although there are many generalizations offered about media use and information acquisition in the United States, it is essential to recognize that there is a significant differentiation in media use behaviors by level of educational attainment.

Before proceeding, it is important to emphasize that there is a difference between descriptive and analytic presentations of data. In Chapters 2 and 3, and the remainder of the book, we provide analytic presentations of data, in which we discuss the effects of factors such as age, gender, and education, on outcomes such as biomedical literacy and interest in health information. In this chapter we provide a description of the use of selected sources of health information, and trust in that information, by different segments of the population. Such a descriptive presentation is useful in finding the best sources of health information to use for targeted groups. Readers should be aware that when we say—in this chapter—that there is a relationship between factors such as age or gender and the use of different media to obtain health information, we are not implying that age or gender causes this use. For example, we will later note that older adults are much less likely than younger adults to have access to the Internet. We do not mean to suggest that it is their age that causes these adults to be less likely to use the Internet. Rather, we are attempting to show that if one wants to communicate with older adults about health information, the Internet would reach only a small portion of the older adult population at this time. We will return to the advantages and disadvantages of using the Internet for reaching selected audiences later in this chapter, but it is important to recognize the descriptive character of many of the results discussed in this chapter.

Broadcast Media

American adults report watching approximately 3 hours of television a day, or slightly more than 1000 hours each year (see Figure 4-1). In 1999, American adults reported watching an average of 1017 hours of television per year, including an average of 431 hours of television news each year (see Figure 4-2). To place these results in context, an average American worker would work approximately 2000 hours per year, which is used as the scale for Figure 4-2. The total number of hours viewed per year ranged from 1404 hours for individuals who did not complete high school to 680 hours for adults with a graduate degree. There was no significant difference in the hours of television viewing per year for men and women. Persons living in households with cable or satellite television service reported slightly more hours of television viewing than individuals without access to this kind of service. Americans 65 years of age and older watched the most television (of any age group), viewing an average of 1389 hours of television per year.

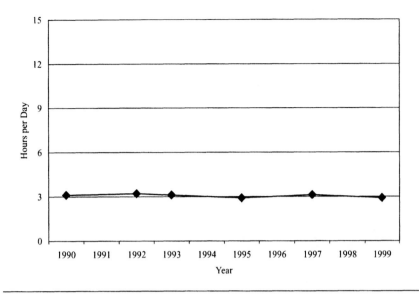

Figure 4-1 Average hours of adult television viewing per day, 1990–1999.

The pattern of television news viewing was similar to the pattern for total viewing, but the ratio of news hours to total hours of viewing was positively associated with education (see Figure 4-2). While the total number of hours of television news viewing declined with higher levels of education, the percentage of total viewing hours devoted to news shows increased steadily from 39 percent for adults who did not complete high school to 51 percent for graduate degree holders. Young adults aged 18 through 24 allocated only 36 percent of their television viewing to the news.

Americans watched an average of 42 hours of science television shows in 1999 (see Figure 4-2). Men watched more hours of science television shows than did women. Individuals who had taken three or more college-level science courses watched more science television shows than did those who had taken fewer college science courses. Adults with children in their home reported watching more science television than did those with no children in the home. Adults aged 65 and older watched about half the amount of science television of any other group of adults. Individuals living in homes with either cable or satellite television service watched more science television shows than those without either service.

Radio is the second major source of broadcast information. In 1999, Americans reported listening to the radio for an average of 918 hours, including 228 hours of radio news broadcasts (see Figure 4-3). It is useful to note that the total number of hours of radio listening is approximately 90 per-

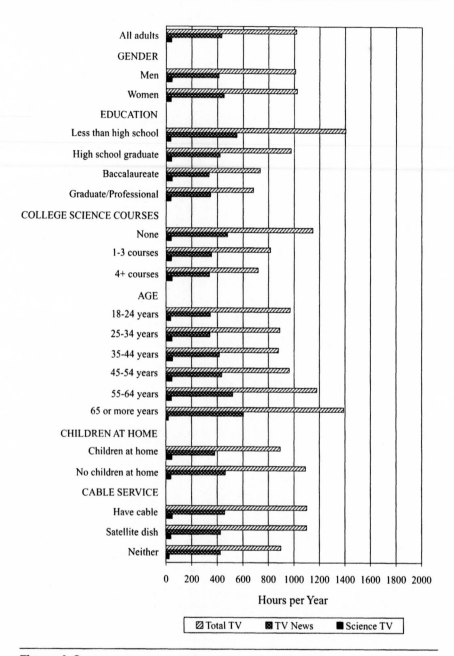

Figure 4-2 Average hours of adult television viewing, 1999.

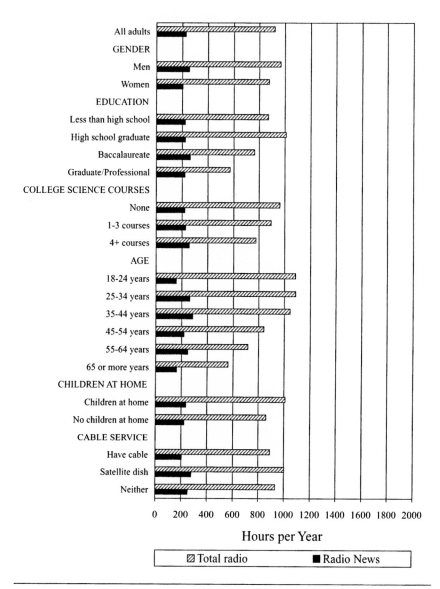

Figure 4-3 Average hours of adult radio listening, 1999.

cent of the total number of hours of television viewing, a relationship that is often lost in media market studies.

Given the diversity of content and format in radio broadcasts, the results suggest that different segments of the population listen to different kinds of radio broadcasts. Younger people reported listening to substantially more total hours of radio broadcasts than older adults, but the proportion of listening hours devoted to news increased from 15 percent among Americans aged 18 through 24 to 35 percent for persons aged 55 to 64, and 29 percent for adults aged 65 and over (see Figure 4-3). Individuals with a college degree listened to less radio broadcasts than other individuals, but devoted a greater proportion of their listening to radio news.

Kubey and Csikszentmihalyi (1990) studied television viewing by members of different demographic groups and found that the viewing tended to be passive and relaxing, with very little concentration. Television viewing was actually a secondary activity in 28 percent of the cases. Donohew *et al.* (1984) reach a similar conclusion. Severin and Tankard (1992) label this view of mass media usage as ritualistic or habitual. Consistent with the data described above, Kuby and Csikszentmihalyi (1990) found that television viewing was negatively correlated with level of education.

Print Media

The percentage of Americans reading a newspaper every day has decreased gradually over the last two decades, from 62 percent in 1983, to less than half of all Americans in 1999 (see Figure 4-4). The decline in newspaper readership has been documented by numerous studies (Nicholson, 1999; Robinson and Levy, 1996). Whereas the total number of hours of television viewing was higher for less well educated adults, the use of virtually all kinds of print media is higher among better educated adults. In 1999, only 36 percent of the adults who had not finished high school reported reading a newspaper on a daily basis, compared to 57 percent of graduate degree holders (see Figure 4-5). It is not surprising that individuals with lower levels of education are less likely to rely on print sources of health information. Baker *et al.* (1997) examined the readability levels of over 250 periodicals, newspapers, newsletters, and pamphlets found on the Health Reference Center on Info-Trac. They found that the readability scores of the items ranged from a low of tenth grade to a high of fourteenth grade, and that every item exceeded the generally accepted reading level of eighth grade. They comment that "although lay medical (and health) materials are being published at a phenomenal rate, little material appears to be aimed at people who read below the eighth-grade level."

Newspaper reading has declined since 1983 for individuals from all levels of education (see Figure 4-6). In 1983, 56 percent of those with less than a high school degree read a newspaper on a daily basis; nearly 20 years later, only 36 percent of those with less than a high school degree reported reading a daily newspaper. Over 70 percent of individuals with a baccalau-

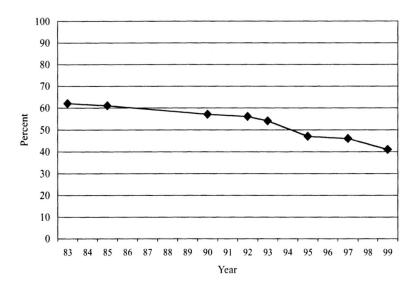

Figure 4-4 Percent of American adults who read a newspaper every day, 1983–1999.

reate degree read a daily newspaper in 1979. By 1999, only 51 percent of those with a baccalaureate degree read a daily newspaper.

Men were more likely to read a newspaper on a daily basis than women in 1999, and older respondents were significantly more likely to read a newspaper every day than younger respondents, despite a generally lower level of educational attainment among older adults (see Figure 4-5). Approximately three-quarters of adults aged 65 and older reported reading a newspaper every day in 1999, over three times the percentage of adults less than 35 years old.

Magazines are the second major print source of health information. Over half of Americans have reported reading some type of magazine on a regular basis for most of the last two decades (see Figure 4-7). While there is a growing number of magazines focused primarily on health and medical issues, a wide array of other magazines now include either a regular section on health and medical news or include numerous stories on health and medical topics. Both *Time* and *Newsweek,* for example, have a regular health and medical news section, and approximately one-fifth of all Americans reported that they regularly read a newsmagazine during the last 20 years. Most women's magazines include articles on one or more health-related topics in almost every issue, but the percent of adults reading a woman's magazine has declined from 20 percent in 1983 to 10 percent by the end of the

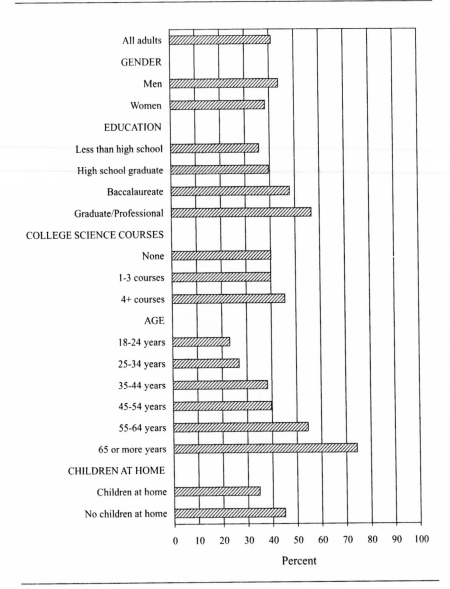

Figure 4-5 Adult daily newspaper reading, 1999.

century. Science magazines also frequently feature at least one article relating to health or medical news; the percent of Americans reading science magazines has dropped slightly from 13 percent in 1983 to 9 percent in 1999.

To estimate the cumulative reach of magazines containing some health information, the magazine reading reports from the 1999 *Science and En-*

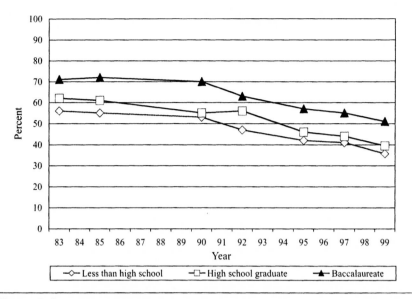

Figure 4-6   Percent of adults who read a newspaper every day by education, 1983–1999.

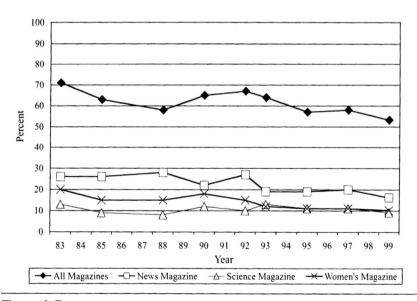

Figure 4-7   Percent of adults who read selected magazines most of the time, 1983–1999.

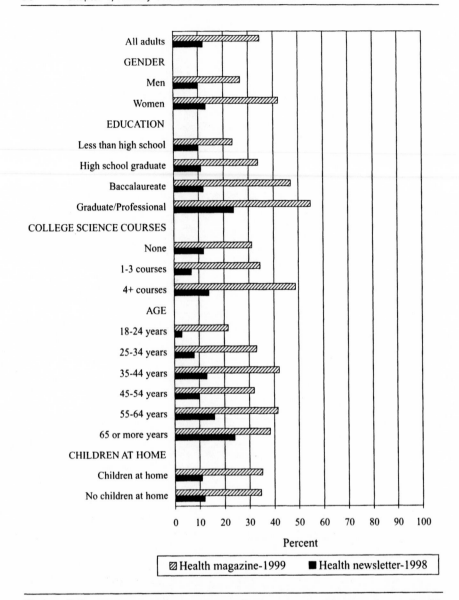

Figure 4-8 Percent of adults who regularly read a health magazine or health newsletter, 1998 and 1999.

gineering Indicators study were divided into those magazines that regularly include some health information[1] and those that do not, or only rarely,

[1]This classification includes news magazines, women's magazines, consumer and nutrition magazines, senior citizen magazines, and magazines focusing primarily on health and medical issues, such as *Prevention.*

include health information. In 1999, 35 percent of adults reported regularly reading a magazine that normally includes some health information (see Figure 4-8). Educational attainment is strongly related to health magazine reading. Fifty-five percent of adults with a graduate or professional degree regularly read a health magazine, which is over twice the percentage of individuals with less than a high school diploma who read health magazines. Women were much more likely than men to read a magazine that includes health information. Young adults were less likely than either middle-aged or older adults to read health magazines. There was no significant difference in health magazine reading based on the presence of children in the family.

Health newsletters are another form of print media used by Americans to obtain health information. In the 1998 Biotechnology Study, respondents were asked whether or not they subscribed to a health newsletter. Twelve percent of the respondents indicated that they subscribed to a health newsletter (see Figure 4-8). Respondents were also asked to provide the name of the health newsletter to which they subscribed. The most frequently mentioned newsletters were those published by senior citizen organizations or health clinics, and those related to a specific disease. Individuals with a graduate or professional degree were much more likely to subscribe to a health newsletter than other individuals. Nearly one-fourth of those 65 years of age and older indicated that they subscribed to a health newsletter, while only 3 percent of adults aged 18 through 24 subscribed.

Computers, the Internet, and Public Libraries

Although most Americans purchase newspapers and magazines, watch their own television sets, or listen to their own radios, it is useful to look briefly at the levels and patterns of utilization of both public libraries and on-line computer access technologies. Traditionally, persons wishing to obtain information not available within their own household have turned to a public library to borrow books, to read newspapers and magazines, and, more recently, to borrow video tapes and CD-ROMs. The recent emergence of the Internet as a source of information has been described as the library of the future, but is currently limited to a relatively small —but rapidly growing—segment of the population.

A 1998 study by the U.S. Department of Commerce Census Bureau, while noting that access to the Internet has expanded for all groups in recent years, speaks of the "persistence of the *digital divide* between the information rich (such as Whites, Asians/Pacific Islanders, those with higher incomes, those more educated, and dual-parent households) and the information poor (such as those who are younger, those with lower incomes and education levels, certain minorities, and those in rural areas)." (U.S. Department of Commerce, 1999, p. xiii). The report further notes that "access to information resources is closely tied to one's level of education. Households at higher education levels are far more likely to own computers and access the Internet than those at the lowest education levels." (p. 6). This study also found that older adults were the least likely to own home computers or have access to the Internet.

Many medical professionals have raised concerns about the quality of health information sites on the World Wide Web (Coelho, 1998; Marwick, 2000; Silberg *et al.*, 1997). A 1997 content analysis of Web sites about fever in children lent credibility to these concerns, finding that:

> *Variability in both content and quality of medical information to the public is not the exclusive of the Internet, as wide differences also exist in other forms of public communication, such as print and broadcast media. However, only a few of the web pages we reviewed gave complete and accurate information for such a common and widely discussed condition as fever in children. This suggests that there is an urgent need to check public oriented healthcare information for accuracy, completeness, and consistency." (Impicciatore et al., 1997, p. 1879)*

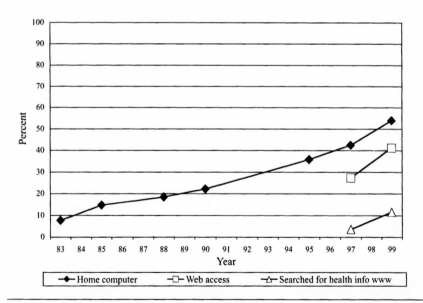

Figure 4-9   Percent of adults reporting a home computer, access to the World Wide Web, and search for health information on the World Wide Web, 1983–1999.

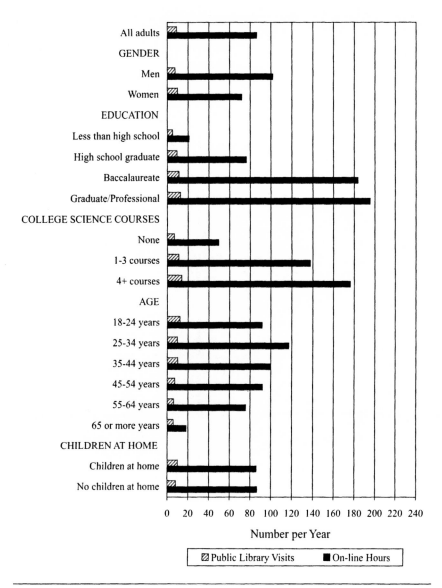

Figure 4-10   Patterns of adult public library and on-line computer use, 1999.

Despite these concerns, the World Wide Web is becoming an important source of health information for an increasing number of Americans (see Figure 4-9).

In 1983, only 8 percent of Americans reported that they had a computer in their home. This number has increased steadily so that half of all Americans reported having a home computer by the end of the century. Access to home computers and the Internet has increased (see Figure 4-10). In 1997, 27 percent of American adults reported that they had access to the World Wide Web either at home or at work. Only 2 years later, over 40 percent of Americans had access to the World Wide Web.

In 1999, American adults reported an average of nine visits to a public library during the previous year and 86 hours of use of an on-line computer service from their home (see Figure 4-10). While better educated citizens were more likely to both visit a public library and use an on-line service than less well educated adults, there was a strong tendency for the best educated respondents to report more on-line hours than library visits. Individuals with a graduate or professional degree, for example, reported in 1999 an average of 13 visits per year to a public library and 195 hours per year of on-line computer usage. Projecting this pattern to the future, it appears that better educated persons are already as likely to use an on-line service as a public library, and we would expect that this trend would continue to expand among the college-educated segment of the population and expand among noncollege groups at a slightly slower pace. Younger adults reported more on-line usage than older adults. Adults aged 65 and older spent an average of only 18 hours on-line in 1999.

Approximately 32 percent of Americans indicated in 1999 that they had tried to get information about a specific topic, and twelve percent of Americans indicated that had looked for information about at least one health-related topic on the World Wide Web (see Figure 4-11). Searching for information about health-related topics on the World Wide Web is strongly related to education. Thirty percent of those individuals with a graduate or professional degree had searched for health information on the World Wide Web, while only 3 percent of those individuals with less than a high school diploma reported making a similar search. Younger individuals were much more likely to search for health information on the World Wide Web than were older individuals. Although men spent substantially more hours on-line than women, they were less likely than women to look for information about health on the World Wide Web.

Looking at the patterns of general information acquisition, a high proportion of Americans devote substantial time each day to reading, viewing, or listening to information about news and current events. People with more formal education tend to rely on print media sources and the Internet more heavily than do others, but they also report regular use of broadcast media as a news source. Older Americans, many of whom may be retired, report high levels of news and information consumption, including both print and broadcast sources. The differences in information acquisition patterns between men and women were minimal.

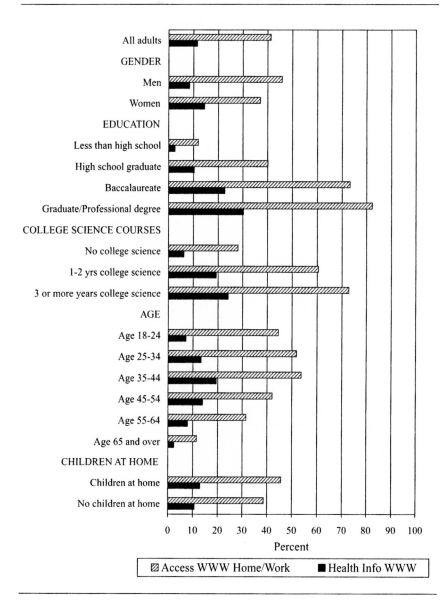

Figure 4-11 Adult access to and use of the World Wide Web for health information, 1999.

PATTERNS OF MEDIA USE
BY SELECTED GROUPS

In the preceding sections, we have described the general patterns of information use among American adults. Sometimes, it is important to communicate information or present a message to a more limited or targeted group. In the following sections, we will provide a set of brief outlines of the media use patterns of segments of the population that are often the focus of specialized health messages.

Media Use Patterns of Young Adults

Young adults are defined as individuals aged 18 through 24. Twelve percent of this group were still in high school in 1999, and 25 percent were enrolled in a college or university. Approximately 45 percent were high school graduates who were not enrolled in school, indicating a decision to enter the work force or, in some cases, begin a family. Only 6 percent of this cohort had completed a baccalaureate degree, and some of these young adults were enrolled in graduate or professional programs. In short, schooling is still an important component of the lives of a majority of these young adults.

Young adults spend more time listening to the radio and watching television than most other adults. There is virtually no differentiation in the number of hours of radio listening among young adults on the basis of gender, although young adults in school listen to slightly fewer hours than do those who are not currently in school (see Table 4-1). There are substantial differences in the number of hours of television viewing for different segments of young adults. Better educated young adults watch significantly fewer hours of television each day than do less well educated young adults. Among young adults, high school dropouts watch an average of 4.4 hours per day, whereas college graduates watch 2.0 hours per day. Young men watch significantly more hours of television each day than do young women.

Only 23 percent of young adults reported reading a newspaper on a daily basis in 1999 (see Table 4-1). Young men were more likely than young women to read a newspaper each day. There is an interesting relationship between educational status and newspaper reading among young adults. Young adults who were no longer in school, including high school dropouts, high school graduates, and college graduates, were more likely to read the newspaper than were students currently enrolled in either high school or college. The low level of reading a newspaper among students probably reflects, at least in part, the time pressures on high school and college students.

Young adults are less likely than all other adults to read a health maga-

Table 4-1 Young Adults Use of Selected Media, 1999[a]

| | Television | Radio | Daily newspaper | Magazine | | | Number |
				Health	News	Women's	
	—Hours per day—		—Percent who read—				
All young adults	2.8	3.1	23	2	12	8	263
Gender							
Men	3.1	3.3	28	2	12	2	125
Women	2.5	2.9	19	3	12	12	138
Educational status							
High school dropout	4.4	3.4	33	0	0	9	34
High school student	2.3	1.2	17	0	16	0	31
High school graduate	2.9	4.0	28	3	11	9	117
College student	2.1	2.4	12	5	12	8	65
College graduate	2.0	2.8	22	0	29	6	17

[a]Source: *Science and Engineering Indicators 2000.*

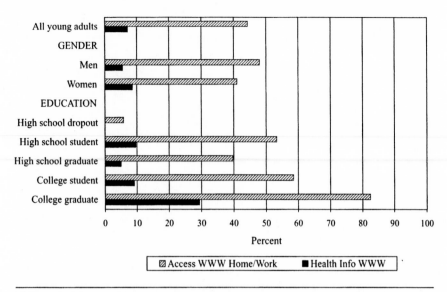

Figure 4-12 Young adults access to and use of the World Wide Web for health information, 1999.

zine. In 1999, only 2 percent of young adults read a health magazine[2] (see Table 4-1). Only 12 percent of young adults reported that they read a newsmagazine, and 8 percent that they read a women's magazine in 1999. Although there were no significant gender differences in reading a health or newsmagazine among young adults, young women were much more likely to read a women's magazine than were young men.

Although young adults are less likely than most other Americans to use the print media, they are among the most likely to use the Internet. In 1999, 44 percent of young adults had access to the World Wide Web, and 7 percent reported having looked for health information on the World Wide Web (Figure 4-12). There were strong differences in the use of the World Wide Web for health information based on educational status. None of the high school dropouts reported looking for health information on the World Wide Web in 1999, but over 10 percent of the college graduates and 18 percent of the current college students looked for health information on the World Wide Web in 1999.

[2]This categorization of health magazines includes magazines devoted to health such as *Health* or *Prevention,* as well as other magazines that regularly include some information about health, such as *Modern Maturity* or *Reader's Digest.* Newsmagazines and women's magazines are not included here as health magazines, but instead are listed separately.

Media Use Patterns of Parents with Children at Home

It is often important to communicate specific health information to the parents of preschool and school-aged children who are living with their families. At the simplest level, information campaigns often seek to alert parents to the need for vaccination for students entering school, while other campaigns have focused on subjects from the use of child-safety seats in automobiles to teenage alcohol use.

Approximately a third of adults in the United States report that their household includes one or more children under the age of 18. Parents reported watching nearly 3 hours of television and listening for approximately 3 hours to the radio each day (see Table 4-2). Parents with baccalaureate degrees spent less time listening to the radio and watching television than did less well educated parents.

Just over a third of parents read a newspaper on a daily basis in 1999 (see Table 4-2). There is a strong differentiation in newspaper reading among parents based on education. Over half of parents with a college degree read a newspaper every day, compared to only 21 percent of parents with less than a high school diploma.

Better educated parents read more newsmagazines than less well educated parents. Nearly one-third of parents with a baccalaureate degree reported reading a newsmagazine regularly, compared to only 12 percent of parents who were high school dropouts. There were significant differences in reading magazines devoted totally to health based on education. However, mothers were significantly more likely than fathers to report reading health magazines and women's magazines.

In 1999, 46 percent of parents had access to the World Wide Web either at home or work, and 13 percent of parents looked for health information on the World Wide Web (see Figure 4-13). Fathers were more likely than mothers to report having access to the World Wide Web, but mothers were more likely than fathers to look for health information on the World Wide Web. Parents with a college degree were much more likely to have access to the World Wide Web and to look for information about health on the World Wide Web than were less well educated parents.

Media Use Patterns of Older Adults

Older adults—persons aged 60 years or more—are another important audience with whom biomedical communicators often need to communicate. Older adults are also a growing segment of the population. In 1999 adults

Table 4-2 Parents Use of Selected Media, 1999[a]

	Television	Radio	Daily newspaper	Health	News	Women's	Number
					Magazine		
	—Hours per day—			—Percent who read—			
All parents	2.6	2.9	35	10	17	12	698
Gender							
Men	2.4	3.2	39	3	18	<1	305
Women	2.7	2.6	31	15	16	21	393
Level of education							
Less than high school	3.4	3.0	21	11	12	6	128
High school	2.5	3.2	33	10	14	15	435
Baccalaureate	1.9	1.9	54	9	29	8	135

[a]Source: *Science and Engineering Indicators 2000.*

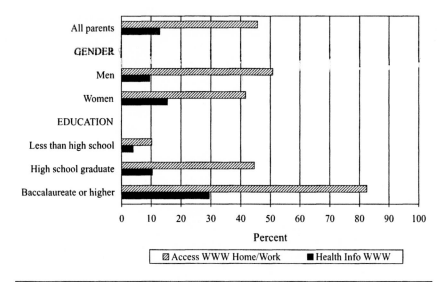

Figure 4-13 Parents access to and use of the World Wide Web for health information, 1999.

aged 55 and older accounted for 29 percent of all adults. The U.S. Census Bureau estimates that by 2025 this group will increase to 40 percent of the total adult population. For this group, information campaigns often seek to provide new information about cancer, heart disease, and other conditions often associated with aging, as well as preventive health information specifically targeted for older adults.

Older adults spent more time watching television and less time listening to the radio than other adults. In 1999 older adults spent an average of 3.9 hours each day watching television and 1.7 hours per day listening to the radio (see Table 4-3). Older adults with less than a high school diploma spent more time watching television than other older adults. There was no difference in the amount of time men and women spent listening to the radio and watching television.

One-fifth of all older adults read a health magazine in 1999, and approximately 15 percent read a newsmagazine or women's magazine. Among older adults, women were more likely than men to read health magazines and women's magazines. Older adults who graduated from college were much more likely to read a newsmagazine than other older adults.

Older adults are less likely to have access to the World Wide Web than younger adults. Only 15 percent of adults aged 60 and older had access to the World Wide Web, and only 3 percent looked for health information on the

Table 4-3 Older Adults Use of Selected Media, 1999[a]

| | Television | Radio | Daily newspaper | Magazine | | | Number |
| | | | | Health | News | Women's | |
	—Hours per day—			—Percent who read—			
All older adults	3.9	1.7	72	21	15	16	361
Gender							
Men	4.1	1.7	77	19	16	2	155
Women	3.8	1.7	68	23	14	27	206
Level of education							
Less than HS	4.8	1.6	63	17	6	19	132
High school	3.7	1.8	74	25	17	16	178
Baccalaureate	2.7	1.5	83	17	31	10	52

[a]Source: *Science and Engineering Indicators 2000.*

World Wide Web in 1999 (see Figure 4-14). Among older adults, men were much more likely than women to look for health information on the World Wide Web. A college education significantly increased the likelihood that older adults would both have access to the World Wide Web, and use it as a source for health information.

Media Use Patterns of Men and Women

For some health and medical issues, it is necessary to communicate primarily to men or women as a separate group. In recent years, for example, a substantial volume of information has been directed to women concerning the identification and treatment of breast cancer. More recently, major information campaigns have focused on alerting men to watch for prostate cancer and providing information about diagnosis and treatment. Although each of the preceding discussions of young adults, parents with children at home, and older adults included some analysis of gender differences, it is useful to summarize in this section the general patterns of media use.

Men and women reported spending nearly the same amount of time watching television and listening to the radio in 1999 (see Table 4-4), and this pattern has remained relatively stable for the past decade (see Figure 4-15). Men were slightly more likely than women to read a newspaper each day. Education was positively associated with newspaper reading for both men and women. Women were more likely than men to read a health maga-

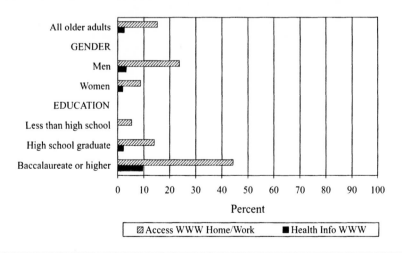

Figure 4-14   Older adults access to and use of the World Wide Web for health information, 1999.

Table 4-4 Men and Women's Use of Selected Media, 1999[a]

	Gender	—Hours per day—		Daily newspaper	Magazine —Percent who read—			Number
		Television	Radio		Health	News	Women's	
All adults	M	2.9	2.8	44	8	18	1	900
All adults	F	2.9	2.5	38	15	16	20	981
Level of education								
Less than HS	M	4.2	2.5	36	8	10	2	94
Less than HS	F	3.8	2.5	36	2	9	7	209
High school	M	2.7	3.2	42	7	17	1	509
High school	F	2.9	2.6	38	16	16	22	602
Baccalaureate	M	2.0	1.9	58	9	30	2	197
Baccalaureate	F	2.0	2.0	43	3	28	6	170

[a]Source: Science and Engineering Indicators 2000.

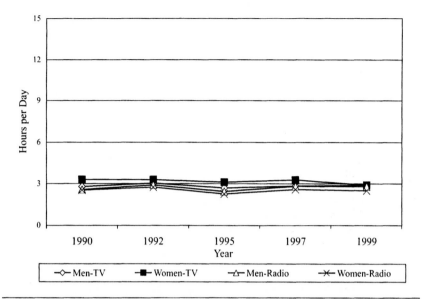

Figure 4-15 Men's and women's hours of viewing television and listening to the radio per day, 1990–1999.

zine or a women's magazine in 1999, whereas there was no significant difference between men and women in reading newsmagazines.

In 1999, 46 percent of men, but only 37 percent of women reported having access to the World Wide Web (see Figures 4-16 and 4-17). However, women were more likely than men to use the World Wide Web to look for information about health, indicating that, when they have access, women are much more likely than men to use the World Wide Web as a source of health information.

TRUST IN HEALTH AND BIOMEDICAL INFORMATION SOURCES

The communications literature[3] suggests that people often trust some sources of information more than others. Anderson (1971) suggests that the credibility of a source serves as a weight to amplify the information received in a message. Numerous studies have found that high-credibility sources of

[3]For recent reports and summaries of the literature, see Atkin and Arkin (1990), Backer *et al.* (1992), Kreps and Thornton (1992), Mileti and Fitzpatrick (1993), and Ratzan (1993). The baseline study in this area is Schramm and Wade (1967).

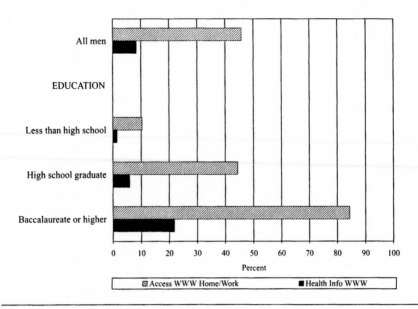

Figure 4-16 Men's access to and use of the World Wide Web for health information, 1999.

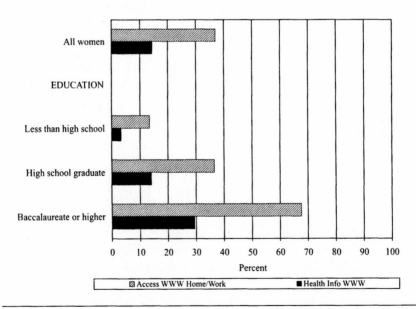

Figure 4-17 Women's access to and use of the World Wide Web for health information, 1999.

information have a greater effect than low-credibility sources (Hovland and Weiss 1951; McGinnies and Ward, 1974; Page *et al.*, 1984).

A series of national studies over the last three decades demonstrate that a high proportion of American adults have a great deal of confidence in physicians and scientists. Since 1973, the General Social Survey has included a series of questions designed to measure the public's confidence in selected institutions, including medicine, the scientific community, the press, and television (Davis and Smith, Annual series). The public has consistently expressed more confidence in the medical and the scientific communities than either the press or television. In 1998, 44 percent of Americans expressed a great deal of confidence in medicine, and 40 percent expressed a great deal of confidence in the scientific community (see Figure 4-18). In contrast, only one in ten Americans expressed a great deal of confidence in the press or television.

Meissner *et al.* (1992) comment that:

> *For most individuals, physicians are one of the most credible sources of information about health and they can strongly influence patient motivation and behavior change. A majority of people state that they are very likely to follow their doctor's advice on ways to reduce possible cancer risks, though they are less likely to report that they have actually talked to their doctor about how to accomplish this." (Meissner et al., 1992, p. 154)*

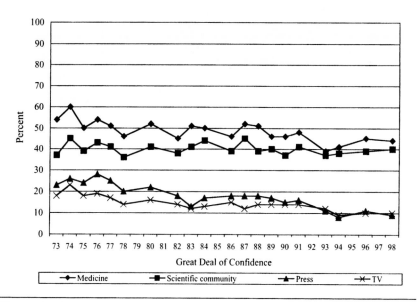

Figure 4-18   **Percent of adults expressing a great deal of confidence in selected institutions, 1973–1998.**

McCallum *et al.* (1991) surveyed individuals in six communities connected to the production or storage of toxic chemicals. They found that physicians were the most trusted source of information about environmental risks, followed by environmental groups and friends or relatives. However, physicians were the least used source of information about environmental risks.

When asked how much they would trust health information from various sources about weight loss, mental illness, or heart disease and cancer, American adults were much more likely to trust physicians and the National Institutes of Health (NIH) than other sources (see Figure 4-19). Three-quarters of Americans expressed a high level of trust in physicians as a source of information about alcoholism, depression, cancer, and heart disease. Two-thirds of adults reported a high level of trust in physician information about weight loss. Information from the National Institutes of Health was the second most trusted source on all three subjects. Three-quarters of American adults indicated a high level of trust in NIH information about alcoholism, depression, cancer, and heart disease, but only 55 percent had an equally high level of trust in NIH information about weight loss.

Approximately 45 percent of Americans said they would have a high level of trust in information about alcoholism, depression, cancer, or heart disease in *Time* or *Newsweek* in a 1998 national study (Miller *et al.*, 1999). Only

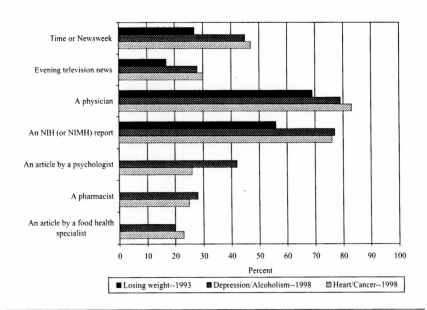

Figure 4-19 **Percent of adults with a high level of confidence in selected sources of health information, 1993 and 1998.**

26 percent said they would have a high level of trust in weight control information in the same magazines in the 1993 Biomedical Literacy Study.

Reflecting the same relatively low regard for television noted earlier, fewer than one in three Americans expressed a high level of trust in information on the television evening news about alcoholism, depression, cancer, or heart disease. Only 17 percent of Americans indicated that they would trust a television news report on weight loss.

Although there was a nearly universal level of trust in information provided by a physician, there was a clear differentiation in media trust by the level of educational attainment (see Table 4-5). College graduates were significantly more likely to trust health information from an NIH report or an article in a newsmagazine. Individuals without a high school diploma were more likely to trust the evening television news for information about cancer or heart disease than were better educated respondents.

IMPLICATIONS FOR BIOMEDICAL COMMUNICATORS

What are the implications of these results for biomedical communicators? How can these results help focus and target messages? First, the basic patterns of media use are strongly influenced by education. Adults without a college education report a significantly higher level of television viewing than college graduates and a lower use of print media of all kinds. There is a growing use of home computers and on-line services, and Americans with a graduate or professional degree reported more hours per year on-line than visits to their local library in 1997. Looking a decade ahead, it is likely that on-line information services will play a major role in the dissemination of health and other information to college-educated Americans.

Second, the level of trust in various sources of health information followed the same general pattern found in media use and was strongly influenced by education. College-educated adults were more likely to express a high level of trust in an NIH report or a magazine article, whereas non-college graduates tended to have a higher level of confidence in information from the evening television news.

Third, different segments of the population—the young, parents, the old, and women—use different media to obtain health information and report different levels of trust in that information. Young adults devote a large amount of time to watching television and listening to the radio, but their rates of reading health and women's magazines are among the lowest of all adults. Although young adults have high rates of access to the Internet, they are less likely than most other adults to use the Internet to obtain health information. Older adults have the highest rates of reading newspapers and

Table 4-5 Trust in Health and Biomedical Information from Selected Media, 1993[a]

	All adults	Less than high school	High school graduate	College graduate
1998: Percent with a high level of confidence in information about heart disease/cancer from . . .				
Time or *Newsweek*	47	47	48	44
Evening television news	30	45	29	22
A physician	83	78	84	85
An NIH report	76	67	76	83
An article by a psychologist	26	37	27	18
A pharmacist	25	37	24	22
An article by a health food specialist	23	34	22	18
Number of respondents	1945	267	1247	425
1998: Percent with a high level of confidence in information about depression/alcoholism from . . .				
Time or *Newsweek*	45	43	45	45
Evening television news	28	40	29	18

A physician	79	71	81	79
An NIMH report	77	67	77	83
An article by a psychologist	42	42	41	44
A pharmacist	28	39	26	27
An article by a health food specialist	20	29	20	14
Number of respondents	1945	267	1247	425
1993: Percent with a high level of confidence in information about losing weight from . . .				
Time or *Newsweek*	27	11	28	39
Evening television news	17	19	18	14
A physician	69	53	72	78
An NIH report	56	40	58	68
Number of respondents	1560	317	937	306

[a]Source: 1993 Biomedical Literacy Study; 1998 General Social Survey.

health magazines. They also spend a large amount of time each day watching television. However, only a small percentage of older adults have access to the Internet, indicating that at present the Internet is not an effective way to reach large segments of older adults. Women are much more likely than men to read health magazines, women's magazines, and to use the Internet to obtain health information. These differential patterns of use and trust serve as guidelines for communicating with various segments of the population.

chapter

5
··········

THE ACQUISITION AND RETENTION OF HEALTH INFORMATION BY CONSUMERS

·················

The ability of individuals to recall reading or hearing about health information is critically important for health communicators. For health communications to be successful, exposure to health information is not adequate; individuals must retain the information for recall and use. This chapter will focus on Americans' retention and recall of health and medical information.

THE RECALL OF HEALTH INFORMATION

On an average day, Americans are faced with a wide array of information about health and medicine. Television and radio newscasts routinely feature the latest dietary recommendations to reduce the risk of cancer and heart disease, as well as the newest genetic linkages to a wide assortment of medical conditions. In 1998, *Time* and *Newsweek* used cover stories on a variety of health and medical topics including cancer and diet, *Escherichia coli*, Viagra, herbal medicines, and the flu. Most women's magazines include at least one regular feature on health and medical information. Beyond the traditional media, the World Wide Web contains an ever-growing number of sites devoted to health and medicine in general, as well as to specific diseases (Akatsu and Kuffner, 1998; Chi-Lum, 1999; Gallagher, 1999; Jadad and Gagliardi, 1998).

The presence of health and medical information in the media is not adequate assurance that Americans will read articles in the print media or listen to stories on television or the radio. Even if they do read or listen to stories about health or medical information, they may not remember the information.

In a 1998 national study,[1] over two-thirds of Americans recalled reading or hearing a story about heart disease or cancer in the last 3 months, while 57 percent of Americans recalled a story about alcoholism or mental health problems (see Figure 5-1). Men were significantly more likely than women to recall news stories or articles about both health topics. Education is positively related to the recall of news stories about both types of health problems. Among those with a graduate or professional degree, 89 percent recalled a story about heart disease or cancer, while 77 percent recalled a story about alcoholism or mental health problems. In contrast, only 63 percent of those with less than a high school diploma recalled a story about heart disease or cancer, and less than half recalled a story about alcoholism or mental illness.

Personal experience with an illness, or class of illnesses, has a direct relationship to the ability of individuals to recall stories about health information. Almost 75 percent of those individuals with a family member who suffered from depression recalled reading or hearing a story about depression, schizophrenia, or alcoholism in the last 3 months. In contrast, only 51 percent who did not have this family experience with depression recalled reading or hearing about a similar story.

In a similar vein, 76 percent of those individuals who either themselves or a family member suffered from heart disease recalled hearing a story about heart disease or cancer. Only 58 percent of those with no personal experience with heart disease recalled hearing a story about heart disease or cancer. As individuals age, they are more likely to suffer from heart disease or cancer themselves, or to have a family member suffer from these illness-

---

[1]Two questions were included in a 1998 Social and Behavioral Indicators Survey to assess Americans' general recall of media coverage of health and medical information (Miller *et al.*, 1999). Respondents were first asked, "Over the last three months, have you heard or read anything about alcoholism or serious mental health problems like depression or schizophrenia?" Later in the interview, they were asked "Over the last three months, have you heard or read anything about heart disease or cancer?" All individuals who indicated that they had heard or read something about one of these conditions were asked "How did you come to know this information?"

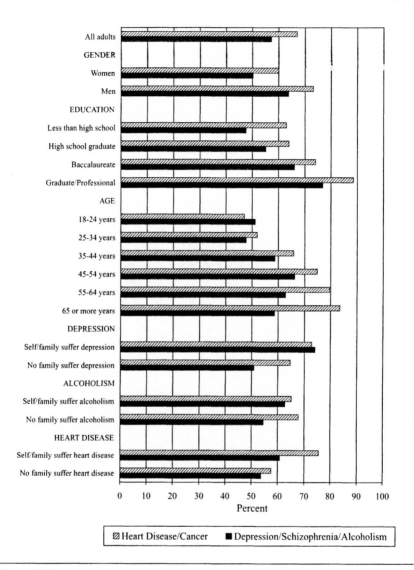

Figure 5-1 The public's ability to recall hearing or reading news about selected illnesses, 1998.

es. This pattern may explain the strong, positive relationship between age and recall of stories about heart disease and cancer. Fewer than half of adults aged 18 to 24 recalled hearing a story about heart disease or cancer, and only 52 percent of those 25 to 34 recalled a similar story. Over 80 percent of adults aged 65 and older recalled reading or hearing a story about heart disease or cancer in the last 3 months.

The 1993 Biomedical Literacy Study went beyond asking respondents whether or not they recalled a story about health information and asked each respondent to describe the subject of at least one piece of health or medical information that they had heard or read in the previous 2 months, and the source of that information. A total of 63 percent of Americans were able to recall a health or medical story, and 61 percent were able to recall the source of the story (see Figure 5-2). These must be considered to be disappointing results, since nearly 40 percent of Americans were unable to recall a single health or medical story.

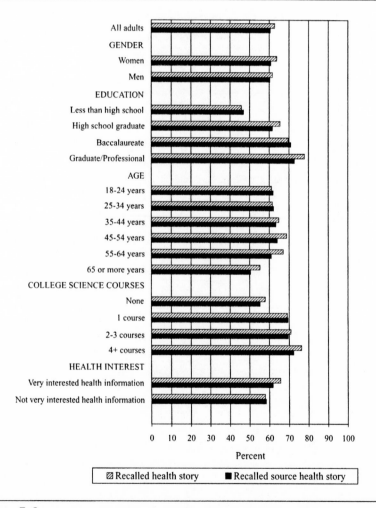

Figure 5-2   Recall of information about health and medicine, 1993.

There is a strong relationship between formal education and the recall of health information. Nearly 80 percent of those with a graduate degree were able to recall a health or medical story, and 73 percent were able to recall the source of the story. Less than half of those who did not graduate from high school were able to recall a health or medical story or the source of the story. There is no significant difference in the ability of men and women to recall health information. Older adults were slightly less likely to recall health information. Individuals who were very interested in health information were slightly more likely than others to recall health or medical information (see Figure 5-2).

CURRENT AND LATENT HEALTH INFORMATION CONSUMERS

For communications purposes, it is useful to distinguish between adults who are active health information consumers and adults who only occasionally or sporadically acquire and retain health information. We classify those adults able to both name a story about health information and recall the source of the story as current health information consumers. In 1993, 56 percent of Americans could be classified as current health information consumers. The 44 percent who could not recall a single piece of health or medical information or could not recall the source of that information should be thought of as latent health information consumers (see Figure 5-3). Given the extensive coverage of health and medical topics in newspapers and magazines and on television, this result points to the filtering role of salience in the communication process.

Simple bivariate tabulations indicate that adults with higher levels of education are more likely to be current health information consumers. Approximately two-thirds of adults with a baccalaureate degree or higher qualified as current health information consumers. Only two-fifths of adults who did not graduate from high school qualified as current health information consumers. The oldest group of adults—aged 65 and older—were slightly less likely to be current health information consumers than younger adults. Nearly 58 percent of those who were very interested in health information qualified as current health information consumers, in contrast to 53 percent of all other adults. There was no difference in the level of current health information consumers between men and women.

Recognizing the limited value of simple bar charts, a structural equation model was constructed to examine the effects of selected factors on the retention and recall of current health information. A variable reflecting current health information retention was added to the basic interest model

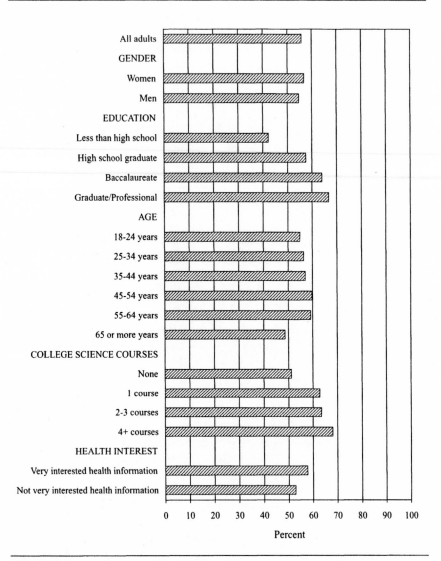

Figure 5-3   Current health information consumers by selected factors, 1993.

used in Chapter 3 (see Figure 3-6). In this new model,[2] all of the variables, including biomedical literacy and interest in health information, are treated as possible predictors of current health information consumption and recall

[2]The model had a good fit with a Root Mean Square Error of Approximation (RMSEA) of .023; 90 percent confidence intervals of .0 and .033; and a chi-square of 52.61, with 29 degrees of freedom. The model accounted for only 13 percent of the total variance in the model.

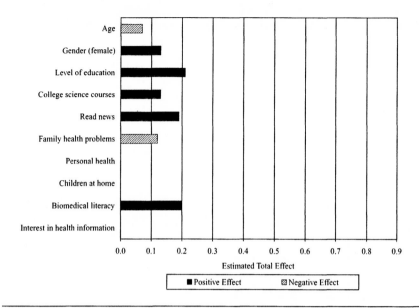

Figure 5-4   **The total effects of selected factors on current health information consumption.**

(Figure 5-4). Unfortunately, the model explains only 13 percent of the total variance in current health information retention and recall, meaning that the remaining 87 percent of the variance either is explained by variables not included in this model or represents noise (or error) in the measurement of the information retention construct. Given the low level of explanation, it is not useful to try to interpret the total effect of each of the variables in the model.

The results are slightly more informative when parallel models are run separately for men and women.[3] In this analysis, the same model described above explained 36 percent of the total variance among women, but only 9 percent of the variance among men. This result suggests that some of the factors that account for the retention and recall of current health information are different for men and for women. Although the predictive power of the model for women is markedly higher than the models of all adults or for men, it is important to recognize that this model leaves 64 percent of the vari-

[3]The model had a good fit with a Root Mean Square Error of Approximation (RMSEA) of .045; 90 percent confidence intervals of .036 and .054; and a chi-square of 145.74, with 57 degrees of freedom. The model explained 36 percent of the total variance among women, but could account for only 9 percent of the total variance in current health information retention among men.

Table 5-1   The Total Effects of Selected Factors on Current Health Information Retention, by Gender, 1993

	Men	Women
Age	−.10	.00
Level of education	.21	.11
College science courses	.19	.00
Read news	.05	.21
Family health problems	.00	−.43
Personal health (excellent)	.00	.13
Children at home	.00	.00
Interest in health information	.00	.62
Biomedical literacy	.29	.00
R^2 (proportion of total variance explained)	.09	.36

ance in current health information retention and recall among women unexplained.

For the third of the variance in women's current health information retention and recall that is accounted for by the model, the results indicate that health interest is the strongest predictor, with a total effect of .62 (see Table 5-1). Women with a family member suffering from a chronic illness were significantly less likely to recall current health information (total effect of −.43) than other women. Women who read newspapers and newsmagazines regularly were slightly more likely (total effect of .21) than other women to be able to recall current health information. Good personal health and level of educational attainment had only slight influence on the recall of current health information (total effects of .13 and .11, respectively). Neither age nor the presence of children in the home had a significant effect on women's recall of current health information.

We report this result because it is what the data tell us, but we do not fully understand the factors that influence the retention and recall of current health information for either women or men. For the third of the variance in current health information recall predicted among women, the relatively strong effect of interest fits into our general model of information acquisition, but the weak influence of education and the negative relationship to having a family member with a chronic illness does not fit our conceptualization of the health communication process.

The full model was run separately for African-Americans, Hispanic-Americans, and Other Americans, to test for possible differential explanato-

Table 5-2   The Total Effects of Selected Factors on Current Health Information Retention, by Race/Ethnicity, 1993

	Other American	African- American	Hispanic- American
Age	—.12	.00	.00
Gender (female)	.19	.00	.00
Level of education	.18	.35	.29
College science courses	.14	.12	.00
Read news	.10	.56	.47
Family health problems	—.27	.00	.00
Personal health (excellent)	.00	.00	.00
Children at home	—.11	.00	.00
Interest in health information	.52	.00	.00
Biomedical literacy	.19	.18	.00
R^2 (proportion of total variance explained)	.24	.38	.22

ry factors based on race and ethnicity (Table 5-2).[4] The model accounted for 38 percent of the total variance in current health information retention and recall among African-Americans, 22 percent of the total variance among Hispanic-Americans, and 24 percent of the total variance among Other Americans. Although these levels of explanatory power are low, they are all higher than the explanatory power of the model for all adults, indicating that the variables included in our core model work differently for these three racial/ethnic groups, producing a higher level of prediction than when the same variables were combined into a single adult model.

For African-Americans, the parallel model accounted for nearly 40 percent of the total variance in current health information retention and recall, and the primary predictors of health information recall were regular news reading (total effect of .56) and educational attainment (total effect of .35). Both the number of college science courses completed and the level of biomedical literacy made smaller additive contributions to the likelihood of recalling current health information (total effects of .12 and .18, respectively). Among African-Americans, age, gender, children at home, and personal health status were unrelated to the ability to recall current health information.

[4]The model had a good fit with an RMSEA of .03 (confidence intervals of .019; .039), and a chi-square of 165.13 with 113 degrees of freedom. The model had an R^2 of .24 for Other Americans, .38 for African Americans, and .22 for Hispanic-Americans.

Because the parallel models for Hispanic-Americans and Other Americans explained less than a quarter of the total variance in current health information recall, it is not useful to examine the influence of individual variables in these models. The important point is that more than three-quarters of the total variance in each of these models is unrelated to the 10 variables included in the basic model described above.

SOURCES OF BIOMEDICAL INFORMATION

Numerous studies have been conducted to examine the primary sources of health information for various groups of individuals. Worsley (1989) has defined three general sources of information about health: (1) formal sources, including family doctors and other health professionals; (2) informal sources, which includes friends and relatives; and (3) commercial and media sources, which includes television, newspapers, and magazines. From a sample of healthy adults, Worsley found that most individuals relied on both informal and formal sources of health information.

Cangelosi and Markham (1994) randomly selected 500 individuals in a seven-county area of the South Central United States and asked them to rate the relative importance of various sources in providing information about preventive health information, and found that personal sources such as physicians, spouses, and nurses, received the highest ratings, while television, magazines, and other media sources received substantially lower ratings.

McCallum *et al.* (1991) examined the primary sources of information about toxic chemical risks in six communities throughout the United States. The communities—Albuquerque, New Mexico; Cincinnati, Ohio; Durham, North Carolina; Middlesex County, New Jersey; Racine, Wisconsin; and Richmond Virginia—were selected on the basis of multiple criteria including the presence of significant industry that used, stored, or released chemicals, the location of a Superfund or other hazardous waste site, and experience with prior emission problems. A total of 3129 individuals in these six communities were interviewed. Respondents were first asked if they had recently heard or read anything about the risks of toxic chemicals in their communities. All those respondents who indicated that they had heard something about toxic chemicals in their community were then asked to name the source of that information. Fifty-two percent of the respondents indicated that they had heard or read something about toxic chemicals in their community. All those who indicated that they had heard or read something in the past week (40 percent of the total respondents) were then asked to name one or more sources of that information. A total of 76 percent of the respondents recalled hearing information about toxic chemicals in a newspaper in the past week, and 62 percent named the local television news.

Meissner *et al.* (1992) used data from the 1987 Cancer Control Supplement to the National Health Interview Survey to examine the relationship between sources of health information and knowledge about and likelihood to have had a cancer screening test. Physicians were rated as the most useful source of information about disease prevention, followed by the print media, and electronic media. Individuals with less than a high school diploma were most likely to mention physicians as the most useful source of information, whereas those with higher levels of education more frequently mentioned the print media. Younger individuals were more likely to mention friends, family, and the electronic media as sources, whereas older individuals more frequently mentioned doctors. Multivariate analyses showed that individuals who relied on the print media were more likely to have heard of the different screening tests than were individuals who relied on physicians or the electronic media for health information.

Johnson and Meischke (1994) note that many studies have combined all media sources when examining health information-seeking behavior. They surveyed 146 women aged 40 and over in one city regarding their preferences for different types and sources of information about cancer. Each woman was asked if she had received any health information in the last year from television, newspapers, or magazines. For each of these sources from which information was obtained, each woman was then asked to rate how likely it was that she would use that medium to get different types of information about cancer. For every type of cancer information, newspapers were the least preferred source of information. Johnson and Meischke comment that:

> *One of the most interesting findings of this study was the generally high scores for magazines across the content domains. Compared with the other mass media, magazines are relatively understudied. But there is a wide range of popular magazines, especially targeted to women, that contain a great deal of specific health information that appears to be useful to them and to which they apparently are likely to turn. (Johnson and Meischke, 1994, pp. 28–29)*

Aaronson *et al.* (1988) interviewed 529 pregnant women in Seattle regarding their major sources of health information regarding their pregnancy and found that health care providers and books were the most frequently cited sources of information. Better educated women were more likely to rely on books and health care providers, whereas less well educated women were more likely to rely on family members. Younger women were less likely to use the print media and more likely to use family members than were older women. Aaronson *et al.* comment that:

> *The information seeking process is influenced by specific and general prior knowledge, and by the costs of the search behaviors. Once knowledge is acquired, decisions about the adequacy and usefulness of the information may be influenced by the level of expertise of the information source and by the relationship of the source to the information seeker. (Aaronson et al., 1988, p. 336)*

Connell and Crawford (1988) studied 182 residents of two counties (one rural and one urban) in Pennsylvania regarding their sources of information about health. They found that women received and retained much more health information than men, and that printed materials (books, magazines, newspapers, and brochures combined) were the most frequently mentioned source of health information for women. No single source of health information was predominant for men. This pattern is consistent with the results of the model of information retention and recall discussed above.

There is an extensive literature regarding the information-seeking behaviors of patients with specific medical conditions (Turk-Charles *et al.*, 1997; Brockopp *et al.*, 1989; Aaroson *et al.*, 1988). However, most of these studies are based on small samples of patients. For example, Turk-Charles *et al.* (1997) surveyed 65 patients at a medical center who had been diagnosed with cancer and found that although older patients were less likely to obtain information from formal schooling, there was no difference based on age in information-seeking from nonformal sources of information.

To improve our understanding of the biomedical information acquisition process, each respondent in the 1993 Biomedical Literacy Study was asked to recall the most important biomedical information that he or she had heard in the preceding 2 months. This open-ended question was designed to elicit a description of a specific item of health or science information. A follow-up probe asked the source of this information, and these responses provide an invaluable insight into the actual information sources used by current health information consumers.

Among current health information consumers, 44 percent recalled a story that they had seen on television, 19 percent mentioned a story they had first read about in a newspaper, and 10 percent cited a story from a magazine (see Table 5-3). Approximately 5 percent of current health information consumers recalled information obtained from a health professional, 12 percent from another person such as a friend, teacher, or parent, and only 6 percent recalled health information from the radio.

The strongest differentiation was by level of education. Approximately half of those persons who did not complete high school recalled a biomedical story from television, and only 18 percent of this group cited a story from a newspaper or magazine. In contrast, 43 percent of graduate degree holders mentioned a story from a print source, and only 29 percent recalled a television story. This pattern is consistent with our previous findings in regard to the strong educational and knowledge base of current health information consumers.

Among current health information consumers, men were significantly more likely to recall a health or medical news item from television than women, and women were significantly more likely to cite a health information item from a conversation with another person, including health professionals. Approximately 30 percent of both men and women cited a story from a print source.

Although latent health information consumers—those individuals who could not recall a health or medical story from the previous 2 months—did not provide the same kind of recall information obtained from current health information consumers, they were asked which information sources they would use if they wanted to obtain some health or medical information. Recognizing that this is a somewhat hypothetical inquiry for individuals who could not recall a single health or medical story in the previous 2 months, the results indicate that nearly 40 percent of these latent health information consumers named a nonmedia source—primarily health professionals (see Table 5-4). A third of latent health information consumers reported that they would look to television for health information, and 28 percent said that they would rely on a newspaper or magazine. Only 2 percent of latent health information consumers indicated that they would rely on the radio for health information.

For purposes of targeting biomedical information and messages, the recalled information sources of current health information consumers are the more reliable guide. These responses are linked to at least one actual piece of relevant information from a defined time period. From the multivariate analyses in the preceding section, we know that current information consumers are more likely to be motivated by a combination of the salience of biomedical issues and a foundation of education and biomedical literacy. The implications of these general patterns will become more apparent as we turn to a discussion of the media use and information acquisition behaviors of selected segments of the population.

More recently, in the 1998 Social and Behavioral Indicators Survey, respondents were asked whether they had heard or read any new information about cancer and heart disease in the last 2 months. Respondents were also asked a similar series of questions about alcoholism or a serious mental health problem such as depression or schizophrenia. Unlike the 1993 Biomedical Literacy Study, respondents were not asked to name the new information that they had heard. Consequently, we cannot provide comparable

Table 5-3 Primary Source of Health Information Recalled by Current Health Information Consumers, 1993

	Percentage of adults recalling an item of health information from . . .							*Number of cases*
	TV	*News-paper*	*Maga-zine*	*Health profes-sionals*	*Other people*	*Radio*	*Other*	
Total adults	44	19	10	5	12	6	4	1737
Gender								
Male	48	20	8	4	9	7	4	815
Female	40	18	12	7	14	5	4	922
Level of education								
Less than high school	49	10	8	5	14	7	7	267
High school	46	20	10	6	11	5	3	1075
Baccalaureate	38	24	11	5	11	7	4	265
Graduate degree	29	26	17	3	13	8	4	130
Age								
18–24 years	45	17	10	2	18	6	2	230
25–34 years	51	17	10	5	9	5	3	408
35–44 years	43	21	9	4	14	6	3	375
45–54 years	39	21	13	8	8	7	4	267
55–64 years	36	23	11	8	13	5	4	207
65 or more years	43	17	10	6	9	7	8	249

Table 5-4 Primary Sources of Health Information of Latent Health Information Consumers, 1993

| | *Percentage of adults recalling an item of health information from . . .* | | | | | | | |
	TV	*News-paper*	*Maga-zine*	*Health profes-sionals*	*Other people*	*Radio*	*Other*	*Number of Cases*
Total adults	32	15	13	21	3	2	12	1374
Gender								
Male	32	19	10	18	4	2	12	674
Female	32	12	16	23	1	2	11	700
Level of education								
Less than high school	30	8	9	32	3	2	12	365
High school	35	14	14	17	2	2	13	795
Baccalaureate	26	30	12	17	4	2	8	149
Graduate degree	24	27	27	12	5	0	5	65
Age								
18–24 years	45	10	6	19	3	1	12	189
25–34 years	36	17	8	17	5	3	12	317
35–44 years	25	22	14	16	3	4	12	283
45–54 years	36	15	15	15	2	2	13	180
55–64 years	37	14	27	8	1	1	10	143
65 or more years	21	12	14	42	1	1	9	263

information about the level of current health information consumers for cancer/heart disease and alcoholism/depression/schizophrenia. However, respondents in the 1998 study were asked to name not only the source of that information, but also the source they would use to obtain additional information about that disease, providing us with valuable information about the different functions that various sources of health information serve for the public.

For the 1998 study, individuals will be considered a current information consumer for heart disease/cancer if they indicated that they had heard some new information about the disease, and if they were able to name the source of that information. All other individuals are considered to be latent information consumers for heart disease/cancer. Current information consumers for mental health/alcoholism were calculated in the same fashion. In 1998, 62 percent of Americans were current information consumers for heart disease/cancer, and 52 percent were current information consumers for mental health/alcoholism (see Figure 5-5). There was a strong relationship between level of education and retention of information about specific health conditions. Over 80 percent of those with a graduate or professional degree were current information consumers for heart disease/cancer, and over two-thirds were current information consumers for mental health/alcoholism. In contrast, 60 percent of those with less than a high diploma were current information consumers for heart disease/cancer, and only 43 percent were current information consumers for mental health/alcoholism.

Over three-quarters of older Americans were current information consumers for heart disease/cancer, in contrast to less than half of those under age 35. This speaks to a strong experiential component of information acquisition for specific illnesses. Further validity is lent to the influence of personal experience on information acquisition by the relationship between the acquisition of information about a specific medical condition and family or personal experience with that condition. Although less than half of the individuals who did not have personal or family experience with depression were current information consumers for mental health/alcoholism, two-thirds of those who did have this personal experience were current information consumers (see Figure 5-5). Similarly, 70 percent of those with personal or family experience with heart disease were current information consumers for heart disease/cancer, whereas only 54 percent without the personal experience were current health information consumers.

The traditional major media served as the source of new information for nearly two-thirds of the current information consumers for heart disease/cancer and mental health/alcoholism in 1998 (see Figures 5-6 and 5-7). Nearly one-quarter of the current information consumers for heart disease/cancer, indicated that they had read about the new information in a maga-

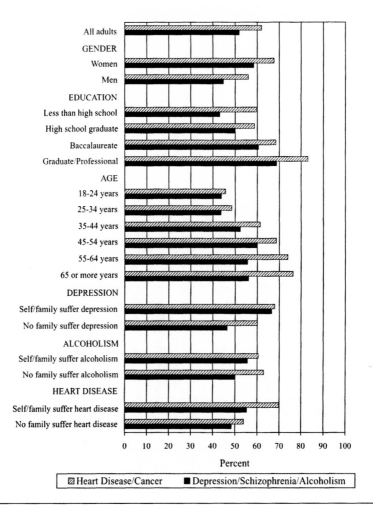

Figure 5-5 Current information consumers for heart disease/cancer and alcoholism/mental illness, 1998.

zine, whereas one-fifth had read about heart disease or cancer in a newspaper. Another 18 percent of current information consumers for heart disease/cancer had heard or seen new information on the television or radio. Current information consumers for mental illness/alcoholism reported nearly identical reliance on the traditional print and broadcast media.

Ten percent of current information consumers for heart disease/cancer reported that they had heard new information from a physician or other health care professional, whereas only 5 percent of current health informa-

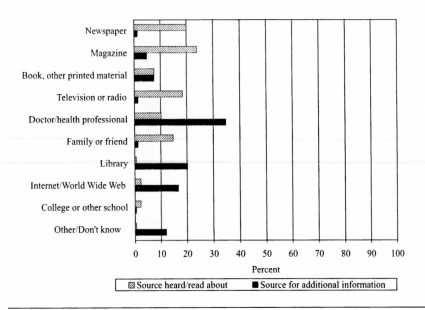

Figure 5-6   **Sources of information about heart disease or cancer, 1998.**

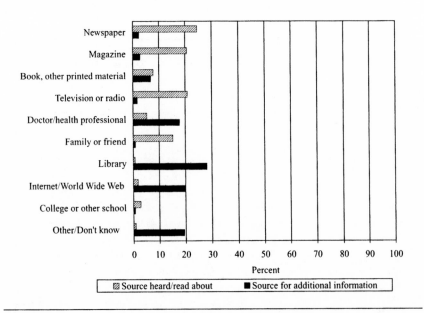

Figure 5-7   **Sources of information about alcoholism or mental illness, 1998.**

tion consumers for mental illness/alcoholism heard new information from a physician or other health care professional. Approximately 15 percent of both groups heard new information from a family member or friend, and 2 percent saw new information on the World Wide Web.

Although the traditional media serve a primary function of alerting the public about new health and medical information, they do not serve as a primary source for additional information. All individuals who indicated that they had read or heard some information about heart disease/cancer or mental illness/alcoholism were also asked where they would go to get additional information. Although nearly two-thirds of current information consumers indicated that they had first heard or read about the new information on television, radio, magazines, or newspapers, fewer than 10 percent said that they would rely on traditional print or broadcast media for additional information.

Over one-third of current information consumers for heart disease/cancer, and nearly one-fifth of current information consumers for mental illness/alcoholism indicated that they would seek out additional information from doctors or other health care professionals. The library would serve as a source of additional information for 20 percent of current information consumers for heart disease/cancer, and 28 percent of current information consumers for alcoholism/mental illness.

Although the traditional print and broadcast media serve as the major source of new information for current information consumers for heart disease/cancer and mental illness/alcoholism, they do not serve as the primary sources for additional information. Fewer than 10 percent of current information consumers for heart disease/cancer and for mental illness/alcoholism indicated that they would rely on the traditional media for additional information. More current information consumers would use the Internet or World Wide Web to obtain additional information than would use all print and broadcast media combined. Nearly 17 percent of current health information consumers for cancer/heart disease and 20 percent of current health information consumers for mental illness/alcoholism would rely on the Internet or World Wide Web for additional information. Use of the Internet or World Wide Web for additional information is strongly related to level of education.

Over one-third of current information consumers for heart disease/cancer and 18 percent of current information consumers for mental illness/alcoholism would rely on doctors or other health care professionals for additional information. The library would serve as the primary source of additional information for 20 percent of current information consumers for heart disease/cancer, and for 28 percent of current information consumers about mental illness/alcoholism.

Throughout this book, we have emphasized the need to target biomedical communications to specific groups. In Chapter 4 we discussed the differential use of selected sources of health information by different groups of Americans. It is also important for biomedical communicators to distinguish between the types of information they want to convey to consumers: do they wish to alert consumers to new health or medical information, or do they wish to provide information that may supplement what the consumer already knows? At the present time, the majority of Americans still obtain new information about health and medicine from traditional media sources such as television and newspapers. In the most recent study in 1998, only a small percentage of Americans first heard or read about new health information from a physician or from the Internet. Thus, for the time being, television, newspapers, and magazines remain excellent sources for alerting the public to new health information. This dependence on the traditional media for new health information may decrease, as access to the Internet becomes more widespread. Indeed, with the introduction of broadband into the majority of homes, the distinction between these media sources may become blurred.

Most Americans do not rely on the traditional media when they want to obtain additional information about health and medical conditions. In the 1998 study, fewer than 10 percent of Americans said that they would use the traditional media to obtain additional information about cancer/heart disease or mental health/alcoholism. Instead, most individuals would look to physicians or other health care professionals, the library, or the Internet to obtain additional information. As access to the Internet expands, reliance on the library may decrease in favor of the more convenient sources of health information available on the World Wide Web.

COMMUNICATING BIOMEDICAL INFORMATION TO SELECTED GROUPS

The preceding sections have focused on the media use and information acquisition behaviors of the total population, although the multivariate models identified group-related factors such as age or gender that influence media use behaviors and information retention. We now turn to four specific segments of the population that are often the subject of targeted biomedical communications and examine the patterns of media use by the individuals in each segment. The analysis will focus on (1) young adults, (2) parents with children at home, (3) older citizens, and (4) gender differences. Within each of these four major groupings, detailed analyses will explore patterns of media use and information acquisition by level of education and for African-Americans, Hispanic-Americans, and Other Americans.

Communicating with Young Adults

A growing volume of health and biomedical information and messages are focused on young adults, defined as individuals aged 18 through 24. Using the data from the 1993 Biomedical Literacy Study, 55 percent of the young adults were current health information consumers, meaning that they were able to recall at least one health or biomedical science information item from the previous 2 months and name the source of that information (see Figure 5-8). Over 80 percent of young adults who had completed a baccalaureate qualified as current health information consumers. Hispanic-American young adults were the least likely to be current health information consumers, with only 42 percent qualifying. Young men and women were equally likely to be current health information consumers.

Among the 55 percent of young adults qualifying as current health information consumers, television was the primary source of health information, with 45 percent of this group recalling information obtained from a television show (see Table 5-5). Approximately 26 percent of young adults recalled a health information story from a newspaper or magazine. Only 2 percent of young adults recalled a piece of health information from a health professional, whereas 18 percent recalled a piece of information from another person such as a parent, friend, or classmate.

Looking at strategies for communicating to specific segments of the young adult population, the primary source of health information for high school students was other people (38 percent), which would include family, teachers, other students, and friends. Television was the source of recalled health information for 23 percent of high school students, newspapers were the recalled source for 18 percent of high school students, whereas magazines were the recalled source for only 13 percent of high school students (see Table 5-5). Only 3 percent of the high school students who were current health information consumers mentioned a doctor, nurse, or other health professional as the recalled source of health information. Contrary to the popular stereotype of high school students and their radios, radio was not cited as a source of health or medical information by any high school students who were current health information consumers.

For young adults who graduated from high school but did not continue into college, television was the dominant source of health information, with 71 percent of this group citing television as the source of a recalled information item. Eighteen percent of this group mentioned information that they read in a newspaper, but only 3 percent cited information recalled from a magazine. Unlike in-school young adults, only 4 percent of this group of recent high school graduates mentioned information from another person, and none mentioned information from a health professional. No recent high school graduates mentioned radio as the recalled source of health information.

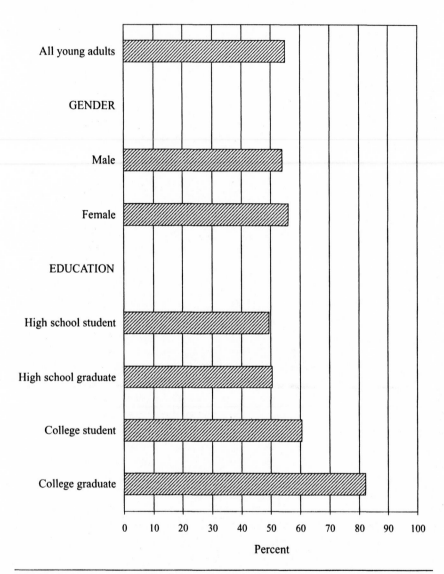

Figure 5-8 Percent current health information consumers among young adults, 1993.

College students who were current health information consumers displayed a diverse set of information sources. Fully 31 percent of this group recalled information obtained from television, and 22 percent from other people, such as friends, teachers, and other students, whereas 4 percent recalled health information from a health professional. Seventeen percent mentioned health information obtained from a magazine, and 14 percent recalled information from a newspaper article. About 11 percent cited information first obtained from radio.

Approximately 10 percent of this age cohort had completed college and were regular health information consumers. Nearly 60 percent of this group recalled an item of health information from a television show, and 23 percent cited information from a newspaper. Given the small size of this group, we would recommend using data from all college graduates for targeting specific messages.

One of the primary components of the design of the 1993 Biomedical Literacy Study was a stratification by race and ethnicity to allow the development of accurate estimates for African-Americans and Hispanic-Americans, two groups often underrepresented in national probability samples in the United States (see Appendix A for sampling information). Looking at only the young adult respondents who are current health information consumers, the results indicate that African-American young adults were most likely to recall health information from a television show (51 percent). Reflecting the school sources discussed above, 17 percent recalled information obtained from another person, 3 percent from a health professional, and 11 percent cited a magazine article as a source of health information. Only 8 percent mentioned health information obtained from a newspaper and only 4 percent cited health information from a radio source (see Table 5-5).

Among Hispanic-American young adults who were health information consumers, 42 percent recalled health information from a television source, whereas 22 percent cited information obtained from another person. No Hispanic-American young adults who were health information consumers recalled information from a health professional. Approximately one in five Hispanic-American young adult health information consumers mentioned information from a newspaper, but only 1 percent recalled information from a radio broadcast.

For other young Americans, television was also the most common source of health information, with 44 percent recalling an item from a television source. Nearly 20 percent of this group recalled a newspaper health item, and 9 percent recalled health information from a magazine article. About 7 percent mentioned information obtained from the radio. Friends, parents, and other people were mentioned as the recalled source of health information by 18 percent of the other young Americans who were current health information consumers, and health professionals were mentioned by another 3 percent.

In summary, the 55 percent of young adults who were current health information consumers in 1993 obtained their information from a variety of sources, but were most likely to recall health information from a television show. Given the high proportion of this age cohort who are full-time high

Table 5-5   Primary Sources for Young Adult Current Health Information Consumers, 1993

	Percentage recalling an item of health information from . . .							Number of respondents
	TV	News-paper	Maga-zine	Health profes-sionals	Other people	Radio	Other	
Total young adults	45	16	10	2	18	6	3	230
Gender								
Male	51	17	5	0	19	4	4	111
Female	40	16	13	4	17	8	2	119
Educational status								
High school dropout	**a	**	**	**	**	**	**	6
High school student	23	18	13	3	38	0	5	39
High school graduate	71	18	3	0	4	0	4	71
College student	31	14	17	4	22	11	1	92
College graduate	59	23	0	0	4	14	0	23
Race/ethnicity								
African-American	51	8	11	3	17	4	6	104
Hispanic-American	42	21	6	0	22	1	8	83
Other American	44	18	9	3	18	7	1	72

a** Too few cases for a meaningful calculation.

school or college students, there was a high degree of reliance on other people—fellow students, teachers, health center personnel, and counselors—for health information, and full-time students were notably less likely to rely on television sources than nonstudents in this age cohort.

The traditional media of newspapers, magazines, and television were the primary source of new information in 1998 for young adults who were current information consumers for heart disease/cancer and mental illness/alcoholism (see Figures 5-9 and 5-10). Only 5 percent of these young current information consumers heard new information about heart disease or cancer from a health care professional, and even fewer heard new information about mental illness or alcoholism from a health care professional. Family or friends served as the source of new information about heart disease or cancer for 19 percent of young adults and as the source of new information about mental illness or alcoholism for 15 percent of young adults.

Although the World Wide Web and public libraries do not serve as primary sources of new information for young adults, they are major sources of additional health information. Although no young adults indicated that they had heard new information about heart disease/cancer or mental illness/alcoholism from a public library, one-third of young adults said that they would

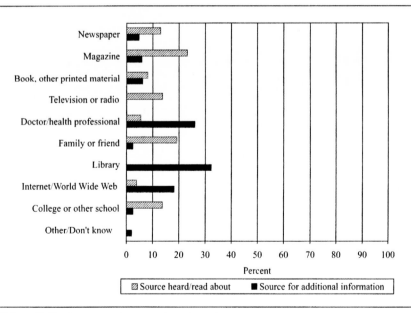

Figure 5-9   Sources of information about heart disease or cancer for young adults, 1998.

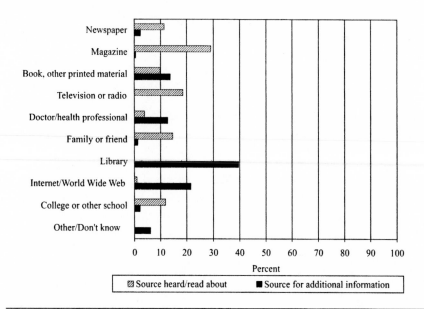

Figure 5-10 Sources of information about mental illness or alcoholism for young adults, 1998.

seek out additional information about heart disease or cancer at a public library, and 40 percent would seek additional information about mental illness or alcoholism at a public library. Only 4 percent of young adult current information consumers for heart disease/cancer named the World Wide Web as the source of their new information, but 18 percent would rely on the World Wide Web for additional information. Similarly, only 1 percent of current information consumers heard new information about mental illness/alcoholism on the World Wide Web, but 22 percent would use the World Wide Web to obtain additional information.

As was noted earlier, doctors and other health professionals do not serve as a major source of new information for young adults who are current information consumers for either heart disease/cancer or mental illness/alcoholism. This pattern undoubtedly reflects, in part, the lower rates of physician visits among young adults. However, one-fourth of these same young adults named doctors or other health care professionals as the source where they would go to obtain additional information about heart disease or cancer. Thirteen percent of young adults said that they would seek out additional information about mental illness or alcoholism from a health care professional.

Communicating with Parents
with Children at Home

In the 1993 Biomedical Literacy Study, parents with children at home represent a third of the adult population of the United States, and 58 percent of this group were able to recall at least one item of health or biomedical information from the previous 2 months, as well as the source of the information, qualifying as a current health information consumer (see Figure 5-11). Parents with a baccalaureate were more likely to be current health information consumers than parents without a college education, and African-American parents were more likely to be current health information consumers than either Hispanic-American or Other American parents. Approximately 60 percent of both mothers and fathers were current health information consumers.

Among parents with children at home qualifying as current health information consumers, television was the primary source of health information, with 44 percent of this group recalling information obtained from a television show (see Table 5-6). Approximately 32 percent of the parents qualifying as current health information consumers recalled a health information story from a newspaper or magazine, and 16 percent cited health information from nonmedia sources such as friends, family members, or a nurse or other health professional.

Looking at strategies for communicating to specific segments of the parent population, there are clear differences in the patterns of media use and recall by the level of educational attainment. Over 70 percent of parents who did not complete high school recalled some health information obtained from television, whereas only 11 percent of this group cited information from a print source (see Table 5-6). In contrast, a third of parents with a college degree recalled health information from a television source, whereas 36 percent of these parents referenced a print medium. Better educated parents were more likely to obtain health information from other individuals than parents without a high school diploma, suggesting a better network of informed resources.

Among African-American parents able to recall at least one item of health information, 60 percent cited an item from a television show, and only 22 percent mentioned an item from a newspaper or magazine. Ten percent of African-American parent health information consumers referenced information from another person, including health professionals. Nearly half of Hispanic-American parent health information consumers recalled an item of health information from a television show, and 22 percent cited a print source, but 13 percent recalled information obtained from another person, including health professionals. Approximately 11 percent of Hispanic-American parent health information consumers recalled an item of information from a radio show, a higher rate of radio use than either of the other two par-

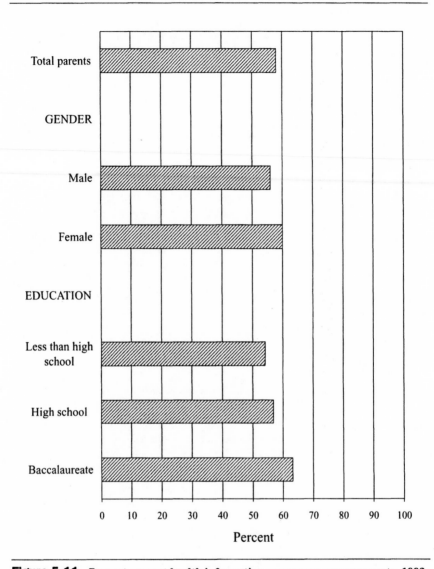

Figure 5-11   Percent current health information consumers among parents, 1993.

ent groups. In contrast, 41 percent of Other American parents recalled an item of health information from a television show, but 35 percent referenced some health information from a print source. Seventeen percent mentioned an item of information obtained from another person or health professional, and only 5 percent cited a radio source.

In summary, 58 percent of parents with children at home are current

Table 5-6 Primary Health Sources for Parent Current Health Information Consumers, 1993

	Percentage recalling an item of health information from							*Number of respondents*
	TV	*News-paper*	*Maga-zine*	*Health profes-sionals*	*Other people*	*Radio*	*Other*	
Total parents	44	21	11	4	12	5	3	610
Gender								
Male	52	21	7	2	7	8	3	286
Female	38	20	15	6	16	2	3	324
Level of education								
Less than high school	72	9	2	8	4	3	2	92
High school	43	22	13	5	11	5	1	342
Baccalaureate	33	25	11	2	18	6	5	176
Race/ethnicity								
African-American	60	12	10	3	7	3	5	198
Hispanic-American	48	12	10	3	10	11	6	227
Other American	41	23	12	4	13	5	2	190

health information consumers. Four of ten appear to rely primarily on television for health information, whereas a third utilize newspapers and magazines. Approximately 16 percent rely on health information from other people—family, friends, co-workers, and health personnel.

In 1998, the traditional media and family and friends served as the primary sources of new information for parents who were current health information consumers about heart disease/cancer and mental illness/alcoholism (see Figures 5-12 and 5-13). Approximately 10 percent of parents heard new information about heart disease/cancer or mental illness/alcoholism from a health care professional, and only 1 or 2 percent from the World Wide Web or a library.

When parents want to obtain additional information about heart disease or cancer, over one-third will seek out that information from a doctor or other health care professional, and one-fifth will look for the information at either a public library or on the World Wide Web. The primary source of additional information about mental illness or alcoholism for parents is the public library. One-quarter of the parents would use the library for additional information about mental illness/alcoholism, and 19 percent would rely on a doctor or health care professional or the World Wide Web. Only 1 percent of current information consumers for heart disease/cancer and mental illness/alcoholism would rely on family or friends for additional information.

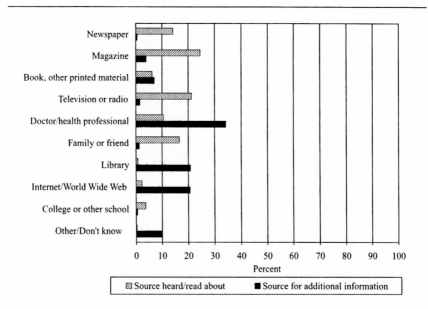

Figure 5-12   **Sources of information about heart disease or cancer for parents, 1998.**

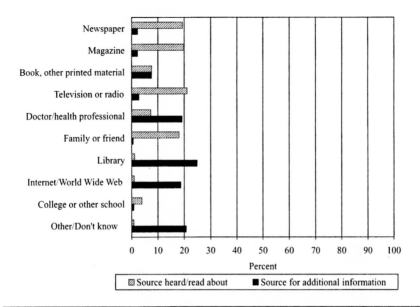

Figure 5-13 Sources of information about mental illness or alcoholism for parents, 1998.

Communicating with Older Adults

Older adults—persons aged 60 years or more—are an important audience for biomedical communicators. For older adults, information campaigns often seek to provide new information about cancer, heart disease, and other conditions often associated with aging. It is important to recall from previous analyses that this age cohort has the lowest level of educational attainment of all of the age cohorts and the highest level of self-reported health problems of any age group. Nonetheless, only 54 percent of this group could recall one or more items of health information from the preceding 2 months as well as the source of the information, qualifying as current health information consumers (see Figure 5-14).

Senior men and women were equally likely to be current health information consumers, but there was a significant variation in health information retention and recall by the level of educational attainment. Only 39 percent of adults who did not complete high school were able to recall any health information from the preceding 2 months, compared to 68 percent of college graduates. This result reflects the cumulative advantages of educational and occupational experiences that have encouraged and enhanced individual skills in information processing, retention, and recall. There were no significant differences by race or ethnicity within the age cohort.

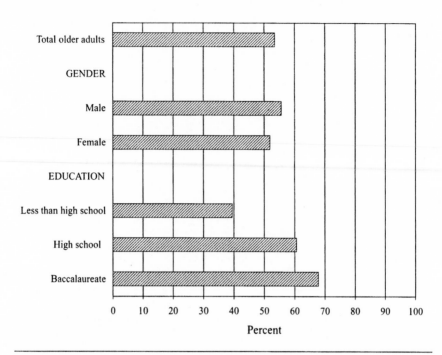

Figure 5-14 Percent current health information consumers among older adults, 1993.

When asked to recall an item of health information from the previous 2 months, 40 percent of older health information consumers cited information obtained from television (see Table 5-7). Nearly 30 percent mentioned information obtained from a newspaper or magazine, and only 6 percent referenced an item from radio. Only 7 percent of older adults cited information obtained from a health professional, despite the relatively high level of physician visits reported by this group. Twelve percent of older adults recalled information obtained from another person, such as a family member or friend.

For older health information consumers who did not complete high school, television was the most common source of health information, with 32 percent recalling one or more information items from a television show (see Table 5-7). Slightly more than 20 percent of this group cited information provided by another person such as a friend or family members, and only 2 percent cited information from physicians or other medical personnel. This level of reliance on one's own family for health information is the highest of the three education strata. Eleven percent of this group recalled health information obtained from the radio.

Table 5-7   Primary Sources of Health Information for Older Adult Health Information Consumers, 1993

	Percentage recalling an item of health information from . . .							Number of respondents
	TV	News-paper	Maga-zine	Health profes-sionals	Other people	Radio	Other	
Total older adults	40	20	8	4	12	6	7	361
Gender								
Male	43	19	11	6	9	4	8	159
Female	37	21	5	7	15	8	7	202
Level of education								
Less than high school	32	11	7	2	21	11	16	99
High school	48	23	5	7	10	4	3	203
Baccalaureate	28	26	17	12	5	5	7	59
Race/ethnicity								
African-American	48	12	1	6	6	3	14	87
Hispanic-American	33	12	4	7	4	26	14	56
Other American	39	21	9	7	13	6	5	129

Nearly half of older health information consumers who completed high school, but not college, recalled an item of health information from television. Nearly a quarter of these older health information consumers referenced information from a newspaper, and 5 percent mentioned health information obtained from a magazine. Only 4 percent of this group cited health information from the radio.

Among college-educated older health information consumers, 43 percent recalled information from a print source, compared to 28 percent who cited information from television. In contrast to the least well educated stratum, 12 percent of this group recalled an item of health information provided by a physician or other health professional, and only 5 percent mentioned information obtained from one's own family or friends. Five percent of this group cited information obtained from radio.

Reflecting differences in education, 48 percent of older African-American health information consumers recalled health information from a television show, whereas only 13 percent cited a print source. Six percent of this group referenced information obtained from a health professional, and 6 percent from another person. Only 3 percent of older African-American current health information consumers mentioned health information obtained from a radio broadcast. Comparatively, 33 percent of older Hispanic-American health information consumers recalled health information from a television show, and 26 percent referenced one or more health news items from radio. Sixteen percent of older Hispanic-American health information consumers cited an item from a print source.

Approximately 40 percent of Other American older health information consumers—87 percent of senior citizens—recalled a health information item from a television source, and 40 percent cited information obtained from a newspaper or magazine (see Table 5-7). About 13 percent mentioned health information obtained from another person, and 7 percent referenced a conversation with a physician or other health professional. Only 5 percent cited health information from a radio source.

In summary, a large part of the variation in health information retention and recall among older adults appears to reflect differences in educational attainment. Older adults who completed a baccalaureate, for example, appear to be less likely to rely on television and more likely to utilize print media or personal contacts than older adults who did not complete college. Older males were slightly more likely to recall a television source, whereas older women were more likely to rely on other individuals for health information.

In 1998, three-quarters of older adult health information consumers had first heard or read new information about mental illness or alcoholism from a newspaper, magazine, or television, and 63 percent had heard new information about heart disease or cancer from the same sources (see Figures 5-15 and 5-16). Only 11 percent of older current health information con-

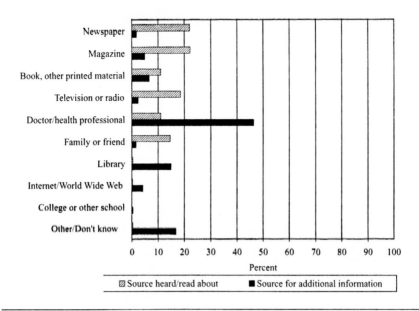

Figure 5-15 Sources of information about heart disease or cancer for older adults, 1998.

sumers for heart disease/cancer and 3 percent for mental illness/alcoholism cited doctors or health professionals as the source of new information. However, 46 percent of these same individuals would rely on doctors or health professionals for additional information about heart disease or cancer, and 18 percent would rely on doctors for additional information about mental illness or alcoholism.

Family and friends served as a source of new information about heart disease or cancer for 15 percent of older current information consumers, whereas 14 percent of current information consumers first heard new information about mental illness or alcoholism from family or friends. Although family and friends informed approximately 15 percent of older adults about new information, they would be relied on for additional information by fewer than 2 percent of older current information consumers.

Nearly a third of older current information users would go to a public library to obtain additional information about mental illness or alcoholism, and 15 percent would do the same for information about heart disease or cancer. Relatively few older adults would go to the World Wide Web to seek additional information about either heart disease/cancer or mental illness/depression.

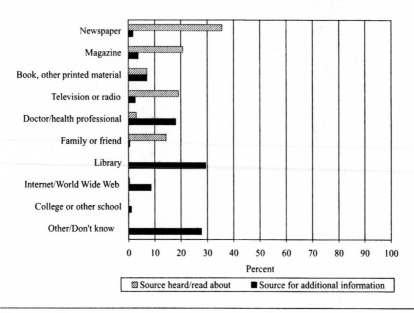

Figure 5-16 **Sources of information about mental illness or alcoholism for older adults, 1998.**

Communicating with Men and Women

Approximately 60 percent of both men and women were able to recall at least one item of health or biomedical information from the preceding 2 months as well as the source of the information, indicating that there is no difference by gender in the likelihood of being a current health information consumer (see Figure 5-17). Even when education, race, and ethnicity were taken into account, there were no statistically significant differences between men and women in their ability to recall health and biomedical information.

Looking at the retention and recall of health information, the similarities between men and women are far greater than the differences. Men were significantly more likely to recall health information from television than women, and women were significantly more likely to recall health information obtained from other people (see Table 5-8). This same set of relationships were not statistically significant for African-American or Hispanic-American men and women. Among college graduates of the three racial and ethnic groups, women were significantly more likely to reference health information provided by other people than were men, but the difference in the recall of health information from television was not statistically different between college-educated men and women.

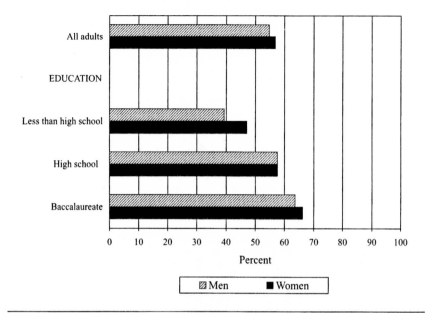

Figure 5-17 Percent current health information consumers by gender, 1993.

On balance, these results from 1993 suggest that there are few significant differences between men and women in the retention and recall of health information or in the sources from which they obtain health information. We would speculate that the differences between men and women in their relative reliance on television and on personal conversations may reflect a greater social acceptance of the discussion of health and medical topics among women and a lesser social acceptance of this kind of discussion among men. Unfortunately, we do not have the kind of data that would be required to explore fully this speculation.

In 1998, men who were current information consumers were slightly more likely than women to report that they had first heard or read information about either heart disease/cancer or mental illness/alcoholism from the traditional media of newspapers, magazines, and television (see Figures 5-18, 5-19, 5-20, and 5-21). However, neither men nor women indicated that they would rely on these traditional media if they wanted to obtain additional information about any of the conditions. A total of 38 percent of women and 30 percent of men who were current information consumers for heart disease/cancer would talk to a doctor or other health care professional if they wanted to obtain additional information. Fewer men (16 percent) and women (19 percent) would seek out a health care professional for additional information about mental illness or alcoholism.

Table 5-8 Primary Health Information Sources for Current Health Information Consumers, by Gender, 1993

	Percentage recalling an item of health information from . . .							Number of respondents
	TV	News-paper	Maga-zine	Health profes-sionals	Other people	Radio	Other	
ALL MEN	48	20	8	4	9	7	4	815
Level of education								
Less than high school	59	6	5	4	12	9	5	130
High school	51	22	7	3	10	5	2	478
Baccalaureate	36	27	12	5	5	10	5	206
Race/ethnicity								
African-American	53	13	8	5	9	5	7	307
Hispanic-American	45	17	8	3	8	15	4	239
Other American	48	22	9	7	13	6	5	129
ALL WOMEN	40	18	12	7	14	5	4	922
Level of education								
Less than high school	38	14	11	6	16	6	9	165
High school	42	18	12	8	12	5	3	569
Baccalaureate	33	23	14	4	18	5	3	188
Race/ethnicity								
African-American	51	14	8	6	11	2	8	344
Hispanic-American	49	12	9	3	10	6	11	265
Other American	37	20	13	7	15	5	3	302

Approximately one-fifth of both male and female current information consumers for heart disease/cancer would go to a public library to obtain additional information. One-quarter of the male and 30 percent of the female current information consumers for mental illness/alcoholism would seek out additional information at the public library. The World Wide Web would be used as a source of additional information by 20 percent of the male and 15 percent of the female current information consumers for heart disease/cancer, and by 25 percent of the male and 16 percent of the female current information consumers for mental illness/alcoholism.

Friends and family served as the source of new information for between 10 and 17 percent of both male and female current information consumers for mental illness/alcoholism and heart disease/cancer. However, neither men nor women would look to friends and family to obtain additional information about these conditions.

A CASE STUDY IN NERVOUSNESS OR STRESS MANAGEMENT

In broad general terms, most Americans believe that they can have a significant impact on their own health through their personal decisions and ac-

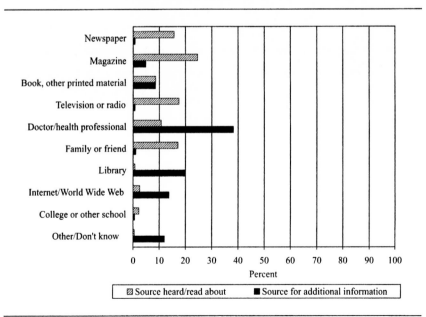

Figure 5-18   **Sources of information about heart disease or cancer for women, 1998.**

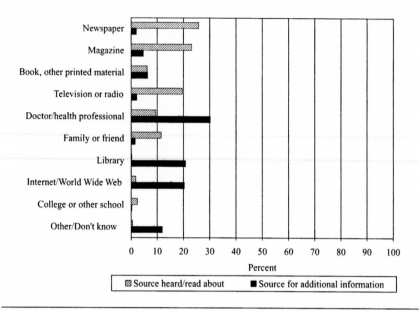

Figure 5-19 **Sources of information about heart disease or cancer for men, 1998.**

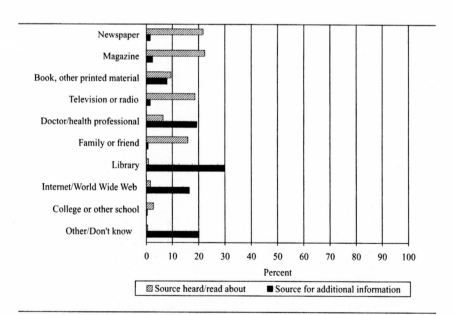

Figure 5-20 **Sources of information about mental illness or alcoholism for women, 1998.**

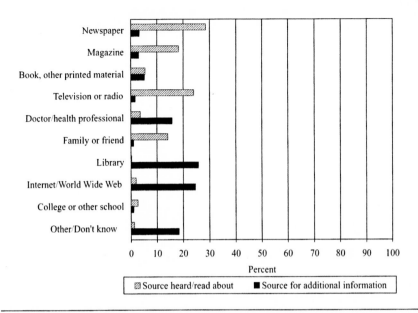

Figure 5-21   Sources of information about mental illness or alcoholism for men, 1998.

tions on diet and exercise. Although many Americans are aware of recent advances in genetic research, which has been covered extensively in the print and broadcast media, they tend to discount the relative importance of genetic factors on their own health. There is a high degree of receptivity to the efficacy of herbs and other natural substances in the treatment of some diseases, and many people apparently see vitamins and other food supplements as being as effective as prescription drugs for general health maintenance.

To place these general views into a more concrete context, each respondent in the 1998 Office of Behavioral and Social Science Research (OBSSR) study was asked the following question:

If you found yourself feeling very nervous for a long time and couldn't figure out exactly why, please tell me how likely is it that you would take any of the following actions—very likely, somewhat likely, somewhat unlikely, or very unlikely?

Pray or talk to a religious counselor?

Go to an herbal store and find something that soothes the nerves?

Go to a physician and ask for a prescription drug?

Go to a physician and ask for a nonprescription drug?

Find a psychologist or other mental health professional and talk about your condition?

Facing this kind of problem, a third of American adults indicated that they would be very likely to turn to prayer or seek religious guidance, and an additional 23 percent said that they would be somewhat likely to seek help through prayer or religious guidance (see Figure 5-22). Women were significantly more likely to report that they would be very likely to seek religious help than were men (see Table 5-9). Less well educated adults were significantly more likely to turn to prayer than were better educated adults.

Seventeen percent of respondents reported that they would be very likely to seek a prescription from a doctor, and an additional 26 percent said that they would be somewhat likely to seek a prescription drug through a physician (see Figure 5-22). There was little variation in the likelihood of seeking a prescription between men and women (see Table 5-9). Adults who did not finish high school were significantly more likely to have said that they would be very likely to seek a prescription from a doctor than were other respondents.

Only 15 percent of adults indicated that they would be very likely to seek help from a psychologist or other mental health professional, and 23 percent said that they would be somewhat likely to seek professional help for this kind of condition. Women were significantly more likely than men to report that they would be very likely to see professional help.

Although a large majority of Americans were willing to agree that herbs and other natural substances were as effective as prescription drugs for some illnesses, it appears that the nervous condition described in the interview is not one of those conditions. Only 10 percent of adults indicated that they would be very likely to seek relief from an herbal store for this condition, whereas an additional 18 percent reported that they would be somewhat likely to seek help from herbal substances (see Figure 5-22). Women were significantly more likely to indicate that they would be very likely to use an herbal substance than men, and less well educated respondents were significantly more likely to say that they would be very likely to seek an herbal solution than better educated respondents.

Nonprescription or over-the-counter drugs were the least favored alternative treatment for the nervous condition described, with only 7 percent of adults saying that they would be very likely to seek help from a nonprescription drug. A majority of adults indicated that they would be very unlikely to depend on a nonprescription drug for this purpose (see Figure 5-22). Less well educated adults were significantly more likely to turn to a nonprescription drug than were better educated citizens (see Table 5-9).

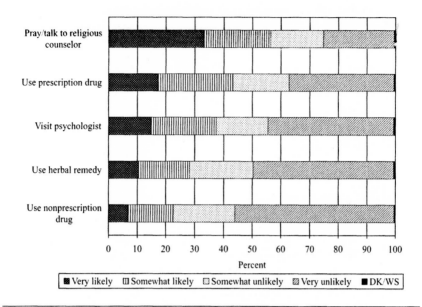

Figure 5-22 Reported response to continuing nervous condition, 1998.

IMPLICATIONS FOR BIOMEDICAL COMMUNICATORS

From this brief exploration of the general structure of biomedical information acquisition, there are several important implications for practicing biomedical communicators.

- First, for a combination of salience and educational reasons, only 56 percent of American adults can recall any health or medical information that they have read or heard in the previous 2 months as well as the source of that information. This finding means that approximately two of five American adults cannot recall a single piece of health or medical information from the preceding 2 months. All adults are exposed daily to a virtual tidal wave of new information from television, newspapers, magazines, and numerous other sources. It is imperative that each individual selects those messages or information that are most salient and ignore—or tune out—other available information. The 56 percent of adults who could recall some health or medical information should be thought of as current health information consumers. The 44 percent of adults who could not recall any health or medical information should be

Table 5-9 Reported Response to Continuing Nervous Condition by Selected Factors, 1998

Percent very likely to _____ in response to a continuing nervous condition . . .

	Pray	Use prescription drug	Visit psychologist	Use herbal product	Use non-prescription drug	Number of respondents
All adults	33	17	15	10	7	1945
Level of education						
Less than high school	44	26	17	16	13	267
High school	33	17	14	11	6	1248
Baccalaureate	26	11	16	5	4	294
Graduate/ professional	28	16	19	6	4	131
Gender						
Men	26	17	11	7	7	934
Women	40	18	18	14	6	1011
Age						
18–24 years	25	11	11	12	7	217
25–34 years	32	13	18	9	9	407
35–44 years	36	14	17	10	6	441
45–54 years	31	19	17	11	3	334
55–64 years	37	27	19	10	9	225
65 or more years	37	23	6	12	7	32

viewed as latent information consumers, meaning that they may read or view various media, but that they currently do not focus on or retain any health or medical information. This differentiation will be an important tool in thinking about and selecting media to reach selected segments of the population.

- Second, although it is often assumed that concern about health information is universal, the results of a 1993 national study demonstrate that approximately 44 percent of American adults could not recall a single piece of health or biomedical information that they had seen, heard, or read during the previous 2 months. Because most Americans are exposed to far more information each day than they can absorb and use, virtually all adults develop an elaborate set of schema to filter out low-salience information. This result demonstrates the effective operation of this filtering mechanism. It is essential for communicators to recognize the real size of the effective audience in estimating the impact of information dissemination efforts.

- Using the results from the 1993 Biomedical Literacy Study, it is possible to define the size of the active audience for health and biomedical information in selected segments of the population and to specify the sources from which they can recall health information. For young adults (age 18 through 24), 55 percent were current health information consumers. Within this group, full-time students displayed less reliance on television for health information and more utilization of print sources and other people. Young adults out of school appeared to rely heavily on television for current health information.

- Parents with preschool and school-aged children are an important audience for health and biomedical information. Using the same database, 58 percent of parents were current health information consumers and displayed a relatively high level of reliance on television for health information. College-educated parents, however, were slightly more likely to recall information from print sources than from television.

- Older adults (age 60 and over) are another important audience for health and medical information. Among this age cohort, active acquisition and retention of health and biomedical information was strongly related to the level of educational attainment, with only 39 percent of older citizens without a high school diploma able to recall any recent health information, compared to 68 percent among college-educated senior citizens. It appears that greater experience with the acquisition and recall of information associated with higher levels of educational attainment carry over to health and biomedical information in one's senior years.

- An extensive analysis of health information acquisition and retention by men and women found few systemic differences. Virtually the same proportions of men and women were active health information consumers. Men were slightly more likely to recall health information obtained from television, whereas women tended to recall health news from other persons. The level of recall of health information from television did not differ for African-American and Hispanic-American men and women.

- Analysis of data from the 1998 Social and Behavioral Indicators Survey indicates that the traditional media sources of television, newspapers, and magazines serve an important function in alerting American adults to new health and medical information. In 1998, over 60 percent of Americans heard or read new information about heart disease, cancer, mental illness, or alcoholism from the traditional media. However, when they want to obtain additional information about these same medical conditions, adults rely on entirely different sources of information. Physicians, libraries, and the Internet were the most frequently mentioned sources of additional information. In contrast, less than 10 percent of Americans would use the traditional media to obtain additional information about heart disease, cancer, mental illness, or alcoholism.

6

·· ·· ·· ·· ··

STRATEGIES FOR COMMUNICATING TO CONSUMERS

·· ·· ·· ·· ·· ·· ·· ·· ··

The preceding chapters in this section have analyzed consumer interest in health matters and biomedical information, described the sources of information used and trusted, and explored several examples of biomedical information acquisition. This chapter will summarize the primary characteristics of biomedical communications to consumers and outline a general model of the process. The chapter will conclude with a set of questions that communicators should ask about both individual communications and communications campaigns.

THE NATURE OF BIOMEDICAL COMMUNICATIONS TO CONSUMERS

Biomedical communications directed to consumers may be described in terms of scope, level, intermediaries, and goals.

The scope of biomedical communications to consumers is inherently broad, inclusive, and nonpartisan. In most cases, the intended reach of any biomedical communication is every possible person to whom the substance of the message may be of interest or value. Even in the case of messages about diseases such as leukemia that impact only a small proportion of the total population, the intended scope of messages about leukemia would be all persons with the disease, as well as their families, friends, and caregivers. In some cases such as dietary information about the value, or lack of value, of a specific food additive, the intended scope would normally be the full adolescent and adult population—all individuals capable of making their own dietary decisions. In virtually all cases, the message is oriented to individual interests, problems, or behaviors and are almost always nonpartisan in tone and substance.

Biomedical communications to consumers should be delivered at all levels of language and understanding. Although differences in personal and educational background will define the range of information that any given individual may be able to receive and understand, it is the responsibility of biomedical communicators to try to deliver messages across the full range of consumer sophistication so that each individual within the society receives information at the highest level that he or she is able to utilize. The idea that one message will fulfill the needs of all consumers is as senseless as the notion that one model of automobile will satisfy all consumers.

Numerous theories of communications have recognized that information does not always—or even normally—flow directly from the communicator to the recipient without interpretation, explanation, or reformulation by various intermediaries. We will discuss this idea in more detail later in this chapter, but it is important to note at this point that information released at a press conference or at a congressional hearing will be received and interpreted by the journalists who hear about it first, will be reinterpreted and reformulated by secondary reports in other media outlets (using wire service reports or having read the original story), and may be further reformatted and reinterpreted by interest groups for publication in a newsletter or on a Web site. When some individuals hear or read the information, they may discuss the material with friends, family, or co-workers, and absorb the comments and judgments of these additional interpreters. Direct communicator to recipient transmissions are rarer than commonly thought, and even the growth of the Web and electronic communications has not eliminated the intermediary role of CNN (Cable News Network), WebMD, AARP (American Association of Retired Persons), or a pharmaceutical company—all of whom operate their own Web sites and provide their own interpretations of biomedical information.

The ultimate objective of biomedical communications to consumers is to promote awareness of health information and to promote good health practices. Toward this end, the immediate objective is to provide clear and accurate information in a format and at a level that the consumer can understand. Some biomedical communications may seek to sell a specific product or to promote or discourage a specific practice (i.e., smoking). Since health and biomedical knowledge tends to be cumulative—with new information either replacing, modifying, or expanding previous understandings or attitudes—it is important for messages to be both sufficiently clear and sufficiently linked to other knowledge to allow its integration at the individual level.

A GENERAL MODEL OF BIOMEDICAL COMMUNICATIONS

One useful approach to integrating the several strands of thought and analysis from the preceding chapters is to use a general model of communications, modified to reflect those conditions or circumstances unique to biomedical communications. We note at the outset that this model is a hybrid of several prior models, and we will try to note our intellectual debts for aspects of this model as we move through our description. The schematic presented in Figure 6-1 may be helpful as a general point of reference. Although the question of where to start in a model that includes feedback is a chicken-and-egg question, we adopt the point of view of the communicator and start with the origination of some information.

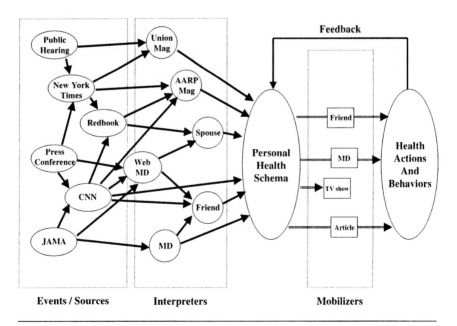

Figure 6-1   A general model of biomedical communications to consumers.

The Pathways of News and Information

New information about health or medicine undoubtedly begins in the minds and laboratories of research scientists, but it first reaches the arena of communication through the publication of a journal article, the conduct of a press conference or briefing, or a public information event such as a Congressional committee hearing. Working journalists attend these events and publish or produce stories based on the original event, including the preparation of wire service and news service stories. Some publications and television shows also serve as sources for other journalists, writers, and producers, who prepare additional pieces for publication, broadcast, or Internet posting.

The number of pathways from the release of a new piece of health or medical information to the individual consumer is complex and may be growing more complex with the expansion of electronic information distribution systems. While the Associated Press, Reuters, and other news services have provided a primary-to-secondary linkage for decades, the growth of Web sites operated by universities, research centers, government agencies, foundations, professional societies, interest groups, and other information reprocessors makes the network of information distribution increasingly complex. Unlike Katz and Lazarsfeld's simple two-step model—which provided an essential metaphor for understanding the increasingly complex communications of subsequent decades—current multistep, multipath patterns provide a significantly greater array of information for journalists, consumers, and decision-makers (Katz and Lazarsfeld, 1955). At the same time, it turns the task of developing a comprehensive model of the full communications process into more of a metaphorical description than a precise mathematical model.

The general model shown in Figure 6-1 provides several examples of the movement of biomedical news and information from its point of origin to the individual consumer. Consider the example of the annual campaigns by the American Lung Association (ALA) and the U.S. Centers for Disease Control and Prevention (CDC) to encourage adults to get a flu shot prior to the beginning of the influenza season. Both the CDC and the ALA hold press conferences on the need for annual flu shots, with the ALA especially emphasizing the high risk from influenza to adults with respiratory disorders. Our schematic shows the flow of information from the press conferences to the *New York Times* and to CNN (as symbols of print and television news coverage). A feature writer for *Redbook* listens to CNN and reads the *New York Times* and writes a piece discussing the health risks associated with not getting a flu shot, which is published in the next issue. The health news editor of WebMD (symbolic of health and medical Web sites) watches the press conference over CNN, reads the *New York Times* report on the electronic edition, and checks for comparable information from other Web sites and news services, then posts a news summary on the WebMD site. A day later, a feature on the flu vaccine is added to the WebMD site. A writer for CNN draws on material from a recent issue of the *Journal of the American Medical Association* (JAMA) in the production of a feature piece on the annual challenge of creating a vaccine that will be effective against the current influenza virus, which is used in a newscast on CNN and posted to the CNN Web site. An editor for *Modern Maturity*, a monthly magazine published by the American Association of Retired Persons (AARP), sees a news report on CNN, reads the influenza story in the *New York Times*, and reads an article in *Redbook* about the medical implications of not being protected. She decides to do a feature piece for *Modern Maturity*, which is published in the next available issue. The number of pathways for the distribution of this information is large, but the point is that the flow of information today is a complex multistep, multimedia process. And, it is likely that the complexity of this process will increase in the decades ahead.

Information Processing at the Individual Level

The point of consumer oriented biomedical communications is to reach and inform individuals about health and medical matters that are, or should be, of concern to them. We want individuals to know the early warning signs of various diseases and conditions, to be able to make sensible personal decisions about diet and exercise and other health maintenance activities, and to know how to treat various kinds of illness and infections that virtually all children and adults encounter at various points in their lives. We know that individuals in modern societies such as the United States are exposed to an extraordinary array of messages every day, ranging from advertisements for foods and medicines to television and news stories about new medical discoveries to discussions with friends and family about health problems. How do individuals handle this array of information and decide which new messages—information, experiences, and exhortations—are important enough to retain and use and which are less important?

There are numerous metaphorical psychological models of this process, but we find the concept of a schema to be most useful in thinking about biomedical communications for both consumer and policy purposes. We will outline our argument for the utility of the schema concept for consumers in this section, and we will return to the use of schemas for thinking about biomedical policy issues in Chapters 9, 10, and 11.

A substantial body of psychology research has identified a schema as a psychological structure that individuals use to receive, filter, and process information and to integrate new information and experiences into coherent clusters. It is a collection of knowledge, previous experience, and attitudes toward a subject (or attitude object) that an individual invokes when confronted with new information or a new event. It is both a storage and organizing device for previous experiences and information and a filter for new information. It is likely that every adult has a schema about his or her personal health that includes retained information about foods, allergies, disease symptoms, and the impact of various lifestyle decisions on one's personal health and well-being. For example, most adults who have ever used alcohol retain a relatively clear memory of the first time that they overindulged and became ill. It is a memory that is available and sometimes invoked when thinking about how much alcohol to consume in some immediate circumstance. Other individuals have acquired and retained information about the impact of fat consumption on their weight and health and they make conscious decisions about which foods to order from a restaurant menu, using this stored set of guidelines about food consumption and health.

A schema also serves as a filter for incoming information. If an individual reads a newspaper story that reports a research finding that extensive use of cell phones can lead to neural damage, the individual may read the story because he or she has a high level of interest in biomedical issues and will seek to evaluate the information in the context of retained information about the effects of radiation on cells in cancer treatment, earlier reports about the possibility of eye damage from computer screens, a discussion with a friend that declined to buy a certain house because it was located close to some power lines, and his or her general recall of biology. This individual may be undecided about the issue, and may retain the information for further thought at a later time. In the same newspaper, this individual may see an advertisement for copper bracelets as a cure for arthritis and reject the idea immediately, based on the content of his or her personal health schema.

Some individuals are more skillful in constructing schemas than other individuals, and psychologists often refer to these differences in information processing and utilization as mental ability. Sternberg and others (Sternberg 1988a,b, 1999; Sternberg et al., 2000) have argued that the ability to utilize abstractions in the conceptualization, storage, and recall of information conveys significant advantages in coping with the challenges of the world. In several of the models reported in previous chapters, the level of education appeared to produce some advantage in biomedical literacy over and above exposure to college-level science courses, and it is possible that one of the major advantages of postsecondary study is the development of general skills in information processing at the individual level.

The scope and quality of personal health schemas undoubtedly vary significantly over the course of the life cycle, and many scholars think that they may differ significantly between men and women. An individual's personal health schema may also reflect an individual's personal and family health history. An adult whose father died at an early age from heart disease may have a greater awareness and sensitivity to dietary, exercise, and hereditary factors than similar individuals without this kind of family history. A woman whose mother or sisters have had breast cancer may be more aware of cancer generally and more inclined to regular examination than another woman with no family history of breast cancer. Similarly, young adults may be more concerned about sexually transmitted diseases than older adults, and older adults may have a much higher level of concern about arthritis, cancer, or Parkinson's disease than younger adults. Although there will undoubtedly be some commonalities among personal health schemas, we should expect systemic variations that reflect real differences in life cycle, lifestyle, biomedical literacy, and family context.

An individual's personal health schema may also be influenced by religious or philosophical views. Some individuals may hold a strong view of a God that governs the daily life of persons and decides how long they will live and when they will die. Other individuals may see the world in deterministic or fatalistic terms. Either perspective may lead to a view that daily decisions about health, diet, or medical care are meaningless. Sometimes this view may lead to unhealthy decisions on the grounds that God will "take me when he is ready and not before." Individuals holding this religious or philosophical perspective may find health or biomedical information to be low in saliency and filter it out by not reading new information on those subjects or not watching television broadcasts focused on health and medical matters. Without seeking to provide a solution to communicating biomedical information to individuals with conflicting religious or philosophical perspectives, it is important for communicators to recognize that this kind of barrier or distortion exists.

Finally, an individual's personal health schema may be reasonably well formed, but it may be in conflict with other lifestyle preferences. Tobacco use is an excellent example. A large number of national studies of children, young adults, and adults have found that more than 90 percent of these groups recognize that tobacco use causes serious health problems. Yet, there has been a small increase in smoking among teenaged students and young adults in recent years, reversing the previous downward trend in tobacco use. The results of many studies suggest that peer pressure and the media portrayal of tobacco use by entertainment stars combine to produce a pattern of behavior that is contrary to the knowledge and attitudinal content of the individual's personal health schema. For most adolescents and young adults, it appears that their awareness of the health dangers associated with tobacco use and their desire for good personal health combine to discourage tobacco use, but the growing number of young smokers illustrates the continuing conflict between the personal health schema and lifestyle preferences at the individual level.

In the schematic model in Figure 6-1, an individual's personal health schema is represented as a large oval that receives information from news and information sources (sometimes modified by intermediaries and interpreters) and processes it. Some incoming information may be filtered out quickly, while other information is retained and integrated into the individual's existing personal health schema. Although the personal health schema is represented by a single oval, it is important to recognize that individual personal health schemas differ substantially in terms of their scope, complexity, organization, and efficiency. Many of the individual differences implicit in the path models presented in preceding chapters reflect this variation in the composition of each individual's personal health schema.

A separate oval is used to represent actual health actions and behaviors, indicating that an individual's personal health schema may influence subsequent behaviors but is distinct from the actions and behaviors themselves. This book has focused primarily on communications rather than behaviors, but the ultimate objective of most communication is some action or behavior. This separate oval for actions and behaviors also recognizes that actions and behaviors provide important feedback to each individual's personal health schema. When an individual consults a physician or spends some days in a hospital, he or she acquires information, experiences, and attitudes that are likely to become a part of his or her personal health schema. Individuals who have had positive experiences in the health care system will be more likely to seek future health care—including preventive services—than individuals who have had negative experiences in the health care system.

The Role of Intermediaries and Interpreters

In a seminal work, Katz and Lazarsfeld (1955) suggested that news and information does not flow from a central point, such as a television tower or a newspaper, directly to the consumer, but rather that it is often discussed with family, friends, and co-workers and that the final acceptance, retention, or use of information is influenced by intermediaries. They characterize the general model of media influence prior to their work in these terms:

> *[The] image . . . was of an atomistic mass of millions of readers, listeners, and movie-goers prepared to receive the Message; and . . . they pictured every Message as a direct and powerful stimulus to action which would elicit immediate response. In short, the media of communication were looked upon as a new kind of unifying force—a simple kind of nervous system— reaching out to every eye and ear, in a society characterized by an amorphous social organization and a paucity of interpersonal relations. (p. 16)*

This was the "model"—of society and of the process of communication—
which mass media research seems to have had in mind when it first began
.... (p. 17)

Katz and Lazarsfeld argued that most adults have a network of family, friends, and co-workers whom they trust on specific topics, but not others, and they referred to this process as the two-step flow of communication. For example, an individual might ask one friend for the name of a good physician to consult, but might ask a different friend for the name of a mechanic to repair her automobile. She might have yet other trusted informants on the use of vitamins, the most interesting movies to see, and the assessment of candidates for mayor of her city. Each of these substantive experts serves as both sources of new information (often repeating what they have read or heard in the media) and as evaluators of information that both parties have heard or read ("Did you read that story about this new genetic research on cancer in yesterday's paper? What do you make of that?"). Katz and Lazarsfeld refer to these local experts as influentials.

It is important to note that Katz and Lazarsfeld were writing in the early stages of the development of television and were reacting—as noted above—to communication theories that viewed information distribution as a series of concentric circles emanating from a central point, such as a television tower. There was a broadly held expectation that the growth of television would give citizens and consumers direct access to products, debates, and leaders—reducing or eliminating the role of newspaper columnists or other information interpreters. The two-step model proposed by Katz and Lazarsfeld was a reflection of that time and reflected a reality prior to the launch of communication satellites, fax machines, the Internet, or Web sites. And, to a large extent, the small city studied by Katz and Lazarsfeld was more influenced by local social groups than by the national interest groups that have become major players in the collection, reanalysis, and redissemination of information in the United States. We read the Katz and Lazarsfeld model as an early recognition of the process of specialization and one of the first explicit descriptions of the role of intermediaries—including intermediaries from everyday life—in the information distribution and interpretation process.

The schematic shown in Figure 6-1 illustrates the roles of various kinds of intermediaries and interpreters in the biomedical communications process. In the classic role of intermediary described by Katz and Lazerfeld, a friend or spouse may serve as an interpreter assessor of validity for new information. In many families, one partner is thought of as more knowledgeable about health than the other—traditionally the woman—and she becomes both the source of information ("Can I take both aspirin and decongestant at the same time?") and an evaluator of new information obtained from other sources ("I read a story in the paper today that said that a glass of red wine every day will reduce the chances of a heart attack. Do you think that there is anything to that?").

In addition to friends and family, there are other important intermediaries that provide new health and biomedical information or reinterpret new or existing health information. Traditionally, an individual's physician has played this role, and the data in the preceding chapters indicate that many individuals still report getting personal health information from their physician and having a high level of trust in that information. For some individuals without ready access to a physician, pharmacists play an intermediary role. For many older adults dependent on home care or institutional care, nurses and other health professionals may play a similar role.

Increasingly, print and electronic media serve as intermediaries in the distribution of biomedical information, including media that represent organizations and interest groups that an individual may trust. In the schematic in Figure 6-1, an AARP magazine or other publication may provide new information about research on specific diseases such as cancer, new pharmaceutical products, or about longer term issues such as the health care implications of genomic research. For an AARP member who does not read a daily newspaper or visit Web sites, a monthly magazine that summarizes health information may be an important and trusted source of information. The number of organizational magazines and newsletters has continued to grow in recent decades and appear to have developed a sufficient audience to be economically viable.

Magazines play a more important role in American society than in Europe or Japan. Reflecting the size of the United States, the absence of strong national newspapers, and a long-standing postage subsidy for magazines, Americans read a lot of magazines and tend to trust a good deal of the information that they read. The number of magazine titles presently exceeds 30,000, reflecting the specialized interests of their readers. Today, there are several monthly health and biomedical magazines without an organizational basis—*Prevention, Men's Health,* and *Health.* More importantly, many magazines with a large national circulation now include either a health section or a large number of health and medical articles. Magazines such as *Redbook, Self, Woman's Day, Time,* and *Newsweek,* all include biomedical information on a regular basis and often have a full-time health or medical editor to acquire and publish biomedical materials.

The rise of the Internet in recent years and the growth of health and biomedical sites injected a new set of intermediaries and interpreters into the system. WebMD is included in our schematic in Figure 6-1 as symbolic of these sites, but it is important to recognize that these sites vary substantially in focus, format, accuracy, and credibility. Because of its linkage to CNN and its relative success in securing visitors and advertisers, WebMD is a good example of a for-profit site that specializes in synthesizing biomedical information for use by both consumers and health professionals. WebMD employs medical editors, reporters, and writers and functions as a newspaper or magazine in terms of information distribution, but it provides interactive opportunities to enter into chat environments and to pose questions via e-mail. While the data are limited at this time, it appears that many individuals trust information from this kind of site, thus it also serves as an interpreter of information for consumers. Similar sites operated by the Mayo Clinic and other distinguished medical institutions attract large numbers of visitors and appear to foster a high level of trust in the biomedical information and advice provided.

In addition to these general focus sites, there are thousands of sites that focus on a single disease or condition, often—but not always—operated by an organization related to that disease. Two examples may be helpful. The Juvenile Diabetes Foundation is an advocacy organization to advance research on and the treatment of juvenile diabetes. It has a record of being influential with the Congress and with executive branch health agencies in securing large appropriations for research in this area, and it obtains private contributions and makes some research grants of its own. It also operates a Web site (www.jdf.org) which provides information for patients and families with juvenile diabetes. Setting aside the policy information that we will discuss in the next part of this book, the site seeks to collect and synthesize information about juvenile diabetes and to provide patient and family oriented information about the diagnosis and treatment of the disease. For individuals and families with this condition, it appears to be a highly trusted site.

Similarly, the National Association for the Mentally Ill (NAMI) is an advocacy organization for the study and treatment of mental illness. NAMI lobbies for higher federal appropriations for mental health research, federal and state legislation to protect the rights of mentally ill individuals, and insurance coverage for the diagnosis and treatment of mental illness on a par with other diseases and conditions. Its Web site (www.nami.org) provides information for patients and families about mental illnesses ranging from depression to schizophrenia. The organization has numerous state and local chapters that provide support groups and services for individuals and families experiencing mental illness. This kind of organization is involved in providing biomedical information, policy information, and actual services through its chapters.

The model also suggests that various individuals, groups, and organizations may serve as mobilizers—encouraging or discouraging specific actions and behaviors. In practical terms, an individual whose personal health schema includes a good understanding of early warning signals may detect a worrisome symptom and discuss it with a friend or a physician, who may either provide strong encouragement to seek medical attention and testing or dismiss it as inconsequential. This encouragement or discouragement may result in a concrete action—making a medical appointment—or not. In this personal health context, mobilization refers to individuals or groups or events that activate a previously existing attitude or understanding in one's personal health schema and converts it into a concrete action. In the schematic in Figure 6-1, an individual watches a television show that seeks to mobilize the viewer to take a specific health action, but it is not sufficiently persuasive to produce the desired action. The same schematic indicates that a conversation with a friend or a physician produced a health-related action, as did the reading of an article in a newspaper or magazine.

The Challenge of New Technologies

During the last three decades, the personal computer has become a part of a majority of American households, as was described in Chapter 4. The growth of the Internet and the Web in the 1990s has had a marked impact on commerce, communications, and education throughout the world. The introduction of broadband communication technologies for business and home use and the continued decline in the cost of high-speed, high capacity microprocessors promises to revolutionize both the delivery and use of information in society. Although these new technologies will not eliminate the traditional media from the twentieth century, there will be substantial convergence among the media and major modifications in the ways that individuals acquire, store, and utilize information in the decades ahead.

Parallel to the revolution in communication technologies, the growth of genomic biotechnology over the next century will be no less dramatic than the communications channels to describe and discuss it. The impact of biotechnology to human disease will be as substantial as the invention of vaccination or antibiotics, and the speed of those changes is likely to be faster than either vaccination or antibiotics. Many new technologies, such as the automobile or television, took decades to reach a majority of American households, allowing time for formal education to introduce related ideas and concepts into the relevant schemas of a large portion of the adult population. The speed of the adoption of personal computers was faster than either automobiles or television, and it is very likely that the introduction and impact of genomic biotechnology to agriculture and medicine will be even faster.

One important implication of the rapid adoption of a new technology is that a substantial portion of the adult population will have to rely on informal learning resources to become and remain knowledgeable about the subject. As noted in Chapter 2, a majority of current adults attended school at a time when biology textbooks would not have included any discussion of

DNA or the modification and recombination of DNA. Yet, there has been a steady growth in the proportion of American adults able to provide an acceptable definition of DNA—at least sufficient to read and understand most newspaper or magazine stories about current genomic research. Fortunately, the parallel growth of communications technologies may provide just the kind of enhanced learning resources that adults will need to stay abreast of the biotechnology revolution.

NINE QUESTIONS TO GUIDE COMMUNICATIONS TO CONSUMERS

The general model of biomedical communications to consumers outlined in the preceding sections of this chapter has important implications for the design, delivery, and assessment of communications to consumers. One useful approach is to frame these implications in the form of a set of questions that might serve as checkpoints or reminders for working biomedical communicators.

- **What information do you want to communicate and what actions (if any) do you want the recipient to take?**
  It is essential to begin with a clear understanding of exactly the message that any given communication is expected to deliver and the response expected from the eventual recipient, recognizing that the pathways to consumers are as likely to be indirect as direct. The announcement of an increase in teenage tobacco use is meant to alert parents, teachers, and local leaders to the reversal of a pattern of declining tobacco use and to encourage these adults to take actions to discourage their children or students to not begin smoking. In contrast, the announcement of the completion of the first draft of a map of the human genome was designed to enhance the public's appreciation and support of biomedical research (which we will examine in the next section) and had little to do with immediate or short-term consumer health interests or behaviors.

- **Whom do you want to receive this message?**
  The target audience for a message or a campaign can be a limited audience, a set of audience segments, or all adults. In some cases, a message may be targeted for school-aged populations. If resources were unlimited, it would be possible to seek to communicate all messages to all adults (or children), but resources are never unlimited and communications have a cost. By focusing on one or more audiences (or even prioritizing possible audiences), it will be possible to utilize the general model outlined above and some of the data-based models in previous chapters to make important communications decisions.

- **What media or sources are likely to transmit the message to the targeted audience?**
  Building on the differentiations in media use and trust outlined in the preceding chapters, communicators should think carefully about which media or vehicles are most likely to be able to deliver the desired message to the targeted audience. Our analyses suggest that television has been overvalued by biomedical communicators, and that a substantial proportion of adults utilize print or electronic media when they want to find reliable health or medical information. Television can serve to alert adults to new developments in an area, but the research reported in Chapters 4 and 5 suggests that most adults turn to print or electronic sources for more definitive information, and our general model suggests that many of these adults will seek additional comment or affirmation of this information from trusted friends and influentials. The exact patterns of media use vary by segment of the public, and it is important to both look at the patterns discussed in Chapter 4 and to seek updated information about media audiences during the year or two prior to the release of a major story or the initiation of a campaign.

- **What is the likelihood that the targeted recipients will hear, read, or view the message?**
  More adults will scan the headline of a news story than will read the full text of the article. Salience appears to be the key factor in determining which stories get read, moderated to some extent by an individual's personal health schema and the time available to read the material. Although most communicators know about the skimming and filtering of media by consumers, there has been relatively little research on this specific factor in regard to the communication of health and biomedical information.

- **What is the likelihood that the targeted recipients of the message will accept (believe) the message and incorporate it into their personal health schema?**
  Some of those individuals who read or hear a news story may decide that the information is not important (or incorrect) and not retain it in their personal health schema. Other adults, however, will read a news story, watch a newscast, read a magazine article, and examine the material on a Web site and integrate it into their personal health schema. The factors that account for individual decisions about the acceptance and integration of information into their personal health schema is not well understood. We expect that this decision will vary substantially among individuals, reflecting their assessment of the degree of personal health endangerment related to the subject of the story and their perception of the degree of influence that they have on the outcome. Because an individual can control his or her diet, for example, but not the deteriora-

tion of the ozone level, it is not surprising that there is more reader or viewer interest in stories about the impact of diet and foods on health than stories about the thinning of the ozone level over Antarctica.

- **What groups or intermediaries might improve the likelihood that a message is received and believed?**
One component of the general model that is overlooked frequently by biomedical communicators is the role of individual and group mediators or interpreters on the acceptance and integration of biomedical information. In the model shown in Figure 6-1, our hypothetical consumer receives biomedical information on a given topic from a union-sponsored magazine, the AARP magazine, his spouse, a friend, his physician, and from CNN. If all of this information is consistent, communication theory would predict a higher likelihood of acceptance and integration of the information into the individual's personal health schema. If there are conflicts between these sources and interpreters, the individual must devise a means of resolving these differences. Often, when individuals receive conflicting information, they interpret the pattern as meaning that there is really little agreement (and therefore expertise) on the issue, and use this conflict to minimize the importance of the information and defer any overt actions. We need more empirical evidence about the factors that drive the acceptance decision for the varied segments of the population on a wide array of issues and information.

- **What is the likelihood that the targeted recipients will take the desired actions?**
Even when members of the targeted audience accept the information and integrate it into their personal health schemas, some proportion of these individuals will subsequently take the desired actions and others will not. For example, most Americans believe that a low-fat diet and regular exercise will reduce the likelihood of heart disease, and many adults have made substantial efforts to select foods that are low in fat and cholesterol. Many fewer engage in a regular exercise program. The process of mobilizing beliefs into actions is an essential part of the biomedical communications process. There is a good literature describing public information campaigns on issues from tobacco use to the fluoridation of water, but relatively few efforts to identify the factors that make this mobilization effective.

- **What groups or intermediaries might improve the likelihood that the target recipients will take the desired action?**
In the same way that individuals and groups interpret information and influence its acceptance, individual and group intermediaries often play an important role in the linkage between beliefs and actions—both positive and negative. In the schematic shown in Figure 6-1, four separate

intermediaries—termed mobilizers—are included to illustrate some of the ways in which the attitudes and information held in a personal health schema might be converted into overt actions. Our hypothetical consumer might believe that she should develop a program of regular exercise, but this does not automatically result in a sustained set of exercise behaviors. In this example, a friend might encourage our hypothetical consumer to join her in an evening walk around the neighborhood. Her physician might strongly encourage her to sign up for an exercise class at the local hospital, and she might read a magazine article about a woman of similar age who was able to remain active at age 90 through a daily program of walking and a weekly exercise class. She may also see a television program encouraging viewers to order some exercise equipment for the home, and she may decide not to undertake that kind of program. Some intermediary encouragement may be effective for some individuals and not for others.

It should also be noted that examples of negative events can be a positive stimulus to action. If a good friend of many years is diagnosed as having breast cancer, for example, an individual may be stimulated to seek a mammogram herself.

- **How will you know how many of the targeted audience hear the message, accepted or believed it, and took the desired action?**
  Finally, it is important to ask how you will know if a particular communication program or campaign was effective in creating the outcome that it was designed to achieve. Too often, biomedical communicators have settled for assessments of the impact of materials at the design stage, using focus groups or small pilot studies. Hopefully, this series of questions illustrates the many opportunities to enhance the effectiveness of communications after the distribution of the original message. We will provide an illustration of this process in the next section.

  Although full assessment studies are often expensive in both time and dollars, there is no substitute for measuring the results of a particular program or campaign empirically. A full description of measurement techniques is beyond the scope of this book, but a listing of major resources that focus on the measurement of outcomes is included in Appendix C.

THE ESTIMATION OF COMMUNICATION IMPACT

The general model of biomedical communications to consumers in Figure 6-1 and the series of questions above suggest a simple approach to estimating the likely impact of a communications program or campaign. For illus-

Line	Instruction	Estimated Number
1	Define the target audience and enter the estimated number of individuals included in this audience in the next column.	32,651,000
2	Estimate the proportion of the target audience that will hear, view, or read the medium (or media) through which you expect this message to be delivered. Enter this proportion (less than 1.0) in the next column.	.83
3	Multiply the number on line 1 by the proportion on line 2 and enter the result on line 3.	27,100,330
4	Estimate the proportion of the target audience that reads the selected media who will read the specific story or information. Enter this proportion on line 4.	.70
5	Multiply the number on line 3 by the proportion on line 4 and enter the result on line 5.	18,970,231
6	Estimate the proportion of the targeted audience that hear, view, or read the message that will accept or believe the message and retain it for possible future use. Enter this proportion on line 6.	.50
7	Multiply the number on line 5 by the proportion on line 6 and enter the result on line 7.	9,485,116
8	Estimate the proportion of the target audience that received and accepted the message that will take the desired action within a defined time period. Enter this proportion on line 8.	.70
9	Multiply the number of line 7 by the proportion on line 8 and enter the result on line 9.	6,639,581
10	Divide the number on line 9 by the number on line 1 and multiply the result by 100. Enter the result on line 10. This is your estimate of the percentage of the target audience that your message will reach and lead to take the desired action.	20 %

Figure 6-2 A worksheet to compute the estimated impact of a message or campaign.

trative purposes, assume that we wish to design a communications program to increase the awareness of prostate cancer among men over age 50 and to encourage these individuals to see a physician and get a diagnostic prostate-specific antigen (PSA) test. Using the form shown in Figure 6-2, we can walk though the process of estimating the likely impact of a specific communications effort.

The first step is to define the target population, and we think that it is important to try to reach men aged 50 and over. We are developing a national program, so we consult the Statistical Abstract online at www.census.gov and find that there were 32,651,000 men in the United States in 1998 who were 50 or more years of age. If our information campaign was focused on a single metropolitan area or state, we would include that parameter in the definition and seek the appropriate population number. In this example, we enter the total target population on line 1.

For our hypothetical communications campaign, we decide to place advertisements and stories in newspapers and newsmagazines. Using available data from national surveys, we find that 83 percent of men aged 50 and over report reading either a daily newspaper most days or a weekly newsmagazine most of the time. We enter 0.83 on line 2 as the proportion of the target population that would be exposed to our messages, and multiply line 1 by this proportion. The resulting estimate (see line 3) is that a comprehensive information program using newspapers and magazines would provide potential message exposure to approximately 27 million men.

We know that newspaper or magazine readers do not read all of the available stories, but tend to scan the headlines and read only selected stories in greater depth. This practice is a reflection of the application of an individual's personal health schema, and stories that are salient to an individual are more likely to be read. We do not have good empirical evidence about the reading rate for biomedical stories among men aged 50 or over (or about any other age group), so we need to make an informed guess. Since there has been a growing media and medical emphasis on prostate cancer, we estimate (perhaps optimistically) that 70 percent of men aged 50 and over who read a newspaper or magazine would read an article about prostate cancer. Obviously, we would make lower estimates for the reading rate for prostate cancer stories among younger men or among women. The important point is that 100 percent of the male readers of these media will not read a prostate cancer story. Biomedical communicators need to think explicitly about how to determine what the real rate is and how they might seek to increase this reading rate. In this example, we enter 0.70 on line 4 and multiply the population on line 3 by this proportion. We enter the result on line 5, which indicates that nearly 19 million men might be expected to read a newspaper or magazine story about prostate cancer as a result of our hypothetical campaign.

We also know that getting individuals to read a story does not mean that they will accept its message and incorporate the new information into their personal health schema. It is sometimes possible to gain some insights into the acceptance rate through the use of focus groups and small pilot studies, but it is essential to recognize that the artificiality of these groups tends to increase the observed interest in and retention of any kind of information over the rate that we would expect to observe without the recruitment and rewards associated with the focus group. For illustrative purposes, we estimate that half of the readers of prostate cancer stories would accept the information and retain it for possible future use. We enter 0.50 on line 6, multiply the population on line 5 by this proportion, and enter the result on line 7. Following the logic of our assumptions so far, we would estimate that our hypothetical information effort would lead about 9.5 million men aged 50 and over to acquire and retain some new information about prostate cancer.

Finally, we know that information alone does not lead to overt actions. In this example, we would expect that some portion of the men would have accepted and retained new information about prostate cancer and would be motivated by the information itself to make an appointment for a physician visit and a PSA test. Other men might accept the information, but require the encouragement of various intermediaries to take the desired action. And, some of this group will resist getting the test despite their recognition of the danger of the disease and the value of the test. For illustrative purposes, we estimate that 70 percent of the men who read and accepted the information would eventually—with or without encouragement—take the desired action. This may be too high, but the point is that only some proportion of those individuals who actually get and accept the information will take the actual behavioral step. We enter 0.70 on line 8, multiply the population on line 7 by this proportion, and enter the result on line 9. We now estimate that our hypothetical information campaign would lead to medical examinations and tests for about 6.6 million men aged 50 or over. By dividing this number by our original population on line 1 (and multiplying by 100), we determine that our hypothetical communication effort would cause about 20 percent of the target population to take the desired action.

The critical point of this exercise for biomedical communicators is that we need to be aware of the steps in the communication process and the probabilities of success at each step in the process. More importantly, by understanding these steps and the associated probabilities, the opportunities to improve the impact of the program by increasing some of the proportions becomes obvious. Let's retrace some of our steps and recall some of the questions posed earlier.

First, we selected two major media for the information program—newspapers and newsmagazines—and we determined the proportion of our target audience reached by these media. This proportion is both empirically determined and relatively high. We could compute the proportion for other media, such as television or radio, and reestimate the same process. By being more rigorous in our definition of the target audience, we are able to select media that are used by this audience and increase our proportion of coverage. It is possible that we could increase this proportion further by utilizing some of the intermediary groups that are trusted by the target population—church groups, unions, chambers of commerce, or social organizations. The use of models and idols from sports or other activities may appeal to some of the members of the target population, especially in advertising or television spots. The analysis of information acquisition patterns in Chapters 4 and 5 may be helpful in thinking about the selection of specific media for specific groups.

Second, the proportion of readers or viewers who examine a particular story carefully is an important part of the equation. Carefully selected pictures or graphics or the involvement of prominent figures may improve this reading rate. For example, it is likely that stories that link prominent political or sports figures to the diagnosis of prostate cancer would be read by a higher proportion of the target audience than straight news reporting. In our example, we estimated the reading rate at 70 percent, but it may be 20 percent. We need more research on both measures of the current reading or attention rates and on factors that might improve that rate.

Third, the rate of acceptance of the message may differ substantially by target audience and by the content of the message. Intermediaries and interpreters can be especially important in increasing or decreasing the acceptance rate. In our schematic shown in Figure 6-1, groups such as the AARP or a trade union or a church can be very influential in promoting or discouraging acceptance.

Finally, the conversion of attitudes and information—collected into a personal health schema—into overt action is a critical and essential step. In our prostate cancer example, we estimated the mobilization rate at 70 percent, but we can find little empirical information about the actual rate. The point is not the accuracy of this estimated rate, but the importance of seeking to understand the factors that cause this rate to increase or decrease.

COMMUNICATIONS TO INFLUENCE PUBLIC POLICY

7

......

CITIZEN PARTICIPATION IN THE FORMULATION OF BIOMEDICAL POLICY

....

One of the two major rationales for promoting biomedical literacy is that it is important in facilitating citizen participation in the resolution of public policy disputes involving health or biomedical policy. Whereas the previous section focused on the role of the individual in regard to his or her personal or family health, this section will examine the role of the individual as a citizen in a democratic political system, seeking to understand the factors that lead some citizens to seek to influence health and biomedical policy while other citizens remain inactive on these issues.

It is essential to recognize that there are some systemic factors that affect the ways in which citizens seek to influence public policy on any issue. In broad strokes, it is useful to differentiate between issues that are largely defined and framed by elections and those issues that are determined almost exclusively outside the electoral process (Rosenau, 1974). In the first half of the twentieth century, national elections tended to focus on a limited set of economic issues, often involving some aspects of collective bargaining legislation, and the two major political parties tended to be organized around a predominately labor perspective and a predominately business perspective, culminating in the election of Franklin D. Roosevelt in 1932 and 1936. This issue polarization tended to erode in the second half of the twentieth century, leading many scholars to declare those decades to be a period of political realignment or dealignment (Beck and Jennings, 1991; Carmines *et al.*, 1987; Carmines and Stimson, 1981; Petrocik, 1987; Stanley, 1988). Setting aside specific arguments about the realignment of the American political system, national elections in recent years have tended to crystallize around a small number of major issues—the stability of the Social Security system, the establishment and continuation of Medicare, or the condition of the economy.

In contrast to these large cross-cutting issues, many issues concerning agricultural policy, transportation policy, health and biomedical policy, and similar matters are salient to only a smaller segment of the total electorate and never become defining issues in electoral contests at the presidential, senatorial, or congressional levels (Almond, 1950; Rosenau, 1974; Miller, 1983b, 1997). Although every candidate is against cancer and disease, specific issues such as the level of funding for the National Institutes of Health (NIH) are rarely discussed in political campaigns. These issues are usually resolved through the legislative process (proposed bills, hearings, and lobbying), with some executive branch influence, especially if the issue is sufficiently important to produce either a presidential veto or the threat of a veto. Rosenau (1974) refers to this process as "politics between elections."

This basic differentiation is made somewhat more complex by a parallel process of political specialization (Miller, 1983b; Miller *et al.*, 1997). In the United States and other industrialized nations, most citizens face a growing number of competing demands for their time. Although the work week has been stable for most industrial occupations for several decades, the effective work week for many professional and technical occupations has been increasing. The number of two-job families has been growing steadily since the 1960s. Most evenings, the typical urban resident of the United States can choose from 20 to 50 television channels, several thousand rental videotapes, several live musical or dramatic performances, several live athletic events, community college or university classes, or a wide array of participant recreations such as aerobics classes or tennis. There has been a growing competition for the individual's time over the last several decades, and the growth of broadband telecommunications in the years ahead will significantly increase both the options available and the pressure on individual time allocation.

In this marketplace for the individual's time, politics and public affairs are but one competitor among many. Each individual citizen must decide how much time, energy, and resources to devote to becoming and remaining informed about politics and to active political participation. The evidence suggests that politics has been losing a portion of its market share of time for many Americans. Although there are many measures of adult interest and participation in political events, a simple and accurate indicator is the proportion of Americans who take the time to vote in presidential and congres-

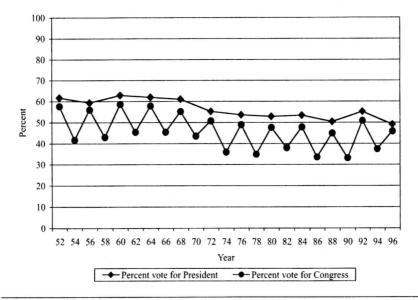

Figure 7-1 Percentage of citizens who voted for president and for congress, 1952–1996.

sional elections. An examination of voter participation data since 1952 points to a steady decline in both presidential and congressional voting during the 1970s and 1980s (see Figure 7-1). Although the rate of voting in congressional contests is higher in presidential election years and lower in nonpresidential election years, a majority of Americans have not voted in congressional elections in nonpresidential election years since the end of the Second World War. In 1994, when the Republican Party gained control of the Congress, only 37 percent of American adults were willing to spend the time and energy to vote for a congressional candidate. The new Republican majority in the House of Representatives was elected with the votes of approximately 19 percent of American adults eligible to vote in that election.

Among those citizens who decide to devote some of their time and energy to public policy issues, there is a second level of specialization involving the selection of issues about which to become and stay informed. The range of issues at the federal level alone is far too broad for any individual to maintain currency, and when state and local issues are included, the full range of potential public policy issues is too vast for any individual to master. Inevitably, all citizens who follow political affairs must focus their attention on a significantly smaller set of issues, and this process of focusing on a limited range of issues is referred to as issue specialization (Miller, 1983b; Miller *et al.*, 1997).

This specialization phenomenon is not new. For decades, both houses of the Congress have conducted their business through a complex network of more than 300 committees and subcommittees, served by more than 20,000 professional staff. Most members of the House and Senate seek seniority on one or two committees and become legislative experts on those substantive areas. For the citizen who is not a full-time political leader, it is necessary to focus one's attention on a much smaller range of issues, usually two or three. Despite the stereotype of single-issue voters, previous studies suggest that few citizens follow a single issue or more than three major issue areas (Almond, 1950; Rosenau, 1974; Miller, 1983b; Miller *et al.*, 1997).

The selection of issues to follow is rarely an overt conscious decision, but rather a reflection of the occupational, educational, religious, racial, ethnic, and geographic factors important to any given person. For example, a person with family and friends living in Belfast may have a stronger interest in the continuing dispute over Northern Ireland than citizens with no ties to the area. And, one's personal and family religion may influence substantive policy views about the role, if any, that the United States should play in this dispute. For similar reasons, a citizen who is a farmer may have a stronger interest in agricultural policy and foreign trade policy than many other citizens, whereas a person who is employed as a teacher may have a stronger interest in education policy than persons who are not involved in the educational system as employees or parents. In all of these examples, interest in a given policy area would appear to the individual as "natural" and not as a conscious selection from a menu of policy areas. Because the selection of areas of policy interest tend to flow from personal characteristics important to the individual, the policy areas to which a citizen pays the most attention tend to be relatively stable over time.

PARTICIPATION IN THE POLICY FORMULATION PROCESS

How, then, does this specialization process affect the formulation of public policy and the resolution of disputes involving health and biomedical issues? Although issues such as the costs and financing of health care will continue to be framed largely by electoral results, the determination of medical research priorities, the use and regulation of new health and medical technologies, and the regulation and monitoring of the health care system itself are almost totally out of the electoral process. No congressional, senatorial, or presidential candidate has ever won or lost a race for office on a primarily biomedical issue. Although elected officers do play an essential role in the process, they are rarely elected on the basis of a commitment to support or oppose a specific aspect of biomedical policy.

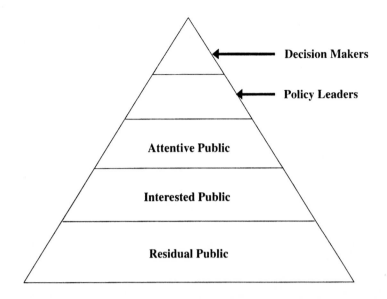

Figure 7-2 A stratified model of public participation in the formulation of public policy.

In his original work, Almond (1950) outlined a pyramidal structure that illustrates the types of public participation in the policy formulation process that are likely to occur under conditions of issue specialization (see Figure 7-2). At the pinnacle of the system, decision makers have the power to make binding decisions on a given policy matter. This group includes executive, legislative, and judicial officers, and in the case of biomedical policy, the officers would be primarily at the federal level. This policy-making stratum of the system includes approximately 100 individual office-holders.

The second level of the system is a group of nongovernmental policy leaders. In the case of biomedical policy, this group of nongovernmental policy leaders would include leading biomedical scientists and engineers; leaders of major corporations active in biomedical science and health-related areas; the officers and leaders of scientific, biomedical, and professional societies; the presidents and relevant deans of major research universities and medical schools; the members of the National Academy of Sciences and the Institute of Medicine; and various business, academic, and other leaders interested in health and biomedical issues. Although the leadership group for biomedical policy has not been listed or counted precisely, comparable measurements of the leadership group for science and technology policy suggest that the leadership for biomedical policy includes between 7000 and 10,000 individuals. Rosenau (1961, 1963, 1974) and others have noted that there is some movement of policy leaders into decision-making posts and of decision makers into the leadership group from time to time.

When there is a high level of concurrence between the decision makers and the policy leadership group, policy is made and there is no wider public participation in the policy process. In fact, most biomedical policy is formulated through this interaction between policy leaders and policy makers. For this reason, we will return to the communication of biomedical policy messages to policy leaders in Chapter 11, but it is important to note now that one important part of biomedical communications for policy purposes is communications to biomedical policy leaders.

On some issues, however, there may be a division of views among the policy leaders themselves, or between policy leaders and policy makers. In those circumstances, there may be appeals to the attentive public to join in the policy process and to seek to influence policy makers by direct contact and by persuasion.

The attentive public—the third level of Almond's model—is composed of those individuals who are interested in a given policy area, are knowledgeable about that area, and are regular consumers of relevant information. To be classified as attentive to a given policy area, individuals must indicate that they are very interested in a given issue area, report that they are very well-informed about it, and be a regular reader of a daily newspaper or relevant national magazines. Although the definition and measurement of attentiveness to biomedical policy will be discussed in more detail later, it is useful to note that 16 percent of American adults were attentive to biomedical research issues in 1999 and that approximately one in six Americans have been attentive to biomedical research issues since 1985.

Although the contacts and processes through which leadership groups mobilize attentives in various policy areas are only now being studied, it would appear that there is a flow of appeals from leaders to attentives through professional organizations, specialized magazines and journals, and employment-related institutions. Contacting of public officials—the policy makers—by attentives appears to use the traditional avenues of letter writing, telephone calls, and personal visits. Recent events suggest that the use of e-mail and other electronic communications is becoming more widely used as a method for contacting political leaders on pending issues (Bimber, 1998; Davis, 1999).

Those citizens who display a high level of interest in an issue area, but who do not think that they are very well-informed about it, are classified as the interested public. This group displays a high level of information consumption on the issue(s) in which they are interested, but is less likely to actually participate in the contacting or other political processes due to their perception that they are not well-informed. It is possible that some of the individuals in the interested public would become attentive during a particular controversy if they were to become convinced that they knew enough about the issue. In the case of the explosion of the space shuttle Challenger, however, a panel study by Miller (1987a) found that virtually no members of the interested public for space exploration moved into the attentive public for that issue as a result of the accident or during the 6 months after the explosion in which numerous public hearings and investigations were held. Further study of the potential role of the interested public is needed.

At the bottom of the pyramid is the residual public. These individuals display a low level of interest in and knowledge about a given policy area. It is important, however, to understand two points about this group. First, the general population always retains a political veto if they should become sufficiently unhappy about the policies that the decision makers, policy leaders, and the attentive public have fostered in any area. The role of the public in ending the wars in Korea and Vietnam illustrates the operation of this veto power. Second, it is important not to equate nonattentiveness to any specific policy area with ignorance of any other policy area or public affairs generally. All citizens are nonattentive to a vast number of areas and issues. Many individuals not attentive to one specific issue area may be attentive to other issues.

In summary, this model of policy formulation in specialized issue areas outlines a stratification of levels of issue interest and a sense of understanding that is linked to differential types of public affairs involvement. It is neither an endorsement nor a criticism of the present system, but a realistic description of the present policy process. It is a useful framework for the analysis of public attitudes toward health and biomedical issues in the United States.

THE ATTENTIVE PUBLIC FOR BIOMEDICAL RESEARCH ISSUES

Given the important role that the attentive public can play in the formulation of biomedical policy, it is important to review the definition and measurement of the attentive public for biomedical research. Although a high level of interest in an issue is a necessary prerequisite for effective citizen participation, it is not sufficient. Professor Gabriel Almond (1950), in a landmark study of public participation in the formulation of foreign policy, argued that it is also necessary for citizens to feel that they are reasonably well-informed and to be continuing consumers of relevant news and information. The primary measurement issue concerns the object of attentiveness, that is, the description of the substantive issues or policy cluster. For example, a series of national studies during the 1980s and 1990s asked individuals about their level of interest in issues about new scientific discoveries and issues about the use of new inventions and technologies. A parallel set of questions asked individuals to assess their own level of knowledge about these two sets of issues, allowing the construction of a measure of attentiveness to science and technology policy.

The problem of defining a comparable issue measure for biomedical research or policy is that these terms are not commonly used outside professional circles. Since 1985, a series of national studies has asked respondents about their level of interest in and knowledge about issues about new medical discoveries, and these items were repeated in the 1993 Biomedical Literacy Study and the 1997–1998 Biotechnology Study. Although issues about new medical discoveries is not a perfect match for biomedical research, it does capture the issue dimension—differentiating it from personal health applications—and new medical discoveries may be seen as a popularized version of biomedical research.

Following the general approach outlined by Almond (1950) and employed in the measurement of attentiveness to science and technology policy, individuals with (1) a high level of interest in new medical discoveries; (2) a sense of being well-informed about new medical discoveries; and (3) regular readership of a newspaper, a newsmagazine, a science magazine, or a health magazine were classified as attentive to biomedical research. In 1999, 16 percent of American adults were classified as attentive to biomedical research, and an additional 52 percent of adults were classified as the interested public for biomedical research (see Figure 7-3). It is important to note that each percentage point in a national survey represents approximately 2.0 million adults, thus about 32 million Americans were attentive to biomedical research in 1999, and an additional 104 million adults had a high level of interest in biomedical research but felt less well-informed about the subject than attentive citizens.

Comparatively, the size of the attentive public for biomedical research is

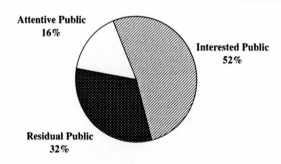

Figure 7-3   The attentive public for biomedical research, 1999.

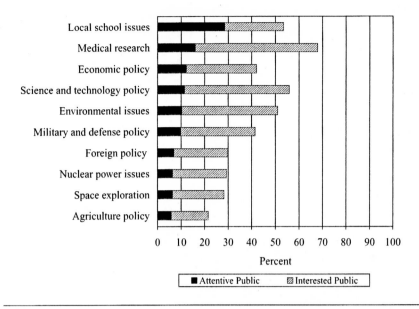

Figure 7-4   **Attentiveness to selected public policy issues, 1999.**

smaller than the attentive public for local school issues, but larger than the attentive publics for economic policy, science and technology policy, environmental issues, military and defense policy, and several other national issues (see Figure 7-4). This distribution of issue attentiveness illustrates some important points about American politics and public policy. Given the multiplicity of national issues, the political attention of the public is fragmented, but issues involving local schools command a larger share of public policy interest and concern than any of the national issues included in a series of national studies during the 1980s and 1990s. Tip O'Neil, the former Speaker of the House of Representatives, has argued that all politics are local politics, meaning that the issues that bring individuals into active political and partisan activity are often local in character. These results demonstrate that national issues do not necessarily command a higher position than local issues on the interest agenda of many citizens.

The proportion of American adults attentive to biomedical research has been relatively stable over the last 15 years for which national measurements are available (see Figure 7-5). From 1985 to 1995, about 16 percent of adults were attentive to biomedical research. This proportion increased to 19 percent in 1997, but returned to 16 percent in 1999 (NSB, 2000). This general pattern is supported by two separate national surveys conducted in 1993 and 1997–1998 (Miller and Pifer, 1995; Miller, 1999, 2001).

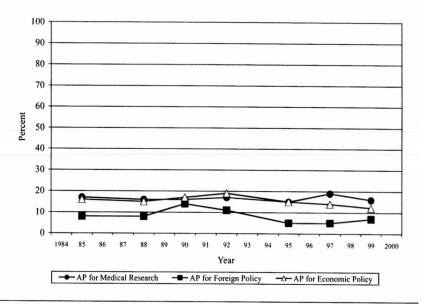

Figure 7-5 Attentive publics for biomedical research, foreign policy, and economic policy, 1985–1999.

From 1985 through 1995, the proportion of adults attentive to economic policy and biomedical research was roughly equal, but the percentage of adults attentive to economic issues has declined slightly to approximately 12 percent in 1999 while the percentage of adults attentive to biomedical research remained at 16 percent in 1999. Traditionally, economic policy has been viewed as the baseline of American politics, and there is substantial evidence that many American voters engage in a kind of retrospective economic voting.

In contrast, the size of the attentive public for foreign policy fluctuates in response to the level of foreign involvement by the United States, especially the engagement of U.S. military forces in actual combat situations in other countries (see Figure 7-5). The size of the attentive public for foreign policy jumped from 8 percent in 1988 to 14 percent in 1990 as the United States moved toward war in the Persian Gulf. By 1995, the size of the attentive public for foreign policy had dropped to 5 percent. With the growth of military activity in the Balkans since 1997, the size of the attentive public for foreign policy increased to 7 percent in 1999. It is reasonable to expect that this percentage might have been higher if U.S. ground troops had been engaged in a military conflict in the Balkans similar to the Persian Gulf War. This pattern illustrates that there is significant variation in the proportion of adults who are attentive to a specific public policy issue, and that changes in attentiveness are related to changes in substantive policy matters. This pattern also illustrates that even military conflicts fail to generate issue attentiveness among a majority of Americans, and it is important to understand the level of attentiveness to biomedical research in this context.

The Distribution of Attentiveness to Biomedical Research

Who are the 30 million Americans who are attentive to biomedical research? What are their backgrounds and what segments of the general population do they represent?

As with most public policy areas, a 1999 national study of adults found that better educated individuals are more likely to be attentive to biomedical research than less well educated adults (see Figure 7-6). Nearly a third of adults with a graduate or professional degree are attentive to biomedical research, compared to 11 percent of adults who did not complete a baccalaureate. Approximately one in five college graduates without an advanced degree were attentive to biomedical research. These differences reflect the greater resources and skills held by most college graduates.

A slightly higher percentage of women are attentive to biomedical research than men. There is a popular stereotype that women have a stronger interest in health due to their roles as mothers and family health monitors, but the magnitude of the differences found in the 1999 study are relatively small. The model testing activity in the next section of this analysis will examine the importance of gender, holding constant differences in age, education, the presence of minor children at home, and other factors.

Thirty percent of adults aged 65 and over are attentive to biomedical research, reflecting in part the greater awareness of and experience with health problems (see Figure 7-6). Slightly fewer than 10 percent of younger adults under age 35 are attentive to biomedical research, whereas nearly 20 percent of middle-aged adults from 35 though 64 years of age are attentive to biomedical research. This pattern conforms to the conventional wisdom that younger adults think that they are immortal, but that the arrival of parenting and family health responsibilities during the middle years increases personal awareness of health and medical information and issues. The greater health problems associated with older age appears to foster a higher proportion of attentiveness to biomedical issues among the adults aged 65 and over.

Finally, it is interesting to note that 55 percent of adults who were attentive to science and technology policy issues in 1999 were also attentive to biomedical research. Comparatively, only 11 percent of adults not attentive to science and technology policy issues were attentive to biomedical re-

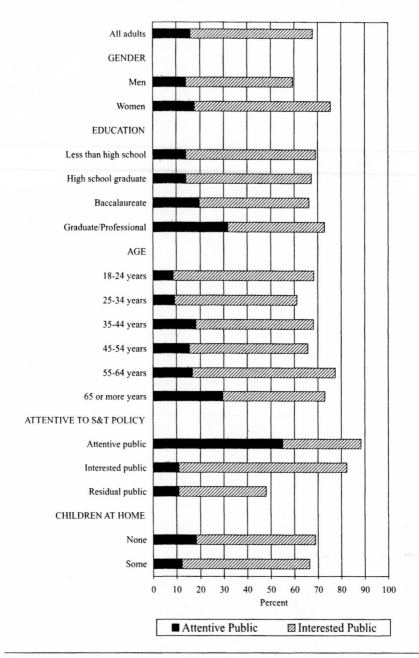

Figure 7-6 Attentive public for biomedical research issues, by selected groups, 1999.

search. This pattern suggests that some interest in and some sense of understanding scientific and technological constructs is important to following and keeping up with biomedical research news and issues.

Some Models to Predict Attentiveness to Biomedical Research

Who is attentive to biomedical research issues? Are some segments of the American population more likely to be attentive to biomedical research issues than other groups? To better understand the relative importance of each of several factors in the development of attentiveness to biomedical research in individuals, it is useful to conduct a multivariate analysis, using a set of independent variables similar to those employed in earlier models. By looking separately at data from the 1993 Biomedical Literacy Study and the *Science and Engineering Indicators 2000* study, it will be possible to obtain two views of the factors that predict attentiveness to biomedical research issues which can help communicators target messages.

Looking first at the data from the 1993 study, the results indicate that an individual's level of general interest in politics (GPI) is the strongest predictor of attentiveness to biomedical research issues, holding constant differences in age, gender, education, exposure to college science courses, biomedical literacy, and personal health status (see Figures 7-7 and 7-8). The

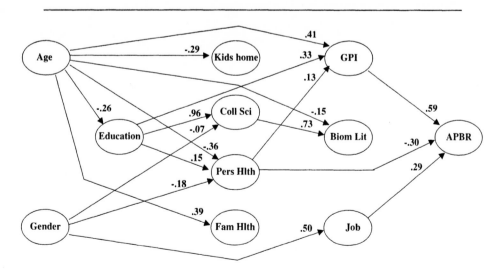

Figure 7-7 A path model to predict attentiveness to biomedical research, 1993.

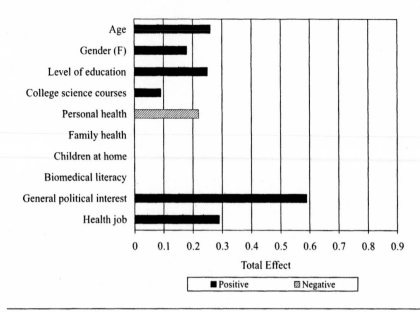

Figure 7-8 Total effect of selected variables on attentiveness to biomedical research, 1993.

total effect of general political interest (.59) is twice as high as the second strongest influence, indicating that biomedical policy issues are not viewed outside a more general framework of politics and public policy. This result stands in sharp contrast to the results reported in the previous section on patient and consumer interest in health information, which tended to be influenced primarily by educational, personal health, and family health concerns.

Employment in a health job was the second strongest predictor of attentiveness to biomedical research issues, with a total effect of .29. Although only 7 percent of the respondents in the 1993 study were employed in health-related jobs, this link to the health care system was a strong predictor of attentiveness to biomedical research issues. This result suggests that policy relevant messages delivered through health care professional societies, employee organizations, or employers may be an efficient means to reach a portion of the attentive public for biomedical research issues.

Age was the third strongest predictor of attentiveness to biomedical research issues (total effect = .26), holding constant all of the other variables in the model, including the measures of personal and family health status. This result suggests that interest in and knowledge about biomedical research issues increase with years of age, regardless of the health experiences of the individual respondent or his or her family. Although the respondent's own health status had a small negative relationship to attentiveness (total effect = −.22), the health status of the respondent's family was unrelated to attentiveness to biomedical research issues. This pattern is an important finding for biomedical communicators, who often assume that it is the experience of health problems—personal or family—that fosters a higher level of interest in and knowledge about biomedical research. This result would suggest that biomedical research messages channeled through publications, such as *Modern Maturity*, that focus on older adults would be an effective means to reach the attentive public for biomedical research issues.

The level of educational attainment is the fourth strongest predictor of attentiveness to biomedical research issues, with a total effect of .25. The number of college science courses completed provides only a small additional amount of explanatory power (total effect = .09), indicating that it is the level of education attained—high school, baccalaureate, graduate or professional degree—that increases the likelihood of becoming attentive to biomedical research issues rather than the exposure to science courses during the college years. Because the use of newspapers, magazines, and other print media is strongly associated with educational attainment within all age groups, this result indicates that the use of print media targeted to older adult populations will be likely to reach a significant number of individuals who are attentive to biomedical research issues.

The 1993 model also provides an important clarification of the role of gender in attentiveness to biomedical research issues. Holding constant age and education, women were slightly more likely to be attentive to biomedical issues than men (total effect = .18). At the same time, the model indicates women are significantly more likely to be employed in a health-related job than men (path = .50), indicating that some of the strong gender effects found in simple bivariate tabulations may reflect differential employment in the health sector. The estimated total effect of .18 is a more realistic description of the real magnitude of the difference between men and women in regard to attentiveness to biomedical research issues.

In summary, looking at the model based on the 1993 Biomedical Literacy Study, attentiveness to biomedical research issues appears to be most strongly associated with a high level of general interest in politics and public policy matters, employment in a health-related job, age, and education. Neither the level of biomedical literacy, the presence of children in the home, nor family health problems were associated with attentiveness to biomedical research issues. It is important to emphasize that each of the total effects described above are additive, thus older, better educated adults with a high level of interest in political matters generally would be the most promising audience for policy-relevant messages about biomedical research issues, and current or prior employment in a health-related occupation or profession would further increase the likelihood of being receptive to biomedical research messages.

By looking at a similar model based on data from the *Science and Engineering Indicators 2000* study, it is possible to explore the stability of the results found in the 1993 model. The 1999 study included most of the same variables included in the 1993 model, but did not repeat the personal or family health status variables.

The 1999 model found the same general pattern observed in 1993, with the level of general political interest being the strongest predictor of attentiveness to biomedical research issues, with a total effect of .68 (see Figures 7-9 and 7-10). Employment in a health-related job was the second-strongest predictor of attentiveness to biomedical research issues in 1999 (total effect = .44), mirroring the pattern found in 1993. Similarly, age was the third strongest predictor of attentiveness to biomedical research issues in 1999, with a total effect of .31. Educational attainment and the number of college science courses were positively related to attentiveness to biomedical research (total effects = .26 and .20, respectively), but biomedical literacy was still unrelated to attentiveness to biomedical research, holding constant all of the other variables in the model. The simplified 1999 model accounted for 75 percent of the total variance in attentiveness in the model, which was a better fit than was found in 1993. This result confirms the general structure of the 1993 model, including the primary role played by a general interest in political or public policy matters.

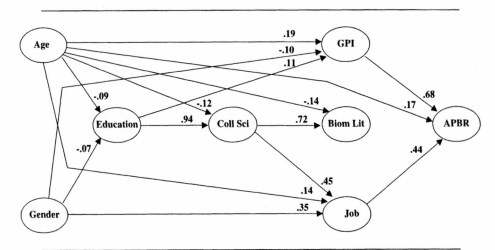

Figure 7-9   A path model to predict attentiveness to biomedical research, 1999.

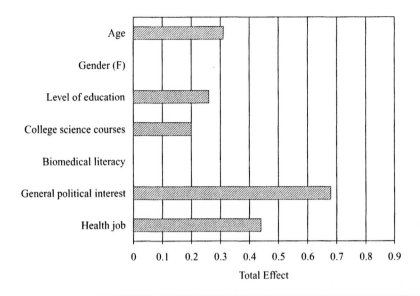

Figure 7-10 Total effect of selected variables on attentiveness to biomedical research, 1999.

Differences by Gender

As demonstrated in previous chapters, it is useful to examine some of these basic relationships in parallel models for men and women, but retaining a common metric for the analysis. Looking first at the 1993 model, the parallel models for men and women show several interesting commonalities and differences. As found in the general model discussed above, general political interest displayed a strong positive relationship to attentiveness to biomedical research issues for both men and women, with a total effect of .64 for both groups (see Table 7-1). Following the same general pattern, neither the presence of minor children in the home nor the level of biomedical literacy was related to attentiveness to biomedical research issues.

   In contrast to the general model, age was the single most important factor for men (total effect = .80), compared to a total effect of .24 for women, holding constant all of the other variables in the model. For men, good personal health was negatively related to attentiveness to biomedical research issues (total effect = −.39), meaning that men who were experiencing some personal health problems were more likely to be attentive to biomedical research than were men with excellent personal health. Family health problems were positively associated with attentiveness to biomedical research issues for men (total effect = .39), indicating that men who experienced serious health problems by other members of their family—spouse or chil-

Table 7-1 Total Effects of Selected Factors, by Gender, 1993

	Total effects	
	Men	**Women**
Age	.80	.24
Level of education	.34	.25
College science courses	.18	.11
Children at home	.00	.00
Personal health	−.39	−.21
Family health problems	.39	.00
Health job	.29	.36
Biomedical literacy	.00	.00
General political interest	.64	.64
R^2	.55	.45

dren—were more likely to be attentive to biomedical research than men without family health problems. Combined, these results indicate that aging is a major factor in encouraging attentiveness to biomedical research issues among men, but that either personal health problems or family health problems appear to increase the likelihood of being attentive to biomedical research issues.

The parallel results for women indicated that personal health was also negatively related to attentiveness (total effect = −.21), but this relationship is somewhat weaker than the relationship found for men. There was no relationship between family health problems and attentiveness to biomedical research issues among women. It may be useful to note that one of the benefits of running parallel models is that all of the path and total effects coefficients are based on the same metric and are therefore comparable. The overall pattern for women suggests that although aging is important in encouraging attentiveness to biomedical research issues for women, it is less important than for men. The experience of personal health problems also encouraged attentiveness to biomedical research issues among women, but the experience of serious health problems by other family members was not related to attentiveness among women.

Looking at the 1999 model to predict attentiveness to biomedical research issues, the models for men and women have substantial commonalities, with only minor differences (see Table 7-2). The level of general politi-

Table 7-2   Total Effects of Selected Factors, by Gender, 1999

	Total effects	
	Men	*Women*
Age	‑.28	‑.28
Level of education	.34	.28
College science courses	.21	.16
Health job	.42	.43
Biomedical literacy	.68	.59
General political interest	.00	.00
R^2	.72	.53

cal interest remained the major predictor of attentiveness to biomedical research issues for both men and women. As in the 1993 model, formal education and college science courses were slightly more influential in encouraging attentiveness to biomedical research issues among men than women. The omission of the personal and family health variables from the 1999 study eliminated several intervening factors that helped to explain differences between men and women, and the resulting parallel models indicated that age was equally important to men and women in encouraging attentiveness to biomedical research issues. These contrasting results demonstrate the importance of looking carefully at the variables included in each analysis, since the inclusion or exclusion of variables may have a substantial impact on the results of the analysis. Substantively, the central role played by an individual's general political interest in both models argues strongly for the importance of viewing attentiveness to biomedical research issues as a part of a general interest in public policy and political matters, and not just a reflection of personal or family health problems. The strong gender differential found in the 1993 model suggests that the experience of illness—personal or family—appears to influence men and women differently.

Differences by Race and Ethnicity

The same general model discussed above was run in a parallel format for African-Americans, Hispanic-Americans, and Other Americans. The results from the 1993 Biomedical Literacy Study show substantial commonality, but some interesting differences.

For all three populations, the level of general political interest was the

Table 7-3   Total Effects of Selected Factors, by Race and Ethnicity, 1993

	Total effects		
	African-Americans	Hispanic-Americans	Other Americans
Age	.16	.05	.26
Gender (female)	.25	.28	.18
Level of education	.31	.30	.36
College science courses	.00	.20	.11
Children at home	.00	.00	.00
Personal health	.00	.00	−.28
Family health problems	.00	.00	.00
Health job	.00	.60	.36
Biomedical literacy	.00	.00	.00
General political interest	.73	.69	.57
R^2	.62	.74	.44

strongest predictor of attentiveness to biomedical research issues (see Table 7-3). The level of educational attainment was also a strong predictor of attentiveness to biomedical research issues for all three groups, but the level of exposure to college-level science courses was more important for Hispanic-Americans and Other Americans than for African-Americans. Women were slightly more likely to be attentive to biomedical issues than men in all three populations, holding constant the other variables in the model. There was no relationship between the level of biomedical literacy or the presence of minor children in the home for any of the three populations.

Employment in a health-related job was most influential among Hispanic-Americans (total effect = .60), less influential among Other Americans (total effect = .36), and unrelated to attentiveness to biomedical research issues among African-Americans. Age had the lowest level of influence on attentiveness to biomedical research issues among Hispanic-Americans (total effect = .05), somewhat more influence among African-Americans (total effect = .16), and the strongest effect among Other Americans (total effect = .26).

The structure of the sample for the *Science and Engineering Indicators 2000* study does not allow the analysis of racial and ethnic differences.

Summary

This analysis has shown that attentiveness to biomedical research issues is strongly related to a general interest in political affairs and is not simply driven by personal or family health concerns. Because many disease-oriented organizations deal with large numbers of patients, families, and health care professionals concerned about personal and family health problems, there is a tendency to assume that these same factors drive the development of interest and attentiveness in the larger population, but these results indicate that it is the level of general political interest, employment in a health-related job, and age that are primarily responsible for attentiveness to biomedical research issues. There are some important differences by gender, with personal and family health experiences being substantially more important to men than women, but there is substantial commonality in structure for men, women, and for racial and ethnic populations.

IMPLICATIONS FOR BIOMEDICAL COMMUNICATORS

What are the implications of these findings for biomedical communicators? What practical conclusions might one draw from these analyses that are relevant to designing and targeting biomedical policy communications?

First, it is essential to recognize that the audiences for policy-related communications are significantly different from the audiences of medical and health information described in Part II. Compared to the audiences for health and medical information, a significantly smaller proportion of adults are interested in policy-related matters and an even smaller proportion are willing to devote the time and energy necessary to become and remain informed about biomedical policy issues. Those adults who are interested in policy-level issues tend to be better educated, and this pattern is stronger for more science-based issues or controversies.

Second, approximately 16 percent of American adults (about 32 million individuals) are attentive to biomedical research issues. These citizens are very interested in biomedical research matters, follow these issues in the media, and feel that they are reasonably well-informed about the area. They are regular consumers of policy-relevant information, and they feel competent to write or contact policy makers or institutional authorities on specific issues. When a piece of legislation is pending, organized interest groups seek to identify, contact, and persuade these individuals to write letters, send e-mail messages, sign petitions, and contribute funds toward some desired objective. These attentive citizens are the foot soldiers for the legislative wars over appropriations and legislation.

Third, 100 million adults in the United States are interested in biomedical research matters, but do not feel sufficiently well-informed to take on contacting or participating in legislative or public policy controversies. These individuals are also frequent information consumers on biomedical research issues and are a good market for health magazines, medical newsletters, and Internet health sites, but they are significantly less likely to become foot soldiers in any dispute or controversy than attentives. It is possible that some individuals from this interested public might become attentive during a prolonged controversy or dispute, but we have no solid data on this point. As Rosenau observed in 1974 in regard to foreign policy controversies, scholars and organizations have focused substantial resources on the study of attitude formation, but relatively little on the study of the processes and dynamics that cause citizens to become active participants in the formulation of public policy generally or in the resolution of specific controversies.

Given the central role of the attentive public in seeking to influence public policy, how can communicators reach these individuals? We now turn to this question in Chapter 8.

chapter

8

••••••••••

THE ACQUISITION OF INFORMATION ABOUT BIOMEDICAL POLICY ISSUES

•••••••••••••••••

The preceding chapter argued for the importance of the attentive public for biomedical research issues. This chapter will seek to define this group in terms of the sources of information that these individuals use to become and remain well-informed. It will also examine the general patterns of information acquisition by the attentive public and the interested public for biomedical research issues as well as the attentive and interested publics for biotechnology policy issues. The chapter will conclude with a discussion of communication strategies to reach these groups.

PATTERNS OF MEDIA USE

The attentive and interested publics for biotechnology policy issues will be defined in greater detail in Chapter 10, but it is sufficient at this point to note that there are some demographic differences from the attentive public for biomedical issues and some overlap. In this section, we will use the most recent national data available for both groups and provide a profile of the kinds of media used on a regular basis.

The Attentive Public for Biomedical Research

Those individuals attentive to biomedical research issues are heavy users of print media and frequent viewers of television news shows, but slightly less frequent users of electronic media. Seventy percent of those individuals attentive to biomedical research issues report that they read a newspaper every day, and an additional 32 percent of those individuals attentive to biomedical research indicated in 1999 that they read a weekly newsmagazine regularly (see Table 8-1). Biomedical research attentives read an average of 276 newspapers and 20 news magazines per year. Approximately 20 percent of these attentives also report reading a science magazine regularly. When all of the different magazines that include a significant amount of health information[1] are combined into a summary category, 53 percent of individuals who are attentive to biomedical research issues report that they read one or more of these magazines on a regular basis. Comparatively, only a third of the interested public for biomedical research issues read one of these magazines regularly, and only a quarter of the residual public reported regular reading of this kind of material.

Because the selection of magazines represents a form of specialization, it is instructive to look at some specific patterns of reported magazine reading. Slightly more than 20 percent of biomedical research attentives indicated that they read *Time* magazine regularly, compared to 13 percent who reported reading *Newsweek*. Comparatively, 13 percent of these attentives reported reading *Reader's Digest* regularly. More than 30 percent of women who are attentive to biomedical research issues indicated that they read one or more women's magazines regularly. *Business Week,* in contrast, was read by only 1 percent of the attentive public for biomedical research in 1999.

Reflecting a general revival of book buying in the United States over the last decade, 44 percent of biomedical research attentives claimed to have purchased a science or health oriented book during the previous year, and nearly 80 percent of these attentives indicated that they visited a public library at least once during the previous 12 months. Nearly a quarter of individuals attentive to biomedical research issues reported visiting a public library more than once a month.

---

[1]This classification includes newsmagazines, science magazines, women's magazines, senior citizen's magazines, health and fitness magazines, and parenting magazines. Although there are undoubtedly some individual magazines that carry some information about biomedical research and new medical discoveries, this combined classification provides a good indicator of the level of reading of this kind of material.

Although print media are undoubtedly a major source of biomedical research information for this attentive public, these individuals are also frequent viewers of television generally and of television news shows in particular. In 1999, individuals attentive to biomedical research issues reported watching approximately 1100 hours of television, including 559 hours of television news (see Table 8-2). They also watched about 47 hours of science television shows during the previous 12 months. Although the existing literature includes no panel studies to document the interaction between print and broadcast media, a short panel study that included media information prior to the explosion of the space shuttle Challenger in January 1986, and two additional measurements during the following 6 months, found that television pictures of the initial disaster stimulated increased reading about the event in newspapers and magazines—as well as increased conversations with other people about the event, its causes, and its consequences—and that the two sources were mutually reinforcing during the months after the accident (Miller, 1987). Although most biomedical research news will be less dramatic than the explosion of a space shuttle, it is likely that television reports of a new treatment or therapy for a disease will stimulate increased reading and, perhaps, trips to a public library to obtain more information on the subject.

Although 60 percent of individuals attentive to biomedical research have access to a computer at home or at work, this group is slightly less wired than the interested or residual publics for biomedical research (see Table 8-3). Although nearly half of the biomedical research attentives have a home computer and 43 percent have access to the Web from home or work, these levels of electronic access are slightly lower than the adult population of the United States generally. This pattern may reflect the slightly lower age profile of biomedical research attentives, but is unusual in that adults with a high level of print media usage are often frequent users of the new electronic media.

It should be noted, however, that slightly more than 70 percent of individuals attentive to biomedical research indicated that their home is served by a cable or satellite service. As the new broadband communications technologies become commercially available for home use, it is likely that the existing cable infrastructure will be the major backbone for the delivery of these services to the home, and the attentive public for biomedical research is well positioned to take advantage of these resources in their search for new information on biomedical research issues.

On balance, the attentive public for biomedical research issues is a literate population of adults with strong reading habits, regular television news viewing patterns, and a reasonable level of access to electronic communications. Given their age and educational profile, they are slightly less frequent users of electronic media than might have been expected, but they are struc-

Table 8-1 Use of Print Information Sources

	Biomedical research (1999)			Biotechnology policy (1997–1998)		
	AP[a]	IP[b]	RP[c]	AP	IP	RP
Reads newspaper daily	70%	37%	32%	81%	40%	44%
sometimes	17%	29%	27%	16%	30%	26%
rarely or never	13%	34%	41%	3%	30%	30%
Number of newspapers read per year	276	166	146	308	177	189
Reads a newsmagazine regularly	32%	15%	14%	45%	22%	14%
Number of newsmagazines read per year	20	10	10	30	13	10
Reads a science magazine regularly	20%	7%	5%	35%	16%	10%
Number of science magazines read per year	3	1	1	7	3	1
Reads a woman's magazine regularly (all adults)	19%	11%	8%	3%	10%	13%
Reads a woman's magazine regularly (women only)	31%	17%	18%	6%	19%	24%

Reads a magazine with health information regularly	53%	34%	27%	74%	47%	35%
Number of health information magazines read per year	30	15	14	39	19	14
Bought one or more science books in previous year	44%	31%	33%	—	—	—
Number of visits to a public library in previous year	10	8	8	—	—	—
Reads the following magazines regularly (most of the issues)						
Time	21%	9%	8%	31%	11%	9%
Newsweek	13%	7%	7%	19%	10%	7%
U.S. News and World Report	5%	3%	3%	6%	4%	3%
Reader's Digest	13%	6%	4%	5%	12%	8%
Business Week	1%	1%	1%	3%	2%	1%
Scientific American	7%	2%	2%	6%	1%	0%
Woman's Day (women only)	5%	2%	2%	0%	1%	5%
Good Housekeeping (women only)	6%	5%	5%	6%	19%	24%
Number of interviews	301	977	603	80	366	620

[a]AP, attentive public.
[b]IP, interested public.
[c]RP, residual public.

Table 8-2 Use of Broadcast Information Sources

	Biomedical research (1999)			Biotechnology policy (1997–8)		
	AP[a]	IP[b]	RP[c]	AP	IP	RP
Total number of hours of television viewed per year	1089	1077	883	—	—	—
Number of hours of TV news viewed per year	559	439	353	—	—	—
Number of hours of science television viewed per year	47	48	30	—	—	—
Cable or satellite service in the home	72%	67%	62%	—	—	—
Watched some episodes of *Nova* in previous year	6%	6%	4%	—	—	—
Watched some episodes of *National Geographic TV*	6%	10%	6%	—	—	—
Total number of hours of radio listening per year	872	876	1007	—	—	—
Number of hours of radio news listening per year	218	247	263	—	—	—
Number of interviews	301	977	603	80	366	620

[a]AP, attentive public.
[b]IP, interested public.
[c]RP, residual public.

Table 8-3 Use of Electronic Information Sources

	Biomedical research (1999)			Biotechnology policy (1997–1998)		
	AP[a]	IP[b]	RP[c]	AP	IP	RP
Access to a computer:						
No access	41%	34%	33%	13%	22%	45%
Access at home or work	30%	37%	30%	39%	37%	34%
Access at home and work	29%	29%	37%	48%	41%	21%
Has a personal computer in the home	48%	53%	58%	75%	41%	41%
Access to the WWW	43%	40%	43%	70%	60%	36%
Has an e-mail address	38%	39%	45%	—	—	—
Estimated number of hours per year on-line from home computer	54	60	60	—	—	—
Estimated number of hours per year on the Web from home and work computers	65	63	78	—	—	—
Looked for science information on the Web	9%	11%	13%	—	—	—
Looked for health information on the Web	16%	13%	7%	—	—	—
Number of interviews	301	977	603	80	366	620

[a]AP, attentive public.
[b]IP, interested public.
[c]RP, residual public.

turally positioned to take advantage of those resources if they should elect to do so in the future.

The Attentive Public for Biotechnology Policy Issues

The attentive public for biotechnology policy issues is both younger and somewhat better educated than the attentive public for biomedical research issues, and it is half the size of the attentive public for biomedical research issues. These differences are reflected in their media utilization habits. Biotechnology policy attentives are frequent readers of print media of all kinds, with 81 percent of this group reporting that they read a newspaper daily (see Table 8-1). Nearly half of biotechnology policy attentives read a weekly newsmagazine regularly, and 35 percent of biotechnology policy attentives report reading a science magazine regularly. In 1997–1998, biotechnology policy attentives reported reading an average of 308 newspapers per year and 30 newsmagazines per year. Using the same summary measure described above, 74 percent of biotechnology policy attentives read one or more magazines regularly that included a significant level of health and medical news. Comparatively, only 53 percent of biomedical research attentives reported this level of health information reading.

Looking at the use of specific magazines, slightly more than 30 percent of adults attentive to biotechnology policy issues reported reading *Time* magazine, compared to 19 percent who reported reading *Newsweek* (see Table 8-1). Although biotechnology policy involves an emerging field of research, only 6 percent of this attentive public reported reading *Scientific American* regularly. Unlike the attentive public for biomedical research issues, women's magazines reach only about 6 percent of women attentive to biotechnology policy. Three percent of biotechnology policy attentives reported reading *Business Week* regularly.

Unfortunately, the 1997–1998 U.S. Biotechnology Study did not include any television viewing items, and we are unable to make comparisons in this area. There is, however, a strong correlation between attentiveness to biotechnology policy issues and attentiveness to science and technology policy issues, and separate analyses of those data suggest that it is likely that biotechnology policy attentives use television only slightly more than American adults generally, with a slightly higher level of television news viewing. It is also likely that reading and television viewing are mutually reinforcing activities for biotechnology policy attentives, as described above.

In contrast to biomedical research attentives, individuals who are attentive to biotechnology policy issues are far more likely to have access to computers and the Web than other Americans (see Table 8-3). In 1997–1998, 87 percent of biotechnology policy attentives had access to a computer at home or at work, and 75 percent reporting owning a home computer. Fully 70 percent of biotechnology policy attentives have access to the Web, although we have less complete information about how many hours they spend on the Web and how often they overtly seek health and medical information from the Web.

In summary, the attentive public for biotechnology policy issues is slightly younger, somewhat better educated, more likely to be biomedically literate, high-volume users of print media, and electronically active. We have relatively less hard evidence about their television viewing habits, but the strong overlap with the attentive public for science and technology policy—about whom we do have television viewing data—suggests that biotechnology policy attentives are likely to be frequent viewers of television news shows and of specialized science television shows such as *Nova*.

A SUMMARY MEASURE OF BIOMEDICAL INFORMATION ACQUISITION

In the preceding discussion, we have examined several measures of media use, including print, broadcast, and electronic media. It is reasonable to ask whether these activities reflect an eclectic set of individual preferences—a smorgasbord approach—or a more systematic pattern of information acquisition. This is an excellent example of how method may inform practice. Too often, working communicators focus on a single medium or a combination of two or three media without thinking about how individuals use these resources—singly and in combination—to build an understanding of some issue or event.

Using a technique called factor analysis, it is possible to examine this set of information acquisition activities to see if there is an underlying pattern. Looking at the *Science and Engineering Indicators 2000* study,[2] the results indicate that eight kinds of media use are correlated with a single underlying dimension—called a factor—that we will label as biomedical information acquisition. The strongest loading activity was buying one or more science books during the preceding year, with a factor loading[3] of .88. The

---

[2] Because the 1997–1998 U.S. Biotechnology Study did not include a full set of media use measures, it is not possible to examine the comparable information structure within that study.

[3] A factor loading is essentially the correlation between the item (buying a science book) and the underlying factor. For a simple discussion of the logic of factor analysis, see Kim and Mueller, 1978; Loehlin, 1987; Long, 1983; Schumacker and Lomax, 1996.

other items loading of this factor—in order of strength of the loading[4]—included visiting a science or technology museum, owning a home computer, seeking science or health information from the Web, visiting a public library, reading a science magazine, reading a newsmagazine, and watching a science show on television. It is important to note that reading a newspaper did not load on this factor, suggesting that newspaper reading is a more general kind of information acquisition activity that might be associated with a strong interest in sports, foreign policy, or the stock market. In any case, this factor analysis found that it was not related to the level of use of other science-related or biomedical-related kinds of information seeking behaviors.

A factor score was computed for each individual in the *Science and Engineering Indicators 2000* study to reflect the overall pattern of science information acquisition, and this score was converted into a zero to 100 index. For all adults, the mean score on the 1999 Index of Scientific and Biomedical Information Acquisition was 30 (see Table 8-4). Looking at the bivariate tabulations, individuals with higher levels of educational attainment, more exposure to college science courses, and a higher level of biomedical literacy were more likely to have a higher score on the Index. Individuals who were attentive to biomedical research issues scored higher than other adults who were not attentive to this issue. The attentive public for science and technology policy—a surrogate for the attentive public for biotechnology policy in the 1999 study—scored even higher on the Index, with a mean score of 46. This pattern suggests that education and literacy are strong factors that predict all forms of information acquisition.

We would expect that individuals who are attentive to biomedical research issues would be regular consumers of scientific information from a variety of sources, and the preceding data concerning the use of major media confirmed this expectation. The moderately higher score by biomedical research attentives on the Index of Scientific and Biomedical Information Acquisition also supports this general expectation. It is important to recognize, however, that there are many individuals who are attentive to energy issues, to environmental and ecological issues, to educational issues, and to agricultural issues who are also regular consumers of scientific information, regardless of their level of attentiveness to biomedical research issues. For example, the Tuesday *New York Times*' Science Times, the science sections of *Time* or *Newsweek,* or *Scientific American* magazine are read by many individuals attentive to one of several scientific or technical issues as well as

---

[4]The loadings of each of the items on this factor were: buying one or more science books (.88), visiting a science or technology museum at least once in the previous year (.66), having a computer in one's home (.61), using the Web to look for science or health information at least once during the previous year (.59), the frequency of visits to a public library (.50), regular reading of one or more science magazines (.40), regular reading of one or more newsmagazines (.38), and the frequency of watching science shows on television (.30).

Table 8-4 Mean Scores on the Index of Science Information Acquisition, 1999[a]

	Mean Index score	Number of interviews
All adults	30	1,881
Gender		
Men	31	900
Women	29	981
Age of respondent		
18–24 years	32	263
25–34 years	35	440
35–44 years	37	395
45–54 years	30	295
55–64 years	26	191
65 or more years	14	296
Level of education		
Less than high school	14	403
High school graduate	29	933
Associate degree	42	177
Baccalaureate	44	239
Graduate/Professional	48	129
College-level science courses		
None	23	1,237
1–3 courses	38	328
4 or more courses	48	316
Biomedical literacy (five levels)		
Lowest level	13	261
Second level	20	357
Middle level	27	324
Fourth level	35	502
Highest level	45	437
General political interest level		
Low	26	805
Middle	30	617
High	37	459
Attentiveness to biomedical research		
Attentive public	36	301
Interested public	29	977
Residual public	29	603
Attentiveness to science and technology policy		
Attentive public	46	216
Interested public	32	836
Residual public	24	830

[a]The Index of Science Information Acquisition reflects the factor score for each respondent, recalibrated so that the lowest factor score was set equal to zero and the highest factor score was set equal to 100.

many individuals who are interested in one or more of these issues, but lack a sufficient sense of being well-informed to be classified as attentive.

From the point of view of communicators interested in getting information to individuals who are attentive to biomedical research issues, it is important to recognize that there are no media categories that uniquely target attentives only. Although there are some specific publications or shows that reach a large number of biomedical research attentives, these publications are also read by other individuals who may be attentive to other issues or to no issues at all. A set of models designed to predict an individual's score on the Index of Scientific and Biomedical Information Acquisition found that educational attainment, college-level science courses, and biomedical literacy were all strong predictors of information acquisition, but that neither attentiveness to biomedical research issues nor attentiveness to any of a set of biomedical and scientific issues were good predictors of information acquisition apart from education, literacy, and general political interest.

TRUST IN INFORMATION SOURCES

To communicate effectively to individuals who are attentive to biomedical research, biotechnology policy, or other scientific and technical issues, it is important to understand the level of confidence or trust that they have in various kinds of information sources. If, for example, attentives expressed a low level of confidence or trust in television talk shows, for example, it would not be a good investment of time and effort for a communicator to work hard to get a particular person or message into one of these shows. Too often, marketing and communications professionals—including individuals and firms devoted to social marketing—place more emphasis on total exposure numbers without any understanding of user confidence or trust in that medium.

Looking first at the attentive public for biomedical research issues, data from the 1993 Biomedical Literacy Study indicate that the attentive public places the highest levels of confidence in information about heart disease obtained from a physician, a report from the National Institutes of Health (NIH), and a scientist (see Table 8-5). Eighty-four percent of individuals attentive to biomedical research issues expressed a high level of confidence in heart disease information obtained from a conversation with a physician, and 76 percent expressed a similar level of confidence in heart disease information provided in an NIH report. A majority of biomedical research attentives reported a high level of confidence in heart disease information found in "an article by a scientist." The interested public and the residual public also indicated high trust in these three sources.

Slightly more than 40 percent of biomedical research attentives indicated that they would have a high level of confidence in heart disease informa-

Table 8-5 Confidence in Selected Information Sources, by Attentiveness to Biomedical Research Issues, 1999[a]

Percent with a high level of confidence in information about heart disease from . . .	Attentiveness to biomedical research issues		
	Attentive public	Interested public	Residual public
A conversation with your physician	84	75	74
A report from the National Institutes of Health	76	67	64
An article by a scientist	56	56	51
An article in *Time* or *Newsweek*	42	51	42
A story on the evening television news	24	33	24
A story in your local newspaper	21	18	13
A television talk show like the *Oprah Winfrey Show* or the *Phil Donohue Show*	15	15	9
Number of interviews	301	997	603

[a]QUESTION:
Earlier, we talked about the sources from which you get your information about various issues. Now, I would like to ask you to tell me how much confidence or trust you would have in various kinds of information about heart disease. Let me read you a short list of news sources that might include some information about heart disease, and, for each one, I would like you to tell me if you have a high level of confidence in information from that source, a moderate level of confidence, or a low level of confidence. OK? First, ...

tion published in articles in *Time* or *Newsweek*. In contrast, only 21 percent of biomedical research attentives expressed a high level of confidence in heart disease information from a story in the respondent's local newspaper. It is not clear whether this differential reflects a national versus a local source of information, or just a lower regard for local newspapers.

Biomedical research attentives expressed the lowest level of confidence in television as a source of heart disease information. Only 24 percent of biomedical research attentives said that they would have a high level of confidence in heart disease information presented on an evening television news show, and only 15 percent of these attentives indicated that they would trust heart disease information provided on "a television talk show like the *Oprah Winfrey Show* or the *Phil Donohue Show*." This result confirms our previous observation that biomedical and other science-oriented attentives tend to trust print sources over broadcast sources.

The data from the 1997–1998 U.S. Biotechnology Study indicate that individuals attentive to biotechnology policy—a significantly smaller and more

Table 8-6 **Confidence in Selected Information Sources, by Attentiveness to Biotechnology Policy Issues, 1997–1998**[a]

Percent with a high level of trust in information about the safty of biotechnology from . . .	Attentiveness to biotechnical policy issues		
	Attentive public	*Interested public*	*Residual public*
The National Institutes of Health	44	35	31
The American Medical Association	34	40	34
Scientists from a university	33	24	28
An article in *Consumers Reports*	29	26	26
The federal Food and Drug Administration	24	22	25
The U. S. Department of Agriculture	19	23	23
An article in *Time* or *Newsweek*	17	15	13
Reporters on a television news show such as *60 Minutes*	8	16	11
Food manufacturers	5	3	6
Number of interviews	301	997	603

[a]QUESTION:

Now, I am going to read you a list of groups. For each of these groups, if they made a public statement about the safety of biotechnology, would you have a lot, some, or no trust in the statement about biotechnology. Would you have a lot of trust, some trust, or no trust in a statement made by the [name of group] about biotechnology?

science-oriented group than the attentive public for biomedical research—have a similar profile of trust in information sources. When asked to assess the level of trust that they would have in various sources of information about "the safety of biotechnology," 44 percent of biotechnology policy attentives expressed a high level of trust in information provided by the National Institutes of Health (see Table 8-6). A third of biotechnology policy attentives indicated a high level of trust in biotechnology safety information from the American Medical Association and "scientists from a university." Nearly 30 percent of biotechnology policy attentives said that they would have a high level of trust in biotechnology safety information published in *Consumers Reports* magazine.

A quarter of biotechnology policy attentives indicated in 1997–1998 that they would have a high level of trust in biotechnology safety information provided by the federal Food and Drug Administration (FDA), and only 19 percent of biotechnology policy attentives reported that they would have a similar level of confidence in biotechnology safety information from the U.S.

Department of Agriculture (USDA). These results contradict the often expressed idea that Americans hold a generally positive view of biotechnology because of the high level of trust that they hold in governmental regulatory bodies.

In sharp contrast to biomedical research attentives, only 17 percent of biotechnology policy attentives indicated that they would have a high level of trust in biotechnology safety information in an article in *Time* or *Newsweek*. Given the results discussed above, this judgment is not a rejection of print media, but a differentiation among sources.

Parallel to biomedical research attentives, only 8 percent of biotechnology policy attentives indicated a high level of trust in information about biotechnology safety obtained from a television news show. In this case, the question referred to a popular television newsmagazine show—*60 Minutes*—known for its investigative reporting and generally considered to offer a more in-depth treatment of issues than the traditional 30-minute news broadcast that seeks to cover all of the major stories of the day, but even this kind of television news reporting was rejected by more than 90 percent of the attentive public for biotechnology policy.

Biotechnology policy attentives expressed the lowest level of trust in biotechnology safety information provided by "food manufacturers," with only 5 percent of these attentives reporting a high level of trust in this information source. It would appear that biotechnology policy attentives found the inherent conflict of interest for manufacturers to be too great to engender confidence in any safety information that they might provide. It is possible that the close association between the USDA and the FDA and the food industry created a slightly low level of trust in those sources.

In general, the level of confidence or trust in all of these information sources is lower than the level of confidence expressed by biomedical research attentives in information about heart disease from similar sources. This differential in trust may reflect the new and rapidly emerging nature of biotechnology information in contrast to decades of research and news stories about heart disease. Citizens—and especially those attentive to an issue—may feel more comfortable with information from major institutions and news sources about an established topic such as heart disease than with information about an emerging area such as biotechnology or "genetic engineering."

IMPLICATIONS FOR BIOMEDICAL COMMUNICATORS

What are the implications of these findings for biomedical communicators? What practical conclusions might one draw from these analyses that are relevant to designing and targeting biomedical and biotechnology policy communications?

First, individuals who are attentive to biomedical research issues or biotechnology policy issues are high-volume consumers of news and information from a wide array of sources, and demonstrate a high degree of selectivity and discrimination in their selection of and trust in information sources. The volume and scope of information consumption by both attentive publics means that these citizens are likely to find, or be exposed to, multiple messages on a specific topic or issue from several major sources. Virtually all of the data point to a strong recognition and acceptance of authoritative information by both attentive publics.

Second, both biomedical research and biotechnology policy attentives are active readers, using newspapers, newsmagazines, science magazines, and books as information sources. To a large extent, this pattern of print utilization reflects the higher levels of educational attainment and biomedical literacy that characterizes both attentive publics. Recognizing the limitations of cross-sectional data, it appears that education produces biomedical literacy that, in turn, encourages greater use of print media. More extensive reading and information acquisition, in turn, enhances the level of biomedical literacy and encourages additional reading and information acquisition. Many of these attentive citizens might be described as self-sustaining learners.

Third, it appears that individuals attentive to biomedical research and biotechnology policy use television news broadcasts to monitor new developments, watching more than 500 hours of television hours of television news each year. At the same time, these attentive citizens report a low level of trust in information provided by television news sources and infrequent use of science television shows such as *Nova* and *National Geographic Specials*. Biomedical research attentives report very low levels of trust in health information provided by television talk shows.

Fourth, individuals attentive to biotechnology policy issues have extensive access to computers and are frequent users of the Web, but we have relatively little information about their use of the Web to search for specific information about biotechnology or other health-related matters. Biomedical research attentives, however, are slightly less likely to have computer or Web access than the modal American adult. It is important to recognize that the 43 percent of the attentive public for biomedical research that have access to the Web includes approximately 13 million adults—a substantial number of citizens for purposes of writing to or contacting public officials. While it is likely that the proportion of biomedical research attentives who use the Web will increase in the years ahead, especially as broadband services make the Web accessible through home television sets, the Web is currently a viable method for communicating to biomedical research attentives. Because half of biomedical research attentives are not current Web users, it is essential to develop non-Web communications programs at the same time.

Fifth, these information acquisition patterns provide useful insights for building programs to communicate with these attentive publics. The information about magazine readership is especially helpful. As noted above, the decision to subscribe to or read a magazine regularly is itself a form of issue specialization. Each individual's time is limited, and there are numerous magazines competing for subscribers within every interest niche. Knowing the patterns of magazine reading of issue attentives can help target freelance writing and advertising, but it is even more important in building direct mail communication campaigns. Virtually all magazine subscription lists are available for purchase or licensed usage. Although a detailed discussion of direct mail campaigns is beyond the scope of this chapter, it is important to recognize the linkage between issue attentiveness, specialized reading habits, and direct persuasion campaigns.

In summary, citizens attentive to biomedical research and to biotechnology are active information consumers, selective in their choice of information sources and discriminating in the level of trust that they accord to various sources. They are active readers and frequent viewers of television news shows and are beginning to use the Web more extensively. Because they are generally better educated and more likely to be biomedically literate, the acquisition of new information becomes a self-sustaining process. In the next two chapters, we will examine the processes through which information is screened, evaluated, retained, recalled, and used, but it is sufficient to note at this point that the volume and scope of information acquisition activities by individuals attentive to biomedical research or biotechnology policy suggests that the primary problem facing attentives is the integration and interpretation of information—not just the acquisition of information.

9

· · · · · · · · · ·

PUBLIC ATTITUDES TOWARD BIOMEDICAL RESEARCH ISSUES

· · · · · · · · · · · · · · · · ·

The attitudes of citizens toward biomedical research are important in democratic societies. Whereas citizens are rarely asked to make a direct decision on a biomedical research issue, a significant number of public policies involving biomedical research issues are decided by governments on a regular and continuing basis. In the United States and many other democratic societies, the policy formulation process is influenced regularly by the interventions of interest groups apart from direct electoral or campaign activities. The general structure of this system was discussed in Chapter 7, and this chapter will focus on the development, maintenance, and change in an individual's attitudes toward biomedical research and related topics. The analysis will also focus on the substantive attitudes held by citizens toward biomedical research generally and about specific issues or controversies. The chapter will conclude with a discussion of communication strategies to influence public attitudes toward biomedical research issues.

As a preface to an examination of attitudes toward biomedical research, it is useful to recall Hennessy's differentiation between opinions and attitudes (Hennessy, 1972). In a landmark review of the literature, Hennessy argued that people have opinions on virtually every subject, but have attitudes toward only those objects that are salient to them. In a survey, for example, an individual might be asked whether he or she thinks that the level of government price support for milk is too high, too low, or about right, and most respondents will select one of those choices as a part of the interview even though they may know little about agriculture and care even less about it. In contrast, a person in the dairy or food processing business may know a good deal about the supply and demand for milk and about the arguments for and against price supports, and this network of knowledge, concern, and preferences constitutes an attitude.

In general, attitudes tend to be stable over a period of time, reflecting their origins in an individual's knowledge and values. In contrast, opinions tend to be fragile and unstable, reflecting the low salience of a particular attitude object. Although there is little theoretical reason to expect opinions to be related to behaviors, there are strong theoretical expectations and substantial empirical evidence linking attitudes to behaviors.

A substantial body of psychology research has identified a schema as a device that individuals use to receive, filter, and process information (Schank, 1977; Minsky, 1986; Lau and Sears, 1986; Milburn, 1991; Pick *et al.*, 1992). In a modern information-rich society such as the United States, most individuals must deal on a daily basis with a massive array of new information, ranging from daily newspapers that sometimes approach 100 pages in size, dozens of television channels and radio stations, hundreds of magazines, and innumerable printed brochures and sales tracts in the mail. A schema is a psychological structure, or mental organizing scheme, that humans use to integrate their information and experiences into coherent clusters. It is a collection of knowledge, previous experience, and attitudes toward a subject (or attitude object) that an individual invokes when confronted with new information or a new event. Some individuals are more skillful in constructing networks of concrete and abstract schemas than other individuals, and psychologists often refer to these differences in information processing and utilization as mental ability.

In practical terms, when an individual opens a daily newspaper and scans the headlines, a series of schema are invoked that help the individual to decide to read one story and skip another, or on reading a story on a topic of interest, to accept or reject the information or arguments offered. For salient topics, an individual's schema will usually continue to grow over time, incorporating new information and experiences and modifying or rejecting older information.

All humans have schemas for simple tasks (such as driving an automobile in traffic) as well as for more complex and abstract tasks (such as understanding the impact of science on society). Schemas help an individual recognize the character of new information and provide an initial filtering or channeling response to the information. For example, when a driver sees lights in the form of an arrow pointing to one side of a highway, it is likely that the driver will assume that he or she will need to turn in that direction and may reason that it will be necessary to slow the vehicle to execute a turn safely. The original observation of the lighted arrow activates various prior experiences and knowledge, bringing into short-term memory a set of alternative explanations and associated behaviors.

Similarly, when an individual hears or reads a news report that a scientist has tested a new drug on a large number of animals and has found that the new drug significantly reduces the development of cancer in those animals receiving the medicine, this information may be recognized as a "scientific study" and one or more schema relevant to this subject may be activated. Although the report involves tests of a drug on animals, the individual may recognize that the importance of the report is that insights gained from animal studies may lead to studies with more advanced animals or with humans, ultimately resulting in a drug that might be useful to this individual, to friends or family, or to humans generally. If the individual holds a positive schema toward biomedical research, he or she may interpret this report optimistically, expecting new medications in the foreseeable future and reinforcing his or her sense that science produces things that make life healthier, easier, and more comfortable. Conversely, if an individual holds a more negative schema toward science, he or she may recall other test reports that have promised results in regard to cancer, but failed to produce major results in recent decades.

Setting aside issues concerning how much, if any, of the ability to develop effective schemas is an inherited trait, it is important to recognize the central role that schemas play in each individual's efforts to receive, organize, and make sense of the wide array of new and complex information encountered daily in the broadcast and print media. The growth and development of schemas during the adult years is an important mechanism in the learning process.

GENERAL SCHEMA TOWARD SCIENCE AND TECHNOLOGY

In previous work, Miller and Pardo (2000) and Miller *et al.* (1997) have found that most adults in the United States and other major industrial nations hold two schemas toward science and technology that operate simultaneously. One schema stresses the promise and potential of science and technology to improve the quality of life and to deal with disease and other problems. The other schema incorporates reservations about the impact of science and technology on the pace of life and on traditional values. It appears that specific stimuli—a news story about a new medical study or a news report on the storage of wastes from a nuclear power plant—may activate one schema or the other.

Although a full discussion of the statistical techniques[1] employed in identifying and measuring these dimensions is beyond the scope of this book, it may be useful to describe briefly the items that are incorporated in each dimension, because the wording of the items may convey a better sense of the substantive composition of each schema. The measure of the promise of science schema is based on agreement or disagreement with each of the following four statements:

1. Because of science and technology, there will be more opportunities for the next generation.
2. Science and technology are making our lives healthier, easier, and more comfortable.
3. Most scientists want to work on things that will make life better for the average person.
4. The application of science and new technology will make work more interesting.

Any individual that expresses strong agreement with all four of these statements may be said to believe in the promise of science. On a zero to 100 scale, the mean score on this Index of the Promise of Science and Technology in 1999 was 70 (see Figure 9-1). This indicator of high expectations for the results of science has been high for at least the last decade for which solid measurements are available, and other items that track attitudes over a 40-year period demonstrate the same pattern.

The measure of the reservations about science and technology schema is based on agreement or disagreement with each of the following four statements:

1. Science makes our way of life change too fast.
2. On balance, the benefits of scientific research have outweighed the harmful results (negatively correlated with the factor).
3. We depend too much on science and not enough on faith.
4. It is not important for me to know about science in my daily life.

Any individual who expressed strong agreement with items one, three, and four and strong disagreement with item two may be said to hold a high level of reservation about science and technology. On a zero to 100 scale, the

---

[1]The two dimensions were identified with a confirmatory factor analysis, using LISREL, a structural equation modeling computer program. The cell entries in the correlation matrix were polychloric correlation coefficients (reflecting the ordinal nature of the variables) and a separate asymtotic covariance matrix was computed by the program. For more information about this procedure, see Jöreskog and Sörbom (1993) and Hayduk (1987).

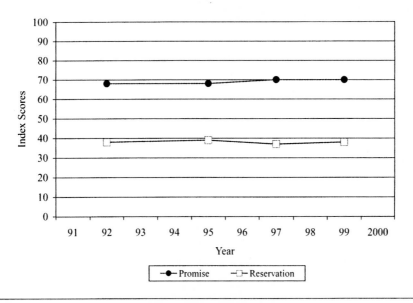

Figure 9-1 Mean scores on the Indices of the Promise of and Reservations about Science and Technology, 1992–1999.

mean score on the Index of Reservations about Science and Technology in 1999 was 38 (see Figure 9-1), and this pattern has been stable over the last decade for which this index can be measured. As noted above, other time-series measures over three or four decades display a similar low level of concern about science and technology among American adults.

In the data for the United States, these two dimensions (schema) are negatively related, meaning that individuals with a strong belief in the promise of science and technology tend to have a lower level of reservation about science and technology. In the United States, the relationship between these two dimensions is −.64, compared to a relationship of −.11 in Europe in 1992 (Miller *et al.*, 1997). Although the Miller *et al.* analysis provides an extended discussion of the social, political, and cultural factors underlying these differences, the pattern found in the United States appears to reflect a more consistent and integrated schema, or set of schema, than the European pattern.

The Distribution of Positive and Negative Schema toward Science and Technology

A quick look at the mean scores on the Index of the Promise of Science and Technology and the Index of Reservations about Science and Technology suggest that education plays a central role in the development of these

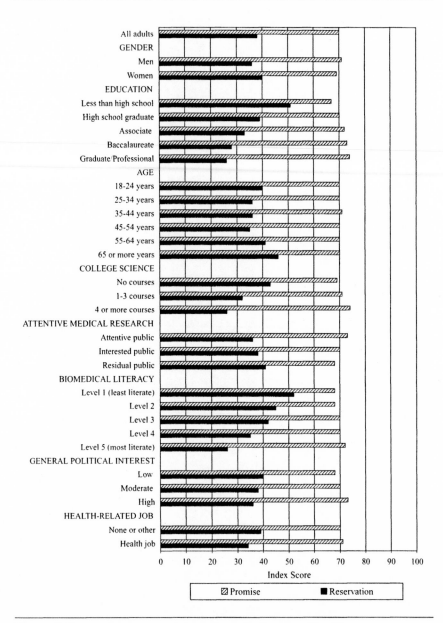

Figure 9-2 **Means scores on the Indices of the Promise of and Reservations about Science and Technology for selected groups, 1999.**

schema (see Figure 9-2). Although the overwhelming majority of American adults hold a strong belief in the promise of science and technology regardless of their level of education, individuals with more formal education have markedly lower levels of reservation—or concern—about potential or actual harmful results from science and technology. Adults who did not complete high school had a mean score of 51 on the Index of Reservations about Science and Technology, compared to mean scores of 28 for baccalaureates and 26 for adults with a graduate or professional degree. Similarly, the level of reservation about science and technology declines substantially with exposure to college-level science courses and with each higher level of biomedical literacy. In contrast, the differences in mean scores on both indices by age and gender were minimal.

Some Models to Predict Schema toward Science and Technology

To provide a more precise estimate of the effect of each of several educational, occupational, and attitudinal variables on each of these indices (schema), a set of models were constructed, building on the models in Chapter 7. Because many of these predictor variables are related to each other (age and education, for example), it is important to examine the net effect of each of these variables on the development of these general schema toward science and technology, which will become an increasingly important set of filters and structures in public thinking about biomedical research. The structure of the model is shown in Figure 9-3.

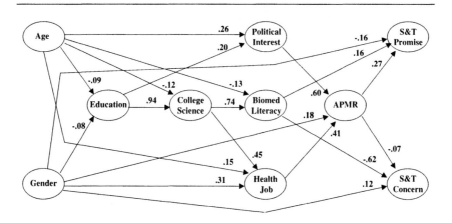

Figure 9-3   A model to predict general attitudes (schema) toward science and technology, 1999.

Substantively, analysis of this model shows that belief in the promise of science and technology is a pervasive cultural phenomenon in the United States, cutting across major educational and occupational and social class groups, but that the level of reservation about science and technology is related to education, college-level courses, biomedical literacy, and other attitudes and experiences. The pervasive nature of the American belief in the promise of science and technology makes the statistical prediction of this attitude (schema) very difficult because there are very few markers to differentiate those adults who do not hold this view. Accordingly, the basic model accounts for only 13 percent of the total variance in belief in the promise of science and technology, and the estimated total effects would be of limited value to a communicator seeking to optimize message delivery or impact concerning the benefits of biomedical research.

On the other hand, reservations or concerns about potential negative consequences from science and technology do vary substantially among American adults, and this basic model provides some very useful insights into the structure and dynamics of these attitudes (schema). The level of biomedical literacy is the strongest predictor of concern about science and technology, with a total effect of $-.62$ (see Table 9-1). This result means that higher levels of reservation about science and technology are associated with lower levels of biomedical literacy, and vice versa. The level of educational attainment and the number of college-level science courses are negatively related to concern about science and technology (total effects $= -.46$ and

Table 9-1   Total Effect of Selected Variables on General Attitudes (Schema) toward Science and Technology, 1999

	Promise of science and technology	Reservations about science and technology
Age	.00	.16
Gender (F)	−.14	.15
Level of education	.19	−.46
College science courses	.17	−.47
Biomedical literacy	.16	−.62
General political interest	.16	−.04
Health-related job	.11	.00
Attentive to biomedical research issues	.27	−.07
R^2 (proportion of variance explained)	.13	.43

−.47, respectively). Women and older adults were slightly more likely to be concerned about possible negative consequences from science and technology than men or younger adults, holding constant the other variables in the model. Citizens attentive to biomedical research were slightly less likely to be concerned about the negative impact of science and technology than nonattentive citizens, again holding constant all of the other variables in the model. Collectively, the model accounted for 43 percent of the total variance in reservations about science and technology among American adults.

Differences by Gender

Following the general strategy outlined in Chapter 2, a pair of models were run for men and women, using a common metric. The results for the separate analyses were generally the same as those found for all adults. Neither the model for men nor the model for women accounted for more than 11 percent of the total variance in belief in the promise of science and technology, reflecting the pervasive acceptance of that view in American society. Conversely, both models provided a moderately good fit for the data on reservations about science and technology, accounting for 34 percent of the variance in reservations among men and 46 percent of the total variance in concerns about science and technology among women (see Table 9-2).

Looking at the model to predict reservations about science and tech-

Table 9-2 Total Effect of Selected Variables on the Prediction of General Attitudes (Schema) toward Science and Technology, by Gender, 1999

	Promise of science and technology		Reservations about science and technology	
	Men	**Women**	**Men**	**Women**
Age	.07	−.04	.04	.25
Level of education	.10	.21	−.41	−.48
College science courses	.06	.17	−.44	−.50
Biomedical literacy	.00	.23	−.59	−.68
General political interest	.19	.22	.00	.00
Health-related job	.13	.00	.00	.00
Attentive to biomedical research issues	.28	.00	.00	.00
R^2 (proportion of variance explained)	.08	.11	.34	.46

nology, educational attainment, college-level science courses, and biomedical literacy were all negatively related to reservations about the impact of science and technology, and these relationships were relatively stronger among women than men (see Table 9-2). Age was also a stronger predictor of reservations about science and technology among women than men (total effects = .25 and .04, respectively), holding constant the other variables in the model. Neither the level of general political interest, employment in a health-related job, nor attentiveness to biomedical research were related to the level of reservation or concern about science and technology.

Summary

The concept of schema is a powerful tool in understanding the formation and maintenance of attitudes. The finding that the primary impact of education and literacy is to reduce reservations about potential negative results from science and technology is important. Educational attainment, college-level science courses, and biomedical literacy may buttress an individual's belief in the promise of science and technology, but—given the pervasive acceptance of the benefits of science and technology in American society—it does not distinguish these individuals from other adults with lower levels of educational attainment and literacy. In the context of the broader literature on attitude formation and the development and maintenance of schema, it is likely that biomedically literate citizens with higher levels of formal education are more firmly committed to the view that science and technology are likely to improve the quality of life, but we cannot test that conclusion empirically in the absence of longitudinal adult data. We will return to the implications of this finding in the concluding section of this chapter and in Chapter 11.

ATTITUDES TOWARD SUPPORT FOR BASIC SCIENTIFIC RESEARCH

Whereas the preceding analysis demonstrated the existence of two schemas concerning the general promise of benefits from science and technology and a general concern or reservation about the possibility of negative consequences from science and technology, it is important to look at individual attitudes toward some specific issues relevant to biomedical policy. This section will focus on the attitudes toward government spending for basic scientific research. The next section will look at attitude toward government spending for biomedical research, and the final section will examine attitudes toward the use of animals in biomedical research.

The conceptualization and measurement of attitudes toward government spending for any specific purpose is complex and difficult (Jacoby, 1994). Most adults in the United States have little information about actual government spending for any specific purpose or program, and Paulos (1988) has demonstrated that most adults have a limited understanding of sums such as million and billion in any case. Some analysts have given respondents a token sum (such as $100) and asked them to distribute it among government programs and purposes to measure the relative priority placed on various activities. In general, all of this work has documented the low level of specific government spending knowledge held by the overwhelming majority of American adults.

To measure the acceptance of government spending in support of basic scientific research, a national study has asked American adults to agree or disagree with the statement that "Even if it provides no immediate benefits, scientific research which advances the frontiers of knowledge is necessary and should be supported by the federal government." Approximately 80 percent of U.S. adults have agreed or strongly agreed with this statement for the last 15 years (see Figure 9-4).

In 1999, 79 percent of American adults agreed or strongly agreed with this statement (see Figure 9-5). Looking at the bivariate distributions by major educational and attitudinal characteristics, biomedical literacy appears to be strongly and positively related to this attitude, whereas age is nega-

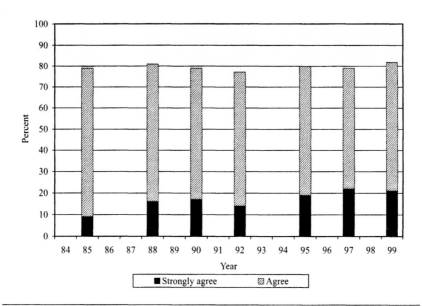

Figure 9-4 Percentage of American adults agreeing that the federal government should support basic scientific research, 1985–1999.

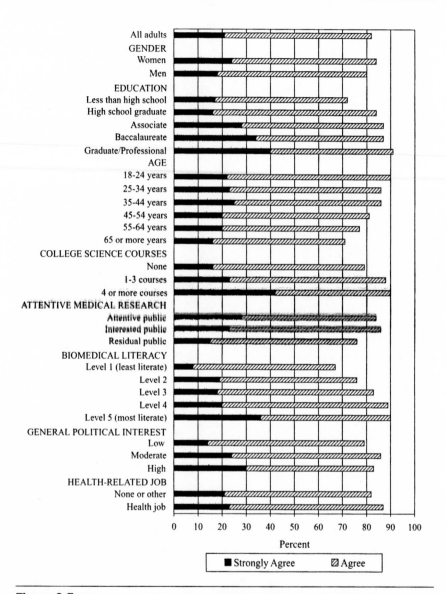

Figure 9-5 Percentage of American adults agreeing that the federal government should support basic scientific research, by selected groups, 1999.

tively related to federal support for basic scientific research. Other variables have less clear patterns of association with support for government spending for basic scientific research.

To assess the relative influence of each of the variables in the cumula-

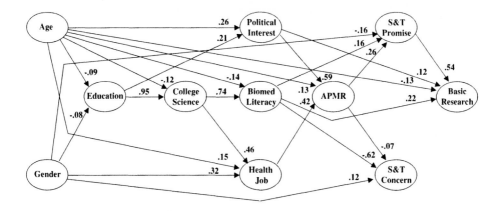

Figure 9-6 A model to predict attitude toward federal spending for basic scientific research, 1999.

tive model that we have employed in the preceding analyses, a model was constructed to examine the structure of public attitudes toward government spending in support of basic scientific research. This model includes the two schema discussed above to explore how these attitudinal constructs might relate to individual attitudes toward government spending for this purpose (see Figure 9-6). All of the other components of the model reflect the cumulative set of variables that we first examined in Chapter 2 and have enlarged in a series of additional analyses. Although we have tried to minimize the use of path models in favor of summary analyses of the total effects, it is important to provide a schematic view of this model since it will be used, with slight modifications, in subsequent analyses in this chapter.

Setting aside the complex set of paths that compose the model, the major finding from the analysis of this model is that schema play an important intervening role between an individual's personal and educational experiences, current knowledge and attitudes, and specific policy preferences, such as the attitude toward government support for basic scientific research. A number of background variables are related to each of the two schema, but the structural model shows that it is only the promise of science schema that is related to the specific attitude or preference toward government spending for basic scientific research. The absence of a path from the reservations about science and technology schema to the attitude toward spending for basic scientific research means that these two variables are unrelated, holding constant the other variables in the model.

This general pattern is reflected in the total effect attributable to each of the variables in the model. The strongest predictor of a positive attitude toward government support for basic scientific research is a strong belief in

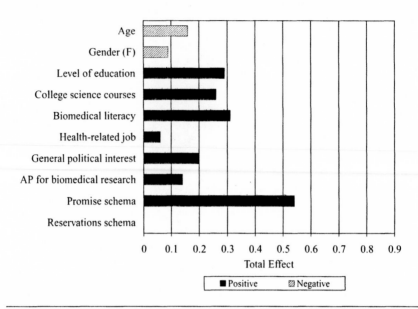

Figure 9-7 Total effect of selected variables on attitude toward federal spending for basic scientific research, 1999.

the promise (or benefits) of science and technology, with a total effect of .54 (see Figure 9-7). The level of educational attainment, the number of college science courses taken, and the level of biomedical literacy are also strong predictors of a positive attitude toward basic scientific research spending, with total effects of .29, .26, and .31, respectively. Attentiveness to biomedical research issues has a positive effect of .14, which is a cumulative effect that is additive to the effects of education, biomedical literacy, and a strong belief in the promise of science and technology. Holding constant all of the other variables in the model, women and older Americans are slightly less likely to support government spending for basic scientific research than men or young adults. Overall, the model accounts for 46 percent of the total variance in attitude toward government support for basic scientific research. This level of prediction can be very useful in designing and targeting messages on this topic.

Differences by Gender

An examination of parallel models for men and for women, using a common metric, found a common attitudinal structure for both men and women, but with a few significant differences (see Table 9-3). The promise of science schema was the dominant predictor for both men and women, and the reservations about science and technology schema had no relationship to attitude

Table 9-3   Total Effect of Selected Variables on the Prediction of Attitude toward Spending for Scientific Research, by Gender, 1999

	Men	Women
Age	−.17	−.11
Level of education	.17	.36
College science courses	.14	.32
Biomedical literacy	.19	.43
General political interest	.20	.25
Health-related job	.00	.00
Attentive to biomedical research issues	.13	.00
Promise schema	.50	.60
Reservations schema	.00	.00
R^2 (proportion of variance explained)	.37	.58

toward federal spending for basic scientific research among either men or women. This pattern suggests that these two schema operate similarly for men and women, as the general literature on cognition and attitude formation would predict.

Educational attainment, college science courses, and biomedical literacy were all substantially more influential among women in regard to attitude toward spending for basic scientific research than among men. In part, this result reflects the fact that there is more diversity of views about support for basic scientific research among women than men, thus these education and knowledge variables are stronger predictors of attitude differential among women than among men.

Attentiveness to biomedical research issues had a small, but significant, total effect (.13) among men in regard to attitude toward spending for scientific research, but no effect among women. Given the similarities in the predictors of biomedical research attentiveness among men and women, we have no immediate explanation for this minor variation.

Summary

This analysis found that positive attitudes toward federal support for basic scientific research are closely associated with a strong belief (schema) in the promise of science and technology to improve the quality of life. This schema, in turn, is positively influenced by higher levels of educational attainment, exposure to college-level science courses, and high levels of biomedical literacy. All of these factors appear to be slightly stronger among women than men, but there is substantial commonality in the structure of men's and women's attitude toward government support for basic scientific research. Attentiveness to biomedical research issues, especially among men, provides some additional support for government spending for basic scientific research. It is important to recognize, however, that the primary communication value of attentiveness to biomedical research is the higher likelihood that an attentive citizen will make the effort to intervene in the policy formulation process when an issue of importance is at stake. The small attitudinal gain is a bonus.

ATTITUDES TOWARD SPENDING TO IMPROVE HEALTH CARE

Whereas a great deal of interest in public attitudes toward spending for biomedical research involves a willingness to support funding for basic scientific research (such as the mapping of the human genome and the mouse genome), it is also useful to look at public support for more traditional medical research. Since 1990, a national study of American adults has asked individuals to indicate whether they think that the government is spending too much, too little, or about the right amount on each of several objectives. One objective is "to improve health care" and another objective is "conduct scientific research." Unfortunately, none of the spending alternatives specifically mentioned medical research. To provide an estimate of public support for medical research, a typology was constructed to identify three levels of the support for government spending for health research:

1. Adults who think that the government is spending too little on improving health care and too little on conducting scientific research will be labeled as having a high level of support for health research spending.

2. Adults who think that the government is spending too little on improving health care but who are satisfied with the level of spending for scientific research will be classified as having a moderate level of support for health research spending.

3. Adults who are satisfied with or think that the government is spending too much on improving health care and conducting scientific research will be defined as having a low level of support for government spending for health research.

Using data from a 1999 national survey of U.S. adults, approximately 30 percent of citizens held a high level of support for health or medical research

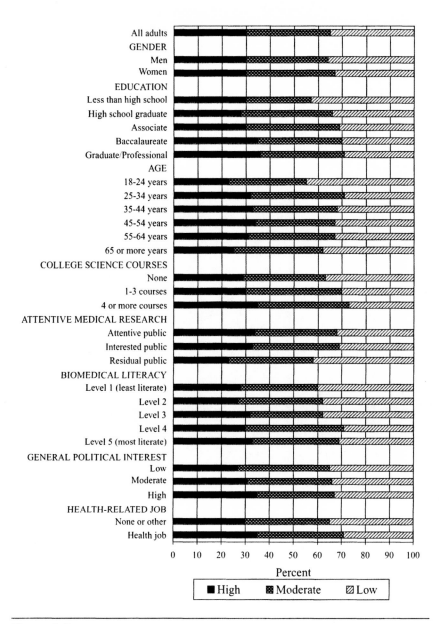

Figure 9-8 Level of support for government spending for health research, 1999.

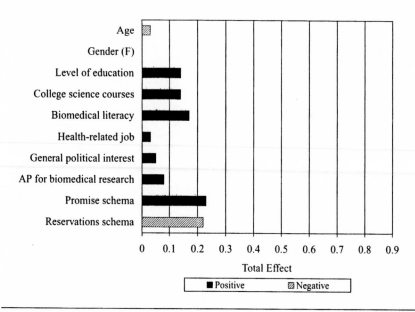

Figure 9-9   Total effect of selected variables on attitude toward federal spending for health research, 1999.

spending, while 35 percent expressed a moderate level of support for health or medical research spending, using the typology described above (see Figure 9-8). An additional 35 percent of American adults indicated a low level of support for health or medical research.

Although this typology attempts to produce some differentiation in regard to public support for health or medical research, it is necessary to recognize that public support for government spending for this purpose is generally high throughout the adult population. Looking at the distribution of this attitude across the major demographic, educational, and attitudinal groupings used in the preceding analyses, there is limited variation—even in this constructed typology.

This general observation is supported by the results of a structural analysis. When attitude toward health and medical research spending is substituted for the attitude toward spending for basic scientific research in the preceding model, only 15 percent of the total variance can be accounted for by the 10 background and attitudinal variables used in the preceding analysis (see Figure 9-9). The low proportion of variance explained is a direct result of the broad support for health research spending that runs across all sectors of the American public.

Table 9-4   Total Effect of Selected Variables on the Prediction of Attitude toward Spending for Scientific Research, by Gender, 1999

	Total effects	
	Men	**Women**
Age	−.01	−.06
Level of education	.10	.17
College science courses	.10	.16
Biomedical literacy	.12	.21
General political interest	.02	.00
Health-related job	.03	.07
Attentive to biomedical research	.04	.00
Promise schema	.16	.33
Reservations schema	−.20	−.20
R^2 (proportion of variance explained)	.10	.23

Differences by Gender

When this same model was run by gender, using a common metric, the model was slightly better at predicting the health research spending attitude of women than men, with 23 and 10 percent of the total variance being explained, respectively (see Table 9-4). As noted in regard to attitude toward government spending for basic scientific research, educational attainment, college science courses, and the promise of science and technology schema were significantly more influential among women than among men. The magnitude of these differences is sufficiently small, however, that one would not want to base an information strategy on these results.

THE USE OF ANIMALS IN BIOMEDICAL RESEARCH

Although more numerous, not all biomedical policy issues are financial or budgetary in nature. One of the continuing nonfinancial issues that impact biomedical research is the level of public concern about the use of animals in laboratory experiments. For more than a decade, the *Science and Engineering Indicators* studies published by The National Science Foundation

(NSF) have asked national samples of American adults to agree or disagree with the statement that "Scientists should be allowed to do research that causes pain and injury to animals like dogs and chimpanzees *if* it produces new information about human health problems." Respondents were asked to strongly agree, agree, disagree, or strongly disagree with the statement. For most of the last decade, Americans have been deeply split over this issue.

Although this statement was written to pose the ultimate tradeoff dilemma—hurting two beloved species in exchange for information to improve human health—some biomedical researchers felt that the statement portrayed the use of animals in draconian terms and suggested that the public held much more approving attitudes toward the use of mice in experiments, which are the most commonly used laboratory animals in the United States. In the 1997 and 1999 NSF *Science and Engineering Indicators* studies, a second question was added that asked each respondent to strongly agree, agree, disagree, or strongly disagree with the statement "Scientists should be allowed to do research that causes pain and injury to animals like mice if it produces new information about human health problems." All respondents were asked both questions, rotated randomly and separated by several other questions. Approximately two-thirds of American adults agreed to the use of mice in biomedical research, but nearly 30 percent of adult respondents continued to voice some level of disagreement concerning the use of animals in research.

To provide a summary measure of attitude toward the use of animals in research, the responses to these two questions—the use of dogs and chimpanzees and the use of mice—were combined. Using a standard Likert technique, the responses were reclassified into individuals who were generally opposed to the use of animals in research, people with mixed feelings (e.g., yes for mice and no for dogs or chimpanzees), and people who were generally supportive of the use of animals in research. In 1999, 26 percent of American adults were generally opposed to the use of animals in biomedical research, 28 percent held mixed feelings about the practice, and 46 percent were generally supportive of animal use in research (see Figure 9-10).

Looking at the bivariate cross-tabulations, men were substantially more likely to support the use of animals in biomedical research than were women. Older adults were more favorable to using animals in research than younger adults. Individuals with higher levels of educational attainment, more exposure to college science courses, and a higher level of biomedical literacy were generally more favorable to the use of animals in research than were other groups. There was no statistically significant difference in attitude to the use of animals by either attentiveness to biomedical research or by employment in a health-related job.

To explore the relative influence of these interrelated factors, a path model was constructed, using the basic model described above and substi-

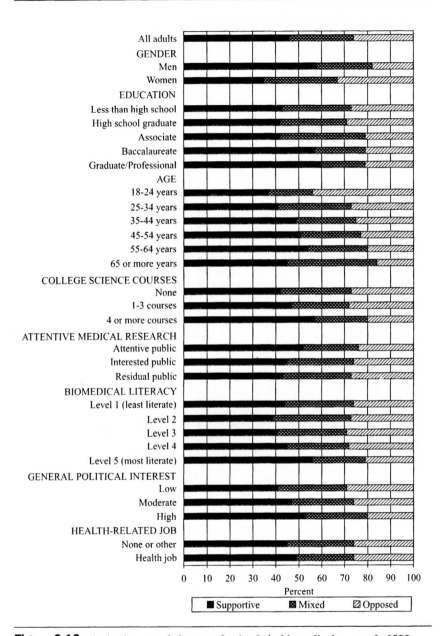

Figure 9-10   Attitude toward the use of animals in biomedical research, 1999.

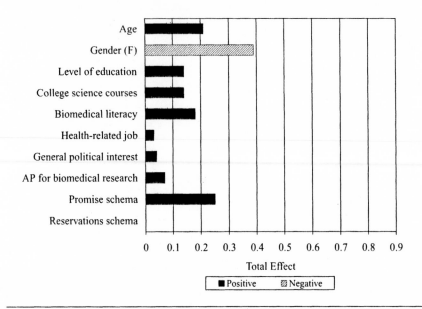

Figure 9-11 **Total effect of selected variables on attitude toward the use of animals in biomedical research, 1999.**

tuting attitude toward animal use in the place of the spending attitude variable. Although the model accounted for only 28 percent of the total variance in attitude toward the use of animals in biomedical research, the results offer some interesting insights into the factors that predict—at least in part—this attitude.

The analysis found that gender, age, and belief in the promise of science and technology were the three primary predictors of attitude toward the use of animals in biomedical research (see Figure 9-11). With a negative total effect of −.39, gender was the strongest predictor of the animal use attitude, with men tending to support the use of animals in research and women being significantly less supportive. It is important to note that this difference takes into account (or holds constant) all of the other variables in the model, indicating that this residual difference is not explained by any of the other factors in the model. This finding is consistent with previous studies that have found that women are more likely to support the animal rights movement and to oppose animal research than men (Bailey, 1994; Bowd and Bowd, 1989; Broida *et al.*, 1993; Gallup and Beckstead, 1988; Galvin and Herzog, 1992; Herzog *et al.*, 1991; Kellert and Berry, 1987; Nibert, 1994; Pifer, 1994, 1996; and Plous, 1991).

Older adults were more supportive of the use of animals in biomedical research, holding constant all of the other variables in the model, with a total effect of .21. This result is not surprising, since aging is associated with increased awareness of health problems and with higher levels of attentiveness to biomedical research issues.

A positive attitude toward the promise of science and technology was also related to support for the use of animals in biomedical research, with a total effect of .25. The linkage is obvious—individuals who expect benefits from science are more willing to allow the use of animals to obtain those results. Interestingly, the level of reservations about science and technology was not related to attitude toward the use of animals in biomedical research.

The relationship between attitudes toward science, and attitudes toward animal research, has been the subject of frequent discussion. Jasper and Nelkin (1992) connect the animal rights movement with broader attitudes about science. They suggest that activists from various social movements in the 1980s began to show opposition to science. Such protest movements formed around an anti-instrumental position and an emphasis on moral rather than instrumental values. Younger activists, according to Jasper and Nelkin (1992), are more likely to question accepted scientific practices.

The level of educational attainment, the number of college science courses, and the level of biomedical literacy were all positively related to support for the use of animals in research, but the total effects were relatively small.

Looking at the full pattern, attitude toward the use of animals in biomedical research appears to be based on a combination of utilitarianism and maternalism. The higher levels of support for the use of animals by older adults appears to reflect their growing interest in and concern about health matters, both personal and family. The clear linkage between support for animal use and a strong belief in the promise of science and technology to improve the quality of life suggests a classic benefit analysis. Although the reasons for the strong resistance to the use of animals in biomedical research by women is not explained by the variables included in the analysis, this result fits into the stereotype that women are more protective of life and that men are more utilitarian.

Differences by Gender

Given the strong gender difference in attitude toward the use of animals in biomedical research, it is useful to look at separate analyses of the structure of these attitudes among men and women, using a common metric. Given the strong gender differential discussed above, it is not surprising that neither of the separate models for men and for women account for as much of the total variance in their respective models as the combined model predicted. The model for men accounted for 23 percent of the total variance in attitude toward animal use among men, but the model for women accounted for only

14 percent of the total variance in this attitude among female respondents. All three models indicate that some significant variables have been omitted from each of the analyses.

Because neither of the gender models account for as much as a quarter of the variance in attitudes toward the use of animals in biomedical research, we will not discuss the nature of the relationships found in each model. It is clear, however, that more research needs to be focused on the origin and maintenance of adult attitudes toward the use of animals in biomedical research.

IMPLICATIONS FOR BIOMEDICAL COMMUNICATORS

The analyses reported in this chapter supports the proposition that schema are useful and functional parts of the process through which adults receive, process, and organize information and form attitudes.[2] Given the high volume of biomedical information included in news reports in newspapers and magazines and on radio and television, the typical citizen needs an organizational scheme to integrate incoming information with previous experiences and his or her existing knowledge base. It is a challenging task, and the very complexity of the task undoubtedly accounts in large part for the growing levels of political and issue specialization found in the United States and other major industrial countries.

Structurally, the evidence points to two major schema that reflect a belief in the promise of benefits from science and technology and a reservation about present or potential dangers from science and technology. The relatively strong negative relationship between these two schema suggest a high degree of integration, but some ambiguity about the benefits and risks of science and technology persists among some Americans. This finding is especially important for communicators. A two-dimensional view of attitude toward science and technology allows the development of messages that address either benefits or concerns, and offers the possibility of targeting messages to segments of the public to address specific concerns or problems.

Substantively, these analyses have found that belief in the promise of benefits from science and technology permeates all levels of American society. Although some groups have slightly higher levels of scientific and technological optimism than others, no major demographic segment of the adult population scored lower than 66 on a zero to 100 scale. A strong belief in the

---

[2]Given the cross-sectional nature of the survey data used in these analyses, we can only infer the role of schema in the dynamic process of attitude development and maintenance, but the inference is reasonably strong when taken across the full set of analyses reported above.

promise of benefits from science and technology is also prevalent among adults in Canada and the European Union, although there is somewhat greater variation among European adults than among North Americans (Miller *et al.,* 1997).

American adults have a lower level of reservation about dangers or problems from science and technology, with a mean score of only 38 on a zero to 100 scale. There is, however, substantially more variation in adult assessments of risk from science and technology. Adults who did not finish high school, for example, have a mean reservation score of 51, compared to a mean reservation score of only 26 for adults with a graduate or professional degree. Similarly, adults with the lowest level of biomedical literacy have a mean reservation score of 52, whereas adults in the highest level of biomedical literacy have a mean reservation score of 26.

The implication for communicators is that there is more to be gained from focusing on the reservations or concerns of the less well educated than trying to persuade them of the potential benefits of science and technology. It is important to try to understand the substantive nature of these concerns and to address those problems in communications targeted to those individuals and groups holding high levels of reservation. Additional messages about the benefits of new scientific work are unlikely to address these reservations because most of the individuals who report concerns already report moderate to high levels of belief in the benefits of science and technology.

Many members of the scientific community, including the biomedical community, hear expressions of concern or reservation about science and technology and worry about the rise of an antiscience movement in the United States. They fail to recognize that the solid record of public support of science and technology over the last five decades is a genuine reflection of belief in the promise of science and technology, and that the expressions of reservation are rooted primarily in the wariness that comes from low levels of understanding or literacy. Although a standard axiom of public relations is to stress the positive and avoid the negative, this analysis suggests that it is important to study the substantive nature of concerns and reservations and to try to address these issues creatively, but forthrightly.

A simple example may be helpful. A substantial body of research shows that most Americans expect that science will "cure" cancer eventually, but research also suggests that many adults believe that people often die in clinical trials. Additional messages about the promise of biomedical science to cure cancer are unlikely to reduce concerns about the risk of clinical trials, given the two-dimensional structure of public attitudes discussed above. In this example, messages that stress the number of patients who have benefited from participation in a clinical trial, and the relatively small number who experience no improvement or die, may be far more effective. There is a need for expanded empirical research on the focus and effectiveness of messages that reduce reservations about science and technology generally and about biomedical research specifically.

Attitudes toward Spending

The issue of public support for government funding of biomedical research continues to worry the biomedical community, despite decades of growing funding and very high levels of public support for federal funding for medical research. Even though the level of biomedical research funding may be debated behind the closed doors of congressional committees, it is a rare legislator that will cast a vote against medical research funding for the record.

The analyses in this chapter have demonstrated the high level of public support for biomedical research funding. Structurally, our analysis found that support for basic scientific research reflects both higher levels of biomedical literacy and belief in the promise of science and technology. Equally important, the same analyses show that reservations about science and technology are unrelated to support for basic research funding. This pattern is consistent with our earlier suggestion that reservations about science and technology are often based on wariness produced by lower levels of understanding. It appears that the sense of uncertainty or wariness inherent in the higher levels of reported concern are not sufficient to lead individuals to conclude that basic research should be reduced or curtailed. We will explore this issue in more detail in regard to biotechnology attitudes in Chapter 10.

Attitudes toward Animal Use

Finally, our analysis found that a plurality—but not a majority—of American adults support the use of animals in biomedical research. Approximately one in four adults hold serious reservations about the use of animals in research. An additional 25 percent have mixed feelings about the issue, indicating that they would support the use of some animals, but not others. Older adults and men were more likely to support the use of animals in research than younger adults or women. Individuals with a strong belief in the promise of scientific research were also more likely to agree with the use of animals in research than other adults. Although the predictive power of the model was low, it is clear that there was a positive linkage between a belief in the promise of science and support for the use of animals in research, and conversely, that there was no linkage between reservations about science and technology and attitude toward animal use.

10

·········

PUBLIC ATTITUDES TOWARD BIOTECHNOLOGY ISSUES

·················

Biotechnology, in contrast to biomedical research, is a new and emerging subject in the public arena. Biotechnology companies have been a favored investment by mutual funds and individual investors and a constant subject of financial analysts and writers in recent years, but most adults in the United States and other industrial nations have a limited understanding—or schema—about biotechnology. Although fewer than one in five adults in all of the major nations of the industrial world have a sufficient grasp of scientific terms, concepts, and processes to follow the stories in the *New York Times'* Science Times and similar publications, the extraordinary advancement of genomics in recent decades means that most adults had limited exposure to these ideas during their formal schooling and are forced to try to keep up with a complex and rapidly expanding subject largely from informal adult learning resources.

The announcement of the completion of a draft map of the human genome by the National Human Genome Research Institute and Celera Genomics marks the beginning of a century of genomic research that will change our conceptions of health, illness, and treatment, but it is still a new and relatively low salience subject for most adults. In making the original announcement, President Clinton observed:

> *Nearly two centuries ago, in this room, President Thomas Jefferson and a trusted aide spread out a magnificent map, a map that Jefferson had long*

prayed he would get to see in his lifetime. The aide was Meriwether Lewis and the map was the product of his courageous expedition across the American frontier, all the way to the Pacific. It was a map that defined the contours and forever expanded the frontiers of our continent and our imagination.

Today the world is joining us here in the East Room to behold a map of even greater significance. We are here to celebrate the completion of the first survey of the entire human genome. Without a doubt, this is the most important, most wonderous map ever produced by humankind. (New York Times, *2000)*

Francis Collins, the director of the National Human Genome Research Institute, spoke of the present and future impact of human genomic research:

*Today we celebrate the revelation of the first draft of the human book of life. Already more than a dozen genes responsible for diseases from deafness to kidney disease to cancer have been identified using this resource in just the last year. . . . (*New York Times, *2000)*

In the context of biomedical communications, the emergence of biotechnology as a new and important subject on the national and international agenda provides a valuable opportunity to examine how adults deal with new and largely unfamiliar scientific subjects. It is an excellent example of an area of scientific research that has been well-known within the biomedical research community for decades, but is just emerging into full public view. There are already interesting and important public policy issues associated with biotechnology—the ownership and patent status of genes and genomic sequences, the protection of personal genetic information, and the use of new therapies such as stem cells in the treatment of human disease. Although a full discussion of the impact of biotechnology or the resolution of policy issues involving biotechnology is beyond the scope of this book, it is important to examine the current levels of public awareness and the structure of attitudes toward biotechnology. The chapter will conclude with a discussion of the implications of public awareness of, understanding of, and attitudes toward biotechnology on biomedical communications.

AWARENESS OF BIOTECHNOLOGY

A substantial portion of American adults have never heard of biotechnology or have only a minimal familiarity with the term. In a national survey of American adults in 1997–1998, 31 percent of adults—about 62 million individuals—indicated that they had never heard the term biotechnology prior to being asked about it in the interview (see Table 10-1). An additional 16 percent of adults reported that they had heard the term, but had never talked to anyone else about the subject, which is an indicator of low salience for most issues. Twenty-eight percent of adults said that they had heard of biotechnology and occasionally talked to other adults about the subject, whereas 8 percent claimed both awareness and frequent conversation about biotechnology.

The likelihood of awareness of biotechnology is strongly associated with educational attainment, college science courses, biomedical literacy, and attentiveness to science and technology policy (see Table 10-1). Half of adults in a 1997–1998 national study who had not completed high school reported that they had never heard of biotechnology prior to the interview, compared to only 6 percent of adults with a graduate or professional degree. Forty percent of adults who have never taken a college-level science course said that they had never heard of biotechnology. Men were more likely to have heard of biotechnology than women, and younger adults were slightly more likely to have heard of biotechnology than older adults.

Unfortunately, there is no solid evidence about the process by which adults who are beyond formal schooling become aware of new subject matters and acquire information about them. From cross-sectional data in our own studies and from other cross-sectional studies reported in the literature, we speculate that there are several viable scenarios for this process. In the simplest scenario, adults who are attentive to a substantively adjacent subject area (such as science and technology policy or biomedical research) may become aware of a new area such as biotechnology because of the increasing frequency of coverage of the subject in information sources already used by a person attentive to one of those issues. Some of the analyses discussed below will demonstrate positive correlations consistent with this scenario.

Another feasible scenario is the media alert model. As noted in Chapter 8, adults with a general interest in public affairs are more likely to read newspapers and newsmagazines regularly and to watch television news shows. Although we have no empirical evidence, it is reasonable to speculate that a *Time* magazine cover story on the announcement of the completion of a draft map of the human genome or a parallel Cable News Network (CNN) Special Report on the likely impact of human genome research on medicine and agriculture may alert an individual to the importance of a new subject and stimulate the person to seek additional information about the matter.[1]

A third possible scenario reflects the impact of occupational exposure

---

[1] For a slightly dated but still accurate discussion of the more general process of political agenda setting, see Kingdon (1984).

Table 10-1 Awareness of Biotechnology by Selected Groups, 1997–1998

	Awareness of biotechnology					Number of cases
	Not heard	Heard, no talk	Heard, min talk	Heard, occ talk	Heard, freq talk	
All adults	31	16	17	28	8	1067
Gender						
Men	24	16	19	33	7	512
Women	38	17	15	22	8	555
Level of education						
Less than high school	51	14	13	18	4	225
High school graduate	35	18	18	22	7	510
Associate degree	19	15	14	40	12	124
Baccalaureate	12	15	20	43	10	137
Graduate/professional	6	16	17	48	13	70
Age						
18–24 years	27	10	23	32	8	145
25–34 years	29	13	20	28	10	237
35–44 years	27	16	15	30	12	223
45–54 years	26	22	14	33	5	171
55–64 years	33	20	22	18	7	105
65 or more years	46	20	10	21	3	185
College science courses						
None	40	18	16	20	6	691
1–3 courses	18	20	20	35	7	186
4 or more courses	11	7	18	49	15	192
Attentive to medical research						
Attentive public	28	11	12	34	15	166
Interested public	30	18	19	26	7	525
Residual public	35	16	16	28	6	375
Attentive to science and technology						
Attentive public	23	8	11	44	14	204
Interested public	27	19	19	28	7	422
Residual public	39	18	18	19	6	440
Biomedical literacy						
Level 1 (low)	55	18	12	14	1	194
Level 2	51	14	18	11	6	208
Level 3	30	20	14	29	7	154
Level 4	28	20	18	27	7	181
Level 5 (high)	7	14	19	47	14	328
General political interest						
Low	38	17	17	23	5	428
Moderate	30	14	19	30	7	347
High	21	18	14	34	13	239
Health job						
No	31	17	17	28	7	1001
Yes	33	8	21	21	17	66

to an emerging subject matter. An adult employed in the financial sector would undoubted be exposed to frequent stories about the growth—and occasional decline—of stock prices for biotechnology companies. An individual investor who is evaluating several alternative mutual funds for possible investment would almost surely be exposed to information about the growth potential of biotechnology companies. Some persons may simply classify biotechnology companies as another form of pharmaceutical company and explore the matter no further, but some individuals may be sufficiently curious about what these new companies are doing to seek additional information and, in the process, become better informed about biotechnology. Some media content studies have found more stories about biotechnology in the business and finance pages than in the news sections of major daily newspapers in the United States and Europe.

A fourth scenario reflects the impact of personal or family experiences on changes in interest patterns. Most 20-year-olds and 30-year-olds have limited interest in Alzheimer's disease, for example, but if an individual's parent or grandparent is diagnosed with the disease and requires assistance in seeking care, the younger adult may develop a need to learn more about this disease. There are hundreds of anecdotes about the extraordinary levels of knowledge and understanding that some individuals without formal medical training have acquired when faced with the need to obtain care for a child, spouse, sibling, parent, or friend. Again, there is limited empirical evidence of the number of adults who have this kind of experience, but there can be no doubt that some adults become aware of and, ultimately, attentive to an issue area through this process.

In Chapters 11 and 12, we will argue that there is a compelling need to develop methodologically solid longitudinal studies of adults to learn more about the origins and structure of interest and attentiveness and the dynamics of information acquisition. At this point, however, it is sufficient to note that it is likely that some proportion of adults are drawn to an emerging issue such as biotechnology through one or more of the pathways described above, but it is also important to recognize that the proportion of adults who will become aware of and attentive to a new subject such as biotechnology will be small in the beginning and grow over time.

The Attentive Public for Biotechnology

Eight percent of Americans were attentive to biotechnology in 1997–1998, using data from the U.S. Biotechnology Study (see Figure 10-1). Comparatively, 16 percent of American adults were attentive to biomedical research and 19 percent of Americans were attentive to science and technology policy in 1999. Unfortunately, there are no time series measures available for at-

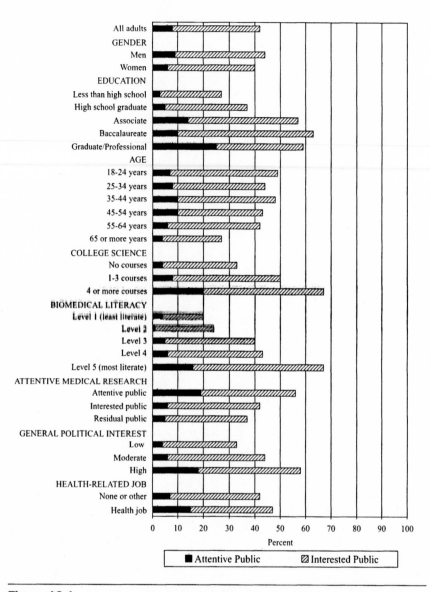

Figure 10-1 Attentive and interested publics for biotechnology, 1997–1998.

tentiveness to biotechnology policy in the United States, but we would expect that this proportion would increase gradually over the next decade to reach the level of attentiveness to biomedical research or science and technology policy.

This pattern is consistent with the general concept of issue attentiveness and the new and emerging nature of biotechnology as a subject of public policy. Because attentiveness to an issue requires that an individual think of the subject as being important and salient and allocate sufficient time and effort to follow the issue in current news sources, the development of attentiveness to an issue often requires some adjustment—perhaps consciously or perhaps not—of other priorities in regard to salience and time use. It is obviously easier to become attentive to a new subject or issue that is logically or substantively adjacent to a subject to which one is already attentive. For example, an individual who is attentive to biomedical research issues might be a regular reader of health and medical articles in newspapers and magazines, and an increasing number of these articles may include new information about the application of biotechnology to various diseases or inherited problems. If the individual were to become more interested, he or she might then buy a popular book or two on the subject or watch a television show reporting on or discussing biotechnology issues. In contrast, an individual who has paid little attention to health or medical issues or to science and technology policy issues might find the development of an initial knowledge base and a continuing information flow to be more burdensome. The marginal effort required to begin to follow a new issue from an adjacent issue will almost always be smaller, and therefore, easier for most individuals.

Looking at the bivariate tabulations of attentiveness to biotechnology policy in 1997–1998, biomedical literacy, formal education, and exposure to college science courses are the three strongest predictors (see Figure 10-1). For example, only 5 percent of high school graduates were attentive to biotechnology policy compared to 25 percent of adults with a graduate or professional degree. Similarly, only 4 percent of adults with the lowest level of biomedical literacy were attentive to biomedical policy, compared to 16 percent of individuals with the highest level of biomedical literacy. These bivariate tabulations also indicate that individuals who were attentive to biomedical research or attentive to science and technology policy were more likely to be attentive to biotechnology policy than other adults. The small difference in the rates of attentiveness to biotechnology policy between men and women is not statistically significant.

When these same variables are examined in a path model, attentiveness to biomedical research is the strongest single predictor of attentiveness to biotechnology policy, with a total effect of .71 (see Figures 10-2 and 10-3). This result is consistent with the general rationale for the development of attentiveness to new and emerging issues discussed above. The level of biomedical literacy was the second strongest predictor of attentiveness to biotechnology policy (total effect = .64), followed by educational attainment and college science course exposure (total effects = .50 and .49, respectively). An individual's level of general political interest was also a strong pre-

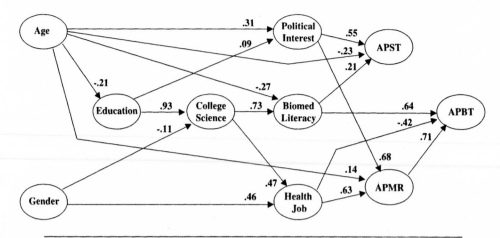

Figure 10-2 A path model to predict attentiveness to biotechnology, 1997–1998.

dictor of attentiveness to biotechnology policy (total effect = .48).

This pattern illustrates the simultaneous role of adjacent attentiveness, substantive knowledge, and general political interest in the development of attentiveness to new and emerging scientific issues. As noted in previous

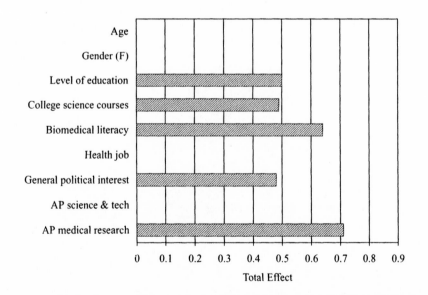

Figure 10-3 Total effect of selected variables on attentiveness to biotechnology.

chapters, the attentive public for biomedical research includes a relatively high proportion of older adults with a strong interest in health and medical developments, some of whom have a high level of biomedical literacy and some of whom do not. The set of predictors of biotechnology policy attentives indicate that it is the combination of a strong adjacent interest and a higher level of biomedical literacy and education and a general interest in politics that lead some individuals to become attentive to biotechnology policy. Because an emerging policy area such as biotechnology requires some specialized knowledge to read and understand a good deal of the available information about it, education and biomedical literacy play an essential catalytic role in the process. The absence of any effect from age, gender, or health job indicate that the combination of skills and interests necessary to identify and follow an emerging subject such as biotechnology are largely independent of traditional demographic factors.

Differences by Gender

Although there were no net differences attributable to gender in the aggregate model, it is useful to examine the structure of factors related to attentiveness to biotechnology policy issues separately for men and women, using a common metric. Although there is a general similarity between the two models, there are some important differences in the strength of various relationships among men and women.

Attentiveness to biomedical research issues is strongly associated with attentiveness to biotechnology policy issues among both men and women, but the strength of this relationship is much stronger among men than women (total effects = .95 and .61, respectively). The influence of educational attainment, college science courses, and biomedical literacy is stronger among women than men (see Table 10-2). In practice, this result suggests that education and biomedical literacy play a relatively larger role in encouraging attentiveness to biotechnology policy among women than men. A high level of general political interest was an important predictor of attentiveness to biotechnology policy issues among both men and women.

Summary

In contrast to attentiveness to biomedical research issues, this analysis indicates that education and biomedical literacy are relatively more influential in the development of attentiveness to biotechnology policy among adults in the United States than personal or family health experiences and needs. Although all of the analyses were limited to existing cross-sectional surveys, the strong inference of these results is that attentiveness to a new and emerging issue area such as biotechnology policy is strongly related to current—and presumably, prior—attentiveness to substantively adjacent sub-

Table 10-2 Total Effect of Selected Factors on Attentiveness to Biotechnology, by Gender 1999

	Total effects	
	Men	*Women*
Age	.13	−.12
Level of education	.41	.61
College science courses	.30	.66
Biomedical literacy	.00	.61
Health job	.36	.51
General political interest	.67	.52
Attentiveness to science and technology	.00	.00
Attentiveness to biomedical research	.95	.61
R^2	.87	.85

jects. In the case of biotechnology policy, these results suggest that prior attentiveness to biomedical research issues is a more likely linkage than prior attentiveness to science and technology policy.

SCHEMAS ABOUT BIOTECHNOLOGY

In Chapter 9 we introduced the concept of a schema as a process that many adults use to receive, screen, evaluate, organize, and retain (or not) new information on salient subjects. The development of a schema—or a set of schema—about biotechnology is an important part of understanding more specific attitudes toward biotechnology. Whereas the previous discussion focused on a parallel set of schema related to the promise of scientific research and reservations about science and technology, the development of a schema, or schemas, about biotechnology offers an opportunity to think about and examine the development of schemas for a new and emerging issue.

Conceptually, if a schema is a collection of previous information, attitudes, and experiences concerning a subject, we would expect that a schema for a new and emerging issue would be smaller and less well-developed. For example, a 50-year-old adult might have a schema—or set of schemas—about biomedical research that incorporates portions of his or her school study of biology, decades of medical care, hundreds of individual appointments or experiences with health care providers, numerous articles read in newspapers and magazines about biomedical research issues, and hundreds (if not thousands) of hours of television news and dramatic shows related to medicine and health directly or indirectly. In this example, the primary challenge may be to organize the large volume of information and experiences into a coherent format that is useful in assessing new information on the same subject.

In contrast, it is unlikely that this hypothetical 50-year-old individual would have studied biotechnology in school and even more unlikely that he or she would have had any personal experiences involving biotechnology or any of its applications. The volume of news coverage about biotechnology has grown in recent years, but the length and depth of prior information, attitudes, and experiences relevant to biotechnology would be markedly smaller, except for a small proportion of adults who have some professional involvement in this area. Although individuals with more recently formed schemas about biotechnology can undoubtedly feel strongly about specific biotechnology-related issues—witness the Greenpeace activism against genetically modified foods in Europe—when the salience of an issue is sufficiently high, this is an unusual event. More commonly, most individuals can be expected to hold smaller, but developing, schema about a new and emerging issue and be somewhat more constrained in their attitudes and activities than individuals with large mature schemas on a subject. It is essential to recognize, however, the critical catalytic role of salience in this process.

To explore the development of schemas related to biotechnology, a small set of items asked of national samples of adults in the United States and the European Union were used to define and measure schemas about biotechnology. An examination of the structure of these eight items found two basic dimensions similar to the structure of the two schema for science and technology described above. One dimension can be characterized as belief in the promise of biotechnology and is defined by agreement that each of the following events is likely to occur within the next 20 years as a result of modern biotechnology:

1. Substantially reduce world hunger.
2. Get more out of natural resources in Third World countries.
3. Substantially reduce environmental pollution.
4. Cure most genetic diseases.

Any individual who believes that biotechnology is likely to create all of these outcomes within the next 20 years may be said to believe in the promise of biotechnology to improve the quality of life, and any individual who thinks that all four of these results are unlikely to occur may be said to have a low level of belief in the promise of biotechnology.

A second dimension can be characterized as concerns, reservations, or fears about the application of biotechnology. This dimension is defined by agreement that each of the following events is likely to occur within the next 20 years as a result of modern biotechnology:

1. Replace most existing food products with new varieties.
2. Produce designer babies.
3. Create dangerous new diseases.
4. Reduce the range of fruits and vegetables we can get.

Any individual who believes that biotechnology is likely to cause all four of these outcomes within the next 20 years may be reasonably characterized as having a high level of concern or reservation about the application of biotechnology, and anyone who reports that all four of these events are unlikely to occur within the next 20 years would appear to have a lower level of concern about or fear of biotechnology.

On a zero to 100 index, the mean score on the Index of the Promise of Biotechnology was 59, and the mean score on the Index of Reservations about Biotechnology was 52 (see Figure 10-4). Comparatively, the mean score on the Index of the Promise of Science and Technology was 70 and the mean score on the Index of Reservations about Science and Technology was 38. Further, the two dimensions—or schema—concerning science and technology have a strong negative relationship of about −0.60, but the two dimensions—or emerging schema—for biotechnology have a small positive correlation of 0.09, meaning that they are almost independent of each other. This pattern suggests that a higher proportion of American adults have developed a stronger set of schema about science and technology generally than about the new and emerging subject of biotechnology. Overall, this result is fully consistent with our expectation that schema toward biotechnology would be less well developed than schema toward long-standing attitude objects such as science and technology.

Looking at bivariate tabulations expressed as bar charts, the level of reservation or concern about biotechnology is lower among better educated citizens, but so is the level of belief in the promise of biotechnology (see Figure 10-4). These patterns reflect the nature of new and emerging issues. A majority of adults who did not complete high school reported that they had not heard of biotechnology prior to the interview, and the mean scores for this group on both biotechnology schemas was higher than either high school or college graduates. Often, respondents who are not familiar with an issue agree to statements presented by an interviewer rather than say that they don't know. Because all of the items in both schemas score for agreement, a tendency to agree without understanding would inflate a respondent's score on both indices, or schemas. This is exactly the pattern observed in

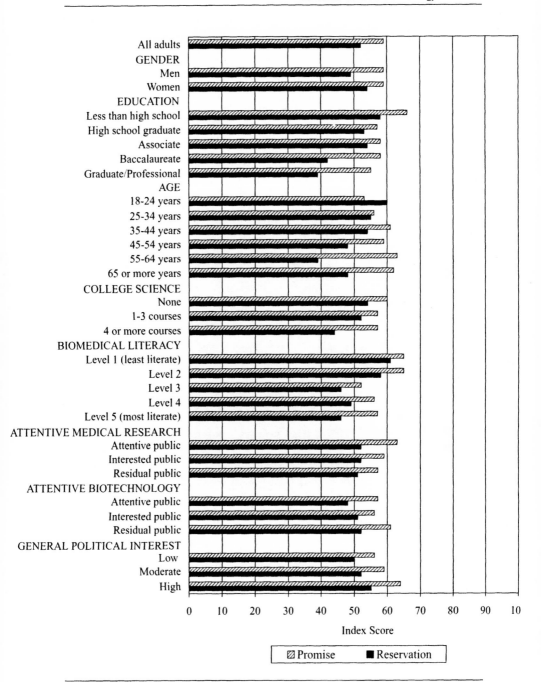

Figure 10-4 General attitudes (schemas) toward biotechnology, 1997–1998.

these data, indicating that there is a good deal of noise (or error) in both measures. Setting aside the high mean score for adults who did not complete high school, the remaining pattern is roughly consistent with the earlier findings in regard to belief in the promise of and reservations about science and technology—better educated adults have fewer reservations about biotechnology than less well educated adults, but the level of belief in the promise of biotechnology is similar for all adults who completed high school or college.

It is also interesting to note that belief in the promise of biotechnology is relatively low among the youngest cohort of adults—aged 18 through 25— and that the level of reservation is relatively high among this group. Because these young adults have a substantially greater likelihood of being exposed to modern biology as a part of their formal education, including college-level science courses, we would have expected a relatively lower level of reservation or concern. We will return to this issue in subsequent analyses.

Given the newer and less well-developed nature of schemas toward an emerging issue such as biotechnology, we would not expect these schemas to be as closely related to attitudes toward specific biotechnology applications as the schema about science and technology were related to specific science policy attitudes, but we would expect some level of linkage in this early stage of issue awareness.

ATTITUDES TOWARD MEDICAL AND AGRICULTURAL APPLICATIONS

The major problem involved in measuring attitudes toward specific applications of biotechnology is that relatively few of these applications are currently available to consumers, and thus there is little concrete recognition or experience with these products or uses. To probe the emergence of attitudes toward actual or potential applications of biotechnology, surveys in the United States and 17 European countries asked individuals to think about five specific applications and to make judgments about the usefulness of each application, any risks associated with the application, the moral acceptability of the application, and whether or not the application should be encouraged. The questions were framed to provide a brief explanation of each application, but even the language used in the descriptions required some familiarity with some scientific concepts. In the U.S. study, each respondent was also asked later in the interview to make a summary judgment about the application of biotechnology for medical purposes and for agricultural purposes.

To provide a summary measure of the acceptability of biotechnology for medical purposes, a scale was constructed, using the following four items:

1. Have you heard of using biotechnology to introduce human genes into bacteria to produce medicines and vaccines, for example, the production of insulin for people with diabetes? [Questions about the usefulness, risk, and moral acceptability of this application followed.] All in all, using biotechnology to introduce human genes into bacteria to produce medicines and vaccines should be encouraged. Do you definitely agree, tend to agree, tend to disagree, or definitely disagree?

2. Have you heard of using biotechnology to introduce human genes into animals to produce organs for human transplants, such as pigs for human hearts? [Questions about the usefulness, risk, and moral acceptability of this application followed.] All in all, using biotechnology to introduce human genes into animals to produce organs for human transplants should be encouraged. Do you definitely agree, tend to agree, tend to disagree, or definitely disagree?

3. Have you heard of using genetic testing to determine whether an unborn child has a genetic predisposition to a serious illness such as cystic fibrosis? [Questions about the usefulness, risk, and moral acceptability of this application followed.] All in all, using genetic testing to determine whether an unborn child has a predisposition to a serious disease should be encouraged. Do you definitely agree, tend to agree, tend to disagree, or definitely disagree?

4. Do you support or oppose the use of biotechnology to develop new medicines to treat human disease?

These four items formed a single dimension, and the responses were converted into a zero to 100 scale, using the same procedures described previously.

To provide a summary measure of the acceptability of biotechnology for agricultural purposes, a scale was constructed, using the following three items:

1. Have you heard of using modern biotechnology in the production of food and drinks, for example, to make them higher in protein, keep longer, or taste better? [Questions about the usefulness, risk, and moral acceptability of this application followed.] All in all, the use of modern biotechnology in the production of food and drinks should be encouraged. Do you definitely agree, tend to agree, tend to disagree, or definitely disagree?

2. Have you heard of using biotechnology to insert genes from one plant into a crop plant to make it more resistant to insect pests? [Questions about the usefulness, risk, and moral acceptability of this application fol-

lowed.] All in all, using biotechnology to insert genes from one plant into a crop plant should be encouraged. Do you definitely agree, tend to agree, tend to disagree, or definitely disagree?

3. Do you support or oppose the use of biotechnology in agriculture and food production?

These three items formed a single dimension, and the responses were converted into a zero to 100 scale, using the same procedures described previously.

Using these scales, American adults display a high level of acceptance and support for both medical and agricultural applications of biotechnology. The mean score on the Index of Support for Medical Applications was 72 and the mean score on the Index of Support for Agricultural Applications was 64 (see Figure 10-5). These results are consistent with two decades of empirical research documenting the broad acceptance of science and technology among American adults, even for new and emerging issues where the depth of prior information and understanding is measurably lower. Without elevating this finding to a general rule, it appears that most American adults tend to be predisposed to accept new scientific and technological developments and to hold positive expectations about the benefits of new science and technology.

The bivariate distribution of positive attitudes toward the use of biotechnology for medical and agricultural uses demonstrates the pervasive nature of this general attitude. No segment of the adult population scored below 68 on the Index of Support for Medical Applications, and only one group—the least biomedically literate—scored below 60 on the Index of Support for Agricultural Applications. Among Americans with the highest levels of formal education and the greatest exposure to college science courses, there was no difference in the level of support for medical and agricultural applications of biotechnology.

Some Models to Predict Attitudes toward Medical and Agricultural Applications

To determine the relative influence of selected variables on attitudes toward the use of biotechnology for medical and agricultural purposes, a path model was constructed and analyzed. Building on the model used to predict attentiveness to biotechnology policy (see Figure 10-2), the two biotechnology schemas (promise and reservation) were added to the model after attentiveness to biotechnology policy, and then the two measures of attitude toward medical applications and agricultural applications were added to the right side of the model, as the outcomes to be predicted (see Figure 10-6).

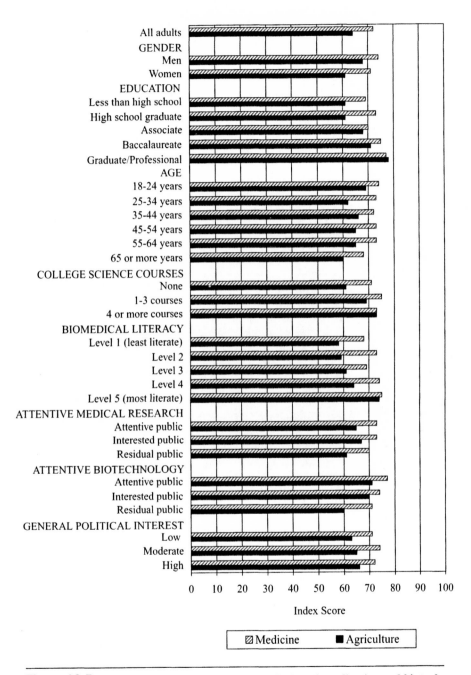

Figure 10-5 Attitudes toward medical and agricultural applications of biotechnology, 1997–1998.

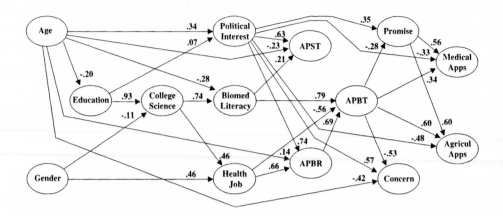

Figure 10-6 A path model to predict attitudes toward medical and agricultural biotechnology applications, 1997–1998.

Predictions and estimates were obtained separately for medical and agricultural applications, using a common metric.

The model to predict attitude toward medical applications explained 31 percent of the total variance, but it is important to recognize that the pervasive patterns of support described above produces relatively little variance. In contrast, there are larger differences in the level of support for agricultural applications, and the model to predict attitude toward agricultural applications accounted for 46 percent of the variance. Although the pervasive character of these attitudes makes prediction somewhat more difficult, the resulting models still provide useful insights into the development of attitudes toward new and emerging subjects such as biotechnology.

Looking first at the prediction of attitude toward the use of biotechnology for medical purposes, belief in the promise of biotechnology was the strongest single predictor with a total effect of .56 (see Figure 10-7). Attentiveness to biotechnology and attentiveness to biomedical research had modest positive effects (.18 and .15, respectively) on attitude toward the medical use of biotechnology. Educational experiences and biomedical literacy had relatively small effects on attitude toward medical use. Holding constant all of the other variables in the model, age had a very small—but statistically significant—negative effect (−.06) on attitude toward the use of biotechnology for medical purposes. It is important to note that the level of general reservation about biotechnology (the schema) was not related to attitude toward medical applications of biotechnology.

Looking at the model to predict attitude toward the use of biotechnology for agricultural purposes, belief in the promise of biotechnology is the

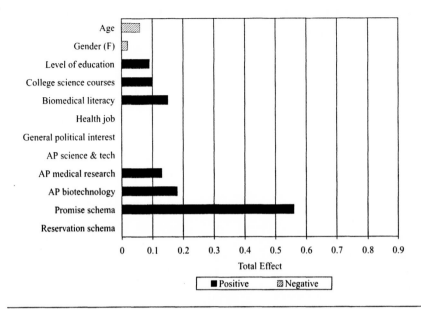

Figure 10-7 Total effect of selected variables on attitude toward medical applications of biotechnology, 1997–1998.

strongest single predictor, with a total effect of .60 (see Figure 10-8). Attentiveness to biotechnology and attentiveness to biomedical research had moderately strong effects (.43 and .30, respectively), and both of these effects are stronger than the comparable relationships to the medical applications of biotechnology. Biomedical literacy (.34), college science courses (.23), and educational attainment (.21) were all positively related to support for agricultural applications of biotechnology. Younger adults were slightly less supportive of the use of biotechnology in agricultural (−.11), holding all other variables in the model constant, and this was a slightly more negative relationship than the comparable effect on attitude toward medical applications. Again, the level of general reservation about biotechnology was not related to support or opposition to the use of biotechnology for agricultural purposes, holding constant all of the other variables in the model.

The combination of the two models indicate that it is the American optimism toward science and technology—the belief in the promise of beneficial results—that produces an initial positive disposition toward a new technology such as biotechnology. Those adults who have become aware of the subject and have started to follow it in the news tend to be more positive about both medical and agricultural applications of biotechnology than citizens who are not attentive to the issue. The models also suggest that prior

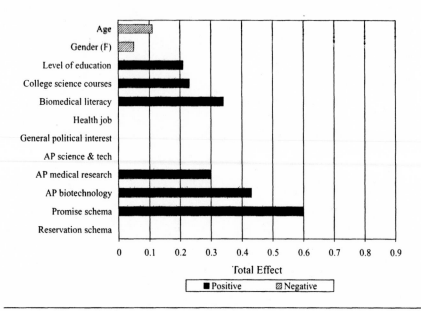

Figure 10-8 Total effect of selected variables on attitude toward agricultural applications of biotechnology, 1997–1998.

interest in biomedical research is strongly related to the development of attentiveness to biotechnology issues, and that it is this linkage to potential health and medical benefits that underlies public awareness and support for biotechnology in the United States.

IMPLICATIONS FOR BIOMEDICAL COMMUNICATORS

These findings have clear and important implications for biomedical communications, especially when viewed in the context of the preceding chapters that looked at the development of biomedical literacy, issue attentiveness, schema, and specific policy attitudes.

First, this analysis demonstrates that new subjects such as biotechnology do not enter the public policy arena independently, but draw initial interest from individuals already attentive to substantively adjacent issues. Our analyses found, for example, that prior attentiveness to biomedical research was strongly related to the development of attentiveness to biotechnology, but that prior attentiveness to science and technology policy was not related to attentiveness to biotechnology. By understanding these linkages, it is possible to target initial communications to those groups most likely to receive and use the information. This approach might be criticized as helping the best informed become even better informed, but, depending on the level of resources available, it may be the most effective way to expand the number of informed citizens within the near term. Given the diversity of issue interests in a complex industrial society, growing the information base from those individuals who already have some level of interest and literacy is not undemocratic.

Second, the development of attentiveness to biotechnology policy appears to involve a combination of prior attentiveness to biomedical research issues, biomedical literacy and formal education, and a general interest in political issues. The linkage between a prior interest in biomedical issues and biotechnology is a reflection of the adjacent issue process. The role of biomedical literacy is more interesting, suggesting that a strong command of basic concepts such as DNA, molecule, probability, antibiotics, and immunity make it easier for an individual to read and understand new information and to incorporate it into his or her schemas for biotechnology. Because a good deal of the initial public discussion of biotechnology has involved some aspects of public policy—the promises of new medical treatments, the possible misuse of human subjects in clinical gene therapy tests, the issues of privacy and insurability, and the competition to complete the first draft of the map of the human genome—it is not surprising that those adults who regularly follow public policy issues generally would be among the first to learn about and become attentive to biotechnology policy issues. This result is fully consistent with the relevant political science literature and with our general understanding of the processes of communication and attitude formation.

Third, the development of schemas about biotechnology appear to follow the general pattern found earlier for science and technology policy issues. A two-dimensional structure was found, with dimensions that appear to represent belief in the promise of biotechnology and concern or reservation about the consequences of biotechnology. As expected, the structure of these general schema, or predispositions, appears to be less well formed for many adults than similar schema pertaining to longer-standing issue areas. For those adults who had not heard of biotechnology prior to the interview or who had only a minimal recall of it, we would not expect separate biotechnology schemas at all, and the results suggest that this is the case for many of the respondents at all educational levels, but especially among those adults who had not completed high school. As discussion of biotechnology continues and expands in the media and among adults generally, we would expect that most American adults would eventually develop schemas about biotechnology. Comparatively, the level of public awareness and understanding of computers in 1970 was minimal, but 30 years later a majority of

American households have a home computer and the idea of dot-com industries has become a part of our language.

Fourth, Americans hold generally positive attitudes toward the use of biotechnology for both medical and agricultural purposes. To some degree, this is a preliminary judgment based on the pervasive American belief in the promise of science and technology and on the absence of any evidence that biotechnology poses a threat to human health or welfare. The glowing endorsement by virtually every major political leader in the United States of the completion of the first map of the human genome and the promise of eminent medical applications will undoubtedly solidify and expand the public predisposition toward biotechnology. Barring a Three-Mile-Island type of genomic event, communicators may assume that this generally positive attitude toward biotechnology will continue, but should recognize that most adults in the United States have had limited exposure to specific products and applications. The point is that there is no need to expect or anticipate hostility in the United States (as one might do in Europe), but, given the emerging awareness and understanding of biotechnology, it is important to continue to seek to provide full information and extensive explanation in regard to both products and policies.

chapter

11

· · · · · · · · ·

STRATEGIES FOR
COMMUNICATING ABOUT
BIOMEDICAL POLICY

· · · · · · · · · · · · · · · · ·

The chapters in Part III have analyzed communications to the public about biomedical policy issues. In contrast to the informational objectives of communications to consumers, virtually all communications to the public concerning public policy are designed to influence the recipients to adopt a specific point of view or to take a specific action to increase the likelihood of a desired policy outcome. This distinction is central to our analysis and to the recommendations included at the end of this chapter and in Chapter 12.

The distinction between communications to consumers and communications to the public to influence public policy is often blurred because they often originate from the same organizations. For example, an organization such as the American Cancer Society (ACS) engages in a significant continuing campaign to educate consumers about the early warning signs of cancer and the best methods for early detection. This is clearly a program to communicate information to consumers. The same organization, however, also seeks to influence citizens and public officials to increase federal appropriations for cancer research each year, and these communications are clearly designed to influence public policy. Without commenting on the communications programs of the ACS (which we have not studied in detail), the logic of our argument is that an effective communications program would recognize the differences in the target audiences for these messages, and seek to channel the messages accordingly. The difference between these two kinds of messages is further clouded because the biomedical community has been so successful in generating broad public support of biomedical research spending that no elected legislator who wishes to seek another term would seriously oppose appropriations for this purpose, thus reducing the necessity for major persuasive campaigns on the spending issue.

We will return to this differentiation in the conclusion of this chapter when we discuss broader strategic issues, but it is important to keep this distinction in mind when thinking about the points raised in this chapter.

THE STRUCTURE OF BIOMEDICAL POLICY COMMUNICATIONS

As first noted in Chapter 7, biomedical policy communications need to function at two levels. One level must focus on biomedical policy leaders and other science and health policy leaders. The other level needs to focus on the public, but particularly the attentive public for biomedical research and, in some cases, other relevant attentive publics. We will look at each of these major components of biomedical policy communications separately, then seek to integrate them into a final discussion of strategies.

Communications to Policy Leaders

In our discussion of the formulation of biomedical policy in Chapter 7, we indicated that most biomedical policy is formulated through negotiations between nongovernmental policy leaders and legislative and executive branch policy makers. This result is inevitable in complex political systems, since vigorous disputes over a large number of biomedical policy issues every year would exhaust the public, the policy leaders, and the policy makers alike. This is not an inherently undemocratic process, but rather it is a reflection of the relatively high degree of consensus among major interest groups and policy makers on biomedical policy. When there is a genuinely important dispute among policy leaders or between policy leaders and policy makers, leaders and groups of leaders will seek to enlist the support of citizens who share their concerns in persuading the policy makers to adopt the policy that they prefer. Some examples may be useful.

By the end of the twentieth century, there was a high level of consensus among policy makers and biomedical interest groups—patient groups, disease groups, educators, researchers, practitioners, insurers, and pharmaceutical companies—that it is important to make a major national investment in biomedical research. The leadership of both political parties have endorsed the idea that the budget of the National Institutes of Health (NIH) should double over a 5-year period. In the context of making budget decisions for the fiscal 2001 budget, both President Clinton and the Republican-led House of Representatives agreed on a budget increase of slightly over $1 billion, but this was short of the rate of increase needed to completely double the NIH budget in 5 years. In the context of this general consensus, it is unlikely that policy leaders and their respective groups will seek to defeat a particular legislator because he or she was unwilling to support a higher NIH appropriation, or that voters would be particularly incensed over the issue of the size of the NIH increase for 2001. Undoubtedly, this disagreement will be negotiated among policy leaders and decision makers in private settings.

In contrast, the 1999 decision of the NIH to reinterpret a federal statute concerning the use of fetal materials in research to allow the limited use of human stem cells in biomedical research provoked deep disagreements in the Congress and among interest groups. Pro-life groups generally reacted negatively to the decision, seeing it as the first step toward the repeal of legislation that they had obtained in previous years. Specific interest groups with a strong commitment to stem cell research—the juvenile diabetes groups, the Alzheimer's and Parkinson's disease groups, and basic biomedical researchers—had been active in promoting the NIH decision and were strongly supportive of it. Religious groups, university groups, and other interest groups not normally involved in biomedical policy matters were alerted to the issue and many became active in the dispute. Given the level and intensity of this dispute, there was little chance that the contending forces would be able to sit down and compromise on the issue. And, given the specialized nature of the issue, there was little chance that it would become a significant stand-alone electoral issue. Undoubtedly, there will be attempts to amend various bills—including appropriations bills—to reverse the NIH decision, and the leaders of the contending forces will appeal to their attentive publics to pressure legislators to support their amendments.

Communications to the Public
on Biomedical Policy Issues

Biomedical policy communications to the public—or to selected segments of the public—may be described in terms of purpose, target audiences, level, intermediaries, and strategies. A systematic comparison of consumer and policy communications in these terms may clarify the differences in these two kinds of communications (see Table 11-1).

The scope of biomedical communications to influence public policy is focused, purposive, and sometimes partisan. As noted above, biomedical poli-

Table 11-1 A Comparison of Consumer Communications and Policy Communications

	Consumer communications	Policy communications
Purpose	To increase the information held by consumers concerning health, including an understanding of diet, disease, early warning signs, sources of medical assistance, and the implications of various choices on future health.	To increase the information about specific policy issues for the purpose of persuading the recipient to hold certain views and take appropriate actions to increase the likelihood of the adoption of those policies within the political system.
Target audiences	Broad, inclusive, and nonpartisan.	Focused, purposive, and sometimes partisan.
Levels of communication	All levels of communication are needed, from the least literate adolescent and adult to the best educated and best informed consumers; multiple messages are needed at various levels of substantive complexity.	Because most biomedical policy is determined outside the electoral process, most communications will be more sophisticated. It is often important to link with other policy interests and messages.
Intermediaries	Media, acquaintances, physicians and other providers, interest groups (especially disease-oriented groups), World Wide Web (WWW).	Media (especially print), interest groups (including unions, sector groups, employers groups, and senior citizen groups), policy leaders, and WWW.
Strategies	Clear comprehensible messages at levels appropriate to consumers in media and through organizations, designed to promote awareness of lifestyle decisions; early warning signs; and local resources for diagnosis, advice, and services.	Focused communications designed to sustain issue interest, strengthen attitude positions, and stimulate actions to influence public policy.

cy issues are rarely decided through elections, and biomedical policy is most often formulated through the legislative process, with substantial policy debate and recommendations from the executive branch. Although many interest groups seek to keep their members and respective attentive publics fully informed about pending issues and negotiations, it is only when this process breaks down or is unable to arrive at an acceptable solution that policy leaders and interest groups begin major communications programs to inform and mobilize their members and their respective attentive publics to overt action on an issue. Since major communications campaigns require time, staff, and resources, the launch of a major mobilization effort is not undertaken lightly by most groups.

Biomedical policy communications are directed primarily to the members of the relevant attentive public or publics, and tend to be more sophisticated in language and content than many biomedical information messages focused on consumers. Although differences in personal and educational background among the members of specific attentive publics will define the range of information and complexity that a message or campaign might include, the general focus of these messages will be on somewhat better educated and more politically alert citizens. Although the idea that one message will serve all policy communications needs is also wrong, the range of message sophistication for policy purposes will undoubtedly be narrower than the range for consumer biomedical communications.

As noted earlier, various theories of communications have recognized that information does not always—or even normally—flow directly from the communicator to the recipient without interpretation, explanation, or reformulation by various intermediaries, and this is as true for policy communications as for consumer communications. The individuals and groups that serve as intermediaries or interpreters for policy communications are markedly different from the intermediaries and interpreters for consumer communications. Individuals who follow politics generally and who are attentive to one or more public policy arenas tend to have more developed political and ideological schemas than other less politically aware adults, and they are more likely to try to integrate new biomedical policy information into existing schemas about science, technology, ecology, and economics than adults who are not attentive to issues related to health, medicine, or science. Further, many of the individuals targeted for biomedical policy messages will be members of interest groups—professional societies, unions, chambers of commerce, and community organizations—that have professional staff that monitor these issues and write periodic reports to members through newsletters, magazines, Web sites, and special reports. Finally, it is likely that most individuals who are attentive to an issue such as biomedical policy already know, work with, and periodically encounter other adults with similar issue interests and concerns, and these linkages provide important opportunities for testing and reconfirming ideas about and interpretations of these issues.

The ultimate objective of biomedical policy communications is to increase the recipient's level of understanding of an issue and, often, to encourage the individual to take some form of overt political action to improve the likelihood that a particular policy outcome will be obtained. Many of the policy leaders and interest groups that may be involved in biomedical policy communications have a continuing and longer term perspective on these issues, recognizing that there will be additional contested issues in future months and years. In this context, biomedical policy communications often seek to build a strong base of well-informed and politically savvy members or supporters who become a "reserve army" for policy battles in the future. It is important, of course, to produce effective short-term pressure on policy makers to obtain favorable policy outcomes in the short term, but it is also essential to not alienate these friends, members, or citizens who are attentive to biomedical policy issues.

A GENERAL MODEL OF BIOMEDICAL POLICY COMMUNICATIONS

In Chapter 6, we introduced a general model of biomedical communications to consumers as a means of integrating several strands of thought and analysis that emerged from our various empirical examinations of actual consumer information acquisition, retention, and use. Although there are significant differences between biomedical communications directed to consumers and communications designed to influence biotechnology policy, the general structure of these communications has a number of similarities. To understand both the differences between and the commonalities among these two kinds of biomedical communications, we now introduce a general model of biomedical policy communications. The schematic presented in Figure 11-1 may be helpful as a point of reference, and the previous schematic in Figure 6-1 may be useful in comparing the functioning of these two general models.

The Pathways of News and Information

New information about biomedical policy most often emanates from biomedical policy leaders, biomedical organizations, or policy makers with responsibility for biomedical matters. Contrary to the ideals of pure democracy, new biomedical policy ideas rarely begin at the grassroots level and grow

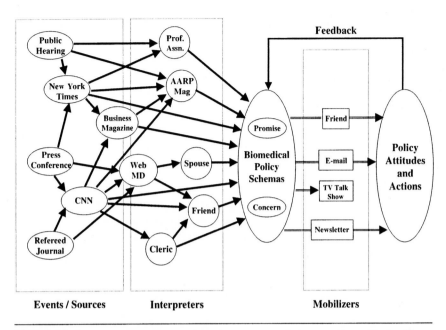

Figure 11-1 A general model of communications to Influence biomedical policy.

to become national agenda issues. Biomedical policy information is usually circulated among policy leaders and policy makers first, as a part of the ongoing discussion and negotiation processes that often result in public policy. Frequently, this information first reaches the arena of communication through organizational newsletters and magazines, conferences and symposia, and organizational Web sites. Eventually, new information relevant to biomedical policy issues may be used in testimony at a congressional hearing, released in a special report by an organization, or presented to the media in a press conference conducted by the organization. For biomedical policy issues that remain on the agenda for some period of time, analytic and discussion articles may appear in popular magazines or refereed journals. Working journalists talk with policy and organizational leaders and may attend events, briefings, and activities sponsored by organizations and groups interested in biomedical policy issues. Occasionally, news coverage of these original events is picked up by wire services and news services and published in daily newspapers such as the *New York Times* and similar upscale papers, but the relatively technical and specialized nature of many biomedical policy matters largely precludes their appearance in regular television newscasts and similar outlets for broad audiences. Biomedical policy information, however, is ideal for distribution from Web-based sites and in subscribed electronic newsletters.

The number of pathways from the release of a new piece of biomedical policy information to policy leaders and to citizens attentive to biomedical policy is complex, and will undoubtedly become more complex with the expansion of electronic information distribution systems. Although the number of biomedical policy leaders is approximately 5000 and only one in five adults can be classified as attentive to biomedical policy issues, the process of interpretation by intermediaries is structurally the same as in the communication of health and biomedical information to consumers. Building on Katz and Lazarsfeld's ideas of intermediaries and interpreters (Katz and Lazarsfeld, 1955; Katz, 1980; Klapper, 1960; Heath and Bryant, 2000), our general model of biomedical policy communications illustrates the important role played by these intermediaries (see Figure 11-1).

The general model shown in Figure 11-1 provides several examples of the movement of biomedical policy news and information from its point of origin inside the biomedical policy leadership community to the wider arena of attentive publics and other interested citizens. Consider the example of the White House press conference featuring Francis Collins and Craig Venter making the announcement of the completion of the first draft of the map of the human genome. The press conference was carried live on Cable News Network (CNN) and was covered by virtually all of the major newspapers, television networks, and news services. Our schematic shows the flow of information from the press conference to the *New York Times* and to CNN (symbols of print and television news coverage). Hypothetically, a feature writer for *Forbes* listens to CNN and reads the *New York Times* and writes a piece discussing the implications of this research for the pharmaceutical industry, which is published in the next issue. The health news editor of Web-MD (symbolic of health and medical Web sites) watches the press conference over CNN, reads the *New York Times* report on the electronic edition, and checks for comparable information from other Web sites and news services, then posts a news summary on the WebMD site. A day later, a feature on the human genome is added to the WebMD site. A writer for CNN draws on material from a recent issue of the *Journal of the American Medical Association* (JAMA) in the production of a feature piece on the medical applications of genomic research, which is used in a newscast on CNN and posted to the CNN Web site. An editor for *Modern Maturity,* a monthly magazine published by the American Association of Retired Persons (AARP), sees a news report on CNN, reads the human genome story in the *New York Times,* attends a congressional hearing on the issue, and reads an article in *Fortune* about the medical implications of this research. She decides to do a feature piece for *Modern Maturity,* which is published in the next available issue. The number of pathways for the distribution of this information is large, but the point is that the flow of information today is a complex multistep, multi-media process. And, it is likely that the complexity of this process will increase in the decades ahead.

Information Processing at the Individual Level

The point of policy-oriented biomedical communications is to reach and inform other biomedical leaders and citizens who are attentive to biomedical policy issues, or substantively adjacent issues. It is important that these individuals know about pending legislative and executive branch issues related to biomedical policy and understand enough about the science associated with those issues to be able to communicate effectively with policy makers, including the ability to answer questions about the science underlying the issue and the implications of the public policy choice that the attentive citizen may be advocating.

Although we may think of consumers as being exposed to a large volume of health-related information, it is more appropriate to think of policy-oriented citizens who are attentive to biomedical policy as being aware of and able to access large volumes of relevant information. For these citizens, a news item about a new federal rule on the use of stem cells in biomedical research may stimulate a decision to pick up the Tuesday *New York Times'* Science Times or to visit some relevant Web sites to obtain additional information. Having read some of the relevant information on this issue, a citizen who is attentive to biomedical issues might then seek the thoughts of friends or co-workers who he or she thinks of as being knowledgeable about this issue. Over the next several weeks following the announcement of a new federal rule about the use of stem cells in research, an attentive citizen may acquire an extensive set of policy relevant information on this issue and become ready to enter into the dispute by writing a legislator or contributing some funds to an interest group active on the issue.

There are useful psychological models of this process of information acquisition and retention. The concept of a schema[1] is most helpful in thinking about biomedical communications for policy purposes and about the retention and organization of policy-related information by citizens attentive to biomedical policy issues.

For the policy-oriented citizen, a schema serves to filter, process, and integrate new information and experiences into existing organizational structures, but it is likely to be more extensively developed and richer in prior

---

[1]We outlined our argument for the utility of the schema concept for consumers in Chapter 6 and will not repeat our discussion of the concept of a schema or its general functions. Readers who skipped Chapter 6 may wish to examine that discussion prior to continuing with the following discussion.

knowledge and detail than the personal health schemas of many consumers. As demonstrated in the preceding chapters, many citizens who are attentive to biomedical policy have a higher level of biomedical literacy and more experience with biomedical issues than other citizens, and this sophistication of knowledge and experience is reflected in the scope and complexity of their schemas. Indeed, it is just this set of integrated information about a subject area such as biomedical policy that marks some individuals as influentials or intermediaries in the Katz and Lazarsfeld (1955) sense, often leading their friends, co-workers, and family to look to them for information and advice on biomedical matters.

Whereas the scope and quality of personal health schemas may vary significantly over the course of the life cycle and by religious or philosophical views, it is likely that the biomedical policy schemas are linked to, if not fully integrated into, an individual's more general schema concerning the political, social, and economic structure of society. Some individuals may see the economic and social stratification of American society in justice or equity terms and favor biomedical policies to redress or minimize these differentials, assuring that all individuals receive the benefits of new medicines and technologies without regard to resources or status. Other adults may believe that differences in social and economic resources are the result of personal effort and abilities and see solutions in generational terms. Some citizens who are attentive to biomedical policy may frame the issues in partisan terms, whereas other attentive citizens may not see the policy choices in partisan terms at all. The range of possible linkages and integrations is as wide as the range of social, economic, and political schemas active in American society.

In the schematic model in Figure 11-1, an individual's biomedical policy schema, or schemas, is represented as a large oval that receives information from news and information sources (sometimes modified by intermediaries and interpreters) and processes it. Some incoming information may be filtered out quickly, while other information is evaluated in terms of prior knowledge and experiences and either retained or discarded, depending on the recipient's assessment of the accuracy, trustworthiness, and utility of the information. As noted earlier, we expect that citizens who are attentive to biomedical policy issues will have larger and more developed schemas than individuals who do not follow health and medical issues at a policy level.

Several studies of public perceptions of science and technology have found that many individuals—and especially citizens attentive to those issues—tend to use two separate, but related, schemas representing the promise of science and technology and reservations about possible harms or dangers from science and technology (see Chapter 9). We saw in Chapter 10 that many Americans who have heard and thought about biotechnology hold separate schemas about this technology that might be characterized as promise and reservation. In our schematic presentation of a general model of biomedical policy communications, we have presented this schema as a large oval, with smaller ovals for promise and reservation imbedded in it. A precise description of the formation and structure of individual schemas toward biomedical policy will require more research, but it is sufficient to recognize at this point that the organization and complexity of policy schemas differ among individuals and that communication efforts and programs need to take this variation into account.

A separate oval is used to represent actual biomedical policy activities or interventions by the individual. These overt actions or behaviors might include communicating a policy view to a member of Congress or an executive branch officer, signing a petition, sending a contribution to an interest group or a political action committee, writing a persuasive article on a biomedical policy issue for publication, or speaking to friends and family about the issue. Although all of these actions and behaviors are generic to a wide array of policy areas, it is the content and purpose of these communications that make them relevant to the formulation of biomedical policy. A letter to a policy maker arguing for the encouragement of stem cell research, for example, is an overt activity designed to influence public policy by persuading a policy maker to support a particular policy or action—vote for a pending bill or issue a favorable regulation or ruling. A letter asking a legislator to expedite the processing of Aunt Martha's Medicare claim is a personal matter, not an effort to influence public policy.

The growth of electronic communications is making the direct participation in the policy formulation process easier for those citizens attentive to an issue and concerned about a particular policy or issue. Traditionally, interest groups have used a combination of magazine articles, newsletters, and direct mail appeals to mobilize individuals to take an overt action to communicate their view to a policy maker. Rosenau (1974) studied this process carefully in regard to a public policy dispute over the ratification of the nuclear testing treaty and concluded that the process of mobilization is difficult and poorly understood by interest group leaders. Prior to the growth of e-mail, communication of one's views to a policy maker required writing (or typing) a letter to the targeted official, getting the title and address correct, and then posting and mailing the message. Petition drives required less effort, but were generally thought to be less effective in persuading policy makers. The growing access to e-mail and the comfort of individuals in using it is beginning to change the policy communication process. An e-mail does not require letterhead stationery, can be typed and spell-checked on a computer, and the same message can be sent to numerous policy makers with minimal effort. The growth of policy-related listservs is one indicator of the greater efficiency of this form of communication. We need to initiate studies to assess the impact of this kind of communication on the policy formulation process.

THE ROLE OF INTERMEDIARIES AND INTERPRETERS

The role of intermediaries and interpreters in consumer communications discussed in Chapter 6 also applies to transmission of biomedical policy information, but with some important substantive differences (see Table 11-1 and Figure 11-1). Following Katz and Lazarsfeld's (1955) general concept that news and information do not flow from a central point, such as a television tower or a newspaper, directly to recipients, but rather that they are often discussed with other adults and compared with previous information and experience. This process is particularly relevant and important for citizens who are attentive to a policy area such as biomedical policy, and it is important to understand some of the aspects of this process that are most relevant for policy-oriented communications.

First, citizens who are attentive to biomedical policy are more likely to rely on print media than broadcast media in assessing the veracity and importance of new information. Television news may provide an early alert of emerging new information relevant to an issue to which a citizen is attentive, but previous studies have found that attentive citizens then turn to print sources for more in-depth information and for confirmation (Miller, 1987b). It is not yet clear how Web-based information will be treated by adults attentive to biomedical policy, but we expect that these policy savvy citizens will make the same kinds of distinctions among Web sources that they make among print sources—trusting some and not trusting others.

Second, citizens attentive to biomedical policy and other issue areas will be more likely to accept and seek policy-related information from organizations and institutions that they already trust, and they will be less likely to turn to friends and family for advice or confirmation. In some work situations, an attentive citizen may seek advice or confirmation from a co-worker who is thought to be especially knowledgeable about a topic, but—on balance—organizations and institutions will be the most trusted and most often consulted sources of biomedical policy information. In some cases, the Web may be the media for obtaining the information, but it is the stature and standing of the institution that makes the Web site credible in the first place.

Third, many citizens who are attentive to a policy area will know the names and locations of policy leaders whose views they trust on any given issue, and it is likely that they will turn directly to one or more of those leaders by looking for newsletter discussions, reports, or Web site information from that source. For example, an attentive citizens reads a story in a magazine that asserts that the U.S. government is not doing enough research to understand the threat from previously unknown viruses, including the development of vaccines and other interventions. This citizen happens to be a high school biology teacher, and she wishes to determine how serious this threat might be. She first looks at the web page for the professional association of biology teachers, where she finds a number of links to the web pages of the American Society for Microbiology, the U.S. Centers for Disease Control and Prevention (CDC), and the international health program at the National Institutes of Health. She also goes to an on-line bookstore, searches for new titles dealing with viruses, and finds two new popular books that she has not seen previously. She orders one of the books, subsequently goes to her local public library to check out the other book, she uses the library's new electronic search facility to find recent articles in *Scientific American* and *Science News* about virus research. Although this sequence of events is hypothetical, it is consistent with the reported patterns of information acquisition and use from citizens attentive to a specific issue or area. We would not expect this individual to do this much reading or thinking about transportation policy or tax policy (unless she was attentive to one of those subjects), but this example illustrates the impact of issue specialization and the ability of an individual with a high level of interest in a subject and a reasonably developed set of schemas about it to access and utilize available resources to acquire more information from which to make a judgment about a particular issue.

Finally, the same individuals, publications, and organizations play an important role in motivating an individual to engage in an overt action or behavior designed to advance the particular policy preference. To continue the previous hypothetical example, if this biology teacher were to become convinced that viruses pose a major threat to the health and stability of the United States, she might contact her federal legislators by e-mail or by letter to convey her views on the issue. She might also feel that the matter is sufficiently important to talk to other teachers about it, to talk to her students about it, and to encourage friends to write letters on the subject. Or, she might decide to use the information to construct a new course module for her high school teaching and not make any policy relevant contacts about the issue. This decision about whether or not to make a contact to advocate a policy may flow from the individual's own knowledge base and biomedical policy schema(s), or it might be fostered by various persuasive messages from friends, the media, or other sources. The process of persuading an individual to take an overt action to influence a public policy is called mobilization, and Rosenau (1974) and others have argued that it is one of the most difficult parts of the communication process.

In the schematic shown in Figure 11-1, several examples of mobilizers are shown. For example, an individual who is attentive to biomedical issues and who is supportive of the use of stem cells in biomedical research may or may not overtly seek to influence pending federal legislation on this topic. One example of mobilization would be the encouragement of a friend or co-worker to sign a petition, write a letter to an undecided senator from their state, or send an e-mail to the entire state congressional delegation on a pending bill. If the friend discusses the messages that he sent, this kind of encouragement may be sufficient to convince our hypothetical citizen to take an overt action.

A second kind of mobilization might come from an e-mail contact. If our hypothetical supporter of stem cell research is on a listserv from an organization that he is affiliated with and he receives an e-mail from the organization saying that a critical committee vote will be held within the next 2 days and that it is important for him to contact Senator X by e-mail immediately, he may be moved to send the requested message. An important component of mobilization is to persuade the citizen that his or her action will make a difference, and this example illustrates how the Internet can be used to distribute appeals on a more timely basis and to generate a sense of urgency that may not be conveyed as convincingly by a traditional letter from an organization requesting support or contacting.

The third example is a television show—perhaps an interview show such as *Larry King Live* or *Meet the Press*—in which someone is interviewed about a pressing biomedical issue. In this case, we might presume that the Surgeon General is interviewed about the spread of the West Nile virus in the United States, and he describes a set of potentially serious outcomes. He also says that additional funds are needed for this work, but does not directly advocate writing a letter or sending a message directly to a congressman or senator. In this case, we show the arrow not connecting to an overt action, indicating that the message was heard but that our hypothetical attentive citizen was not moved to take an action. This is, in fact, the modal case. The schematic shows three of the four possible mobilizing influences resulting in a contact, which is meant to suggest that any individual may experience more than one mobilizing agent on the same issue within the constrained period of time. The schematic is not meant to suggest that three out of four mobilization attempts succeed. Although we have virtually no evidence about the mobilization rate on biomedical policy issues, the existing evidence on mobilization on other issues suggests that the successful mobilization rate is much lower.

The fourth example involves the use of a newsletter from an organization or group that an individual is associated with. It might be a newsletter from a professional organization, an employee retirement fund, or a religious organization. Prior to the growth of the internet, newsletters were a major vehicle for increasing issue awareness among members and for encouraging members to engage in various forms of policy-related contacting. Because only half of the attentive public for biomedical issues reported having e-mail or Web access in our 1999 study, we include this example to remind communicators that newsletters will continue to be a standard way of communicating to members for some years to come. In this example, we show that the newsletter was successful in motivating the individual to make a contact, but we believe that it is imperative that more research be done on the question of the relative efficacy of alternative methods of mobilization on biomedical issues.

Finally, it is essential to note the feedback loop included in the schematic in Figure 11-1. Policy communications are virtually never a onetime shot. Every organization is created to continue to represent an interest or constituency over some period of time, and to seek to influence policy more than once. The development of formal membership procedures, officers, offices, and other infrastructure all imply and demand a longer term view. In this context, each message and each attempt to mobilize an individual, produces some feedback about whether the experience was effective or a waste of time. Most citizens who are attentive to one or more issues tend to be careful with their time, and they are not likely to continue to respond to mobilization calls that are frustrating or produce no understandable results. We observe too many organizations that appear to operate on the principle that more is always better. They do not conserve their mobilization efforts, and, not surprisingly, many of these organizations experience low rates of success in mobilizing their members. Biomedical communicators need to be aware that most of their communication efforts produce some feedback in the schema structure of their audiences, and they need to think carefully about longer term cumulative effects as well as short-term objectives.

The Impact of New Information Technologies on Policy Communications

Throughout the preceding analysis, references have been made to the revolution in information technologies and the likely influence of these new technologies on biomedical communications. At this point, it may be helpful to discuss—briefly—the implications of new information technologies on policy-oriented communications.

Given the general experience of attentive citizens in accessing, evaluating, storing, and recalling information, the emergence of new information technologies will change primarily the speed of information access and the speed and ease of contacting. There may be some expansion of the scope of information sources as these citizens gain more experience with internet technologies and discover new information sources and databases not readily available in print form. As relatively inexpensive higher quality color printers become a standard fixture in upscale homes, it is likely that some newspapers and magazines currently read in print form will be read or searched in electronic form, with articles of interest then printed for subsequent reading or for retention.

The major change emanating from new information technologies may be faster and improved communications between interest groups and their members, or among the members of an interest group. With the rapid growth of e-mail access and listserv technologies during the last decade, millions of Americans now receive periodic—daily in some cases—updates from groups and organizations on selected matters or issues. Education associations can distribute information to college and university presidents, school superintendents, and selected administrators and faculty in hours, alerting members of pending legislative or executive branch actions and urging an immediate intervention on the part of the member. Trade and industry groups have similar rapid access to their members, and many larger corporations have equally fast means of communicating to their distributors and customers. Many major biomedical policy associations and groups operate a membership listserv or post breaking information on their Web site. The power of this new technology is just being discovered by many groups and will undoubtedly grow in the years ahead.

As suggested above, new information technologies are expanding the opportunities for direct communications to policy makers. We have seen some examples of the extensive use of e-mail communications, but it is still unclear as to how legislators are handling and evaluating these inputs. Some federal agencies have initiated on-line opportunities for citizen comment on pending regulations, but are still seeking processes to integrate these comments into the policy formulation process. A recent experiment by the U.S. Department of Agriculture produced approximately 400,000 e-mail comments on pending regulations about the definition of organic foods. Apparently shocked by the volume of responses, funding has been provided to a university grantee to develop software to scan and categorize the contents of the responses. It is clear that we are just beginning to explore the methodologies and the consequences of easier communications from attentive citizens to policy makers, and it is important that communicators seek to understand this process as it develops in the years ahead.

NINE QUESTIONS TO GUIDE COMMUNICATIONS FOR POLICY PURPOSES

The general model of biomedical communications for policy purposes outlined in the preceding sections of this chapter has important implications for the design, delivery, and assessment of communications to attentive and potentially attentive citizens. As observed in regard to biomedical communications to consumers, one useful approach is to frame these implications in the form of a set of questions that might serve as checkpoints or reminders for biomedical policy communicators.

- **What information do you want to communicate, and what actions (if any) do you want the recipient to take?**
Recognizing that many attentive citizens are experienced in information acquisition and evaluation, it is especially important to have a clear understanding of the information that you want to communicate, and an even more precise set of desired actions. It is not useful to urge attentive citizens to contact a legislator to encourage them to be more supportive of research on disease X without reference to a relevant piece of legislation. It is the responsibility of policy leaders to see that the desired legislation is introduced and that there is sufficient legislative interest to push for hearings, committee action, and floor consideration if there is a substantial public push for the legislation. Similarly, urging citizens to contact a congressman or senator to support increased appropriations for research on disease X without reference to the current levels of funding or without some legislative leadership is meaningless and may result in negative feedback experiences for the well-meaning attentive citizen who attempts this kind of contact.

- **Whom do you want to receive this message?**
The target audience for most biomedical policy messages will be the attentive public for biomedical policy issues, which we have defined and discussed in Chapter 7. In general, this is a small and reachable segment of the public. In some cases, it may be important to seek to engage other attentive publics such as senior citizen groups, women's interest groups, or patient and family support groups for a specific disease or condition. In other cases, it may be strategically useful to engage union members, corporate or trade group members, or insurance companies on a specific issue. Communications addressed to other attentive publics should be channeled through the policy leadership groups associated with those interests. It is unlikely that a biomedical policy communications campaign targeted to another attentive public will be successful if the policy leadership in that area is strongly opposed to the objectives of the communication.

- **What media or sources are likely to transmit the message to the targeted audience?**
As noted above, the attentive public for biomedical policy tends to consume a large volume of information from numerous sources. Traditionally, it has been relatively easy to identify a set of magazines that are read by a substantial portion of the attentive public for biomedical policy, and these vehicles have been especially effective because attentive citizens tend to use and trust print media more than broadcast media. Looking to the future, it is likely that citizens attentive to biomedical policy issues (as well as other major policy issues) will make progressively greater

use of electronic communication technologies, especially Web based or broadband delivered versions of trusted information sources such as the *New York Times* or organizational news messages. As with all communications, it is important to think carefully about alternative means for transmitting a message and to assess the reach and credibility of each potential channel for the intended attentive audience.

- **What is the likelihood that the targeted recipients will hear, read, or view the message?**
  Most adults attentive to a public policy area such as biomedical policy are active seekers of information. As noted previously, broadcast news and newspaper headlines may serve as an early alert system for new information, but most attentive citizens bring a well developed set of biomedical schema to the processing of new information and will tend to seek additional information beyond an initial headline or broadcast. Yet, even among attentive citizens, there is a skimming and filtering of information, and not all messages will be read or absorbed. In general, the rate of reading and retention among attentives will be relatively higher than that found among health information consumers generally, but the traditional message enhancements—location, presentation, brevity, conciseness, and utility—will all have some influence on the receipt of the message.

- **What is the likelihood that the targeted recipients of the message will accept (believe) the message and incorporate it into their biomedical policy schema(s)?**
  This is a complex question when applied to issue attentives. On the one hand, they tend to be more selective in accessing information and might be expected to be more trusting of the sources that they have selected. At the same time, the larger and more developed biomedical policy schemas held by biomedical policy attentives means that they bring a more sophisticated set of information and experiences to the evaluation of new information, effectively setting a higher standard for the acceptance, trust, and retention of new information. Biomedical policy attentives may dismiss a message because it is too simplistic and does not address important aspects of an issue that they already understand to some extent. Issue attentives will be more sensitive to the background and other interests of the information source.

- **What groups or intermediaries might improve the likelihood that a message is received, accepted, and incorporated into an individual's biomedical policy schema(s)?**
  As suggested previously, biomedical policy attentives tend to place greater trust in selected organizations and institutions, and these groups play an intermediary role in interpreting new information and suggest-

ing how it relates to previous policy discussions or disputes. In the model shown in Figure 11-1, our hypothetical attentive citizen receives biomedical policy information from her professional association, the AARP magazine, her spouse, a friend, CNN, and her priest. If all of this information is consistent, communication theory would predict a higher likelihood of acceptance and integration of the information into the individual's biomedical policy schema(s), but the degree of intermediary influence will be inverse to the strength and complexity of her existing biomedical schema(s). A biomedically literate attentive citizen with a strong commitment to stem cell research may note the reservations of her priest on this issue, but may not be moved from her previously developed position. In contrast, an attentive individual who has not followed a specific biomedical controversy—such as the use of stem cells in medical research—may still be collecting, evaluating, and assembling his or her views on the subject, and substantial agreement or disagreement among friends, family, and trusted organizations may exert relatively greater influence on the development of a policy view on this issue. Although it is difficult for information campaigns to utilize friends and family in interpreter or intermediary roles, it is possible to enlist various groups and organizations that might be effective in encouraging the acceptance of a policy-related message.

- **What is the likelihood that the targeted attentive citizens will take the desired actions?**
Mobilization—the conversion of attitudes and beliefs into actions and behaviors—is a critical step in the policy communication process, as discussed previously. Numerous political scientists have argued that most policy aware adults use a rough calculus to assess the level of effort required to influence a decision, the likelihood of success in the effort, and the personal and societal benefits that might be expected if the desired policy was adopted (Downs, 1957; Buchanan and Tullock, 1962). In this context, it is important to note that most biomedical policy issues are resolved through negotiations between biomedical policy leaders and policy makers, and that relatively few biomedical issues reach the point where there is a need to mobilize the attentive public to intervene in the policy formulation process. Some biomedical groups annually seek to rally their members to write to legislators to encourage higher appropriations for biomedical research generally or for specific research programs, but it is difficult to create a sense of urgency in the face of strong bipartisan support for biomedical research. It is likely that the current mobilization rate for most biomedical issues is relatively low, due primarily to the lack of meaningful experience in targeting legislators and executive-branch leaders. It is important, however, for biomedical com-

municators to recognize this problem and make realistic estimates of the likely rates of mobilization. It is equally important to study the factors that are associated with higher rates of mobilization on biomedical policy issues.

- **Which groups or intermediaries might improve the likelihood that the targeted recipients will take the desired action?**
  As noted several times previously, citizens attentive to biomedical policy tend to have higher levels of confidence in selected organizations and institutions—the NIH, the CDC, medical schools, and major disease associations—and these groups and organizations can play an important role in encouraging mobilization. Although government agencies such as the NIH and CDC are prohibited from urging congressional contacting on their own behalf, they can provide essential verification of information relevant to the decision to contact a legislator or policy maker. It is possible that the internet and other new information technologies will make the policy contacting process easier and allow greater individuality in the shaping of messages; however, we are just beginning to observe the growth of this practice and its net impact is still unclear.

- **How will you know how many members of the targeted audience hear the message, accepted or believed it, and took the desired action?**
  The good news is that it is not difficult to measure the effect of biomedical policy communications efforts, assuming that the messages seek to promote some form of policy contacting in support of a specific policy preference. The bad news is that almost no one does it.
  Most biomedical groups and organizations define one of their major policy objectives to be increased federal funding for biomedical research, especially for the diseases of special interest to the organization. Since the total level of biomedical spending by the federal government has grown steadily and substantially over the last four decades, numerous organizations and groups can point to this outcome as evidence of the success of their efforts. And many make this claim. Given the large number of organizations that are actively promoting increased federal spending for biomedical research, it may be impossible to identify the unique contribution of any one group to the total outcome.
  The most interesting test will come when groups and organizations seek to influence federal (or state or local) policy on issues other than funding. While the groups opposed to the use of animals in biomedical research have continued their activities in recent decades, the proportion of American adults opposed to the use of animals in research has not increased markedly, although it is higher than many of the leaders of the biomedical research community would like it to be (see discus-

sion in Chapter 9). Although most of the organizations in the biomedical research community have attempted to avoid direct confrontations over the issue and to rely on law enforcement officers to prevent trespass on their property, there is no evidence of successful persuasion or mobilization by the biomedical research community on this issue.

The stem cell issue is just emerging at the time of the publication of this analysis. To a large extent, this issue represents the successful negotiation by biomedical policy leaders of an administrative ruling from the Clinton Administration that is likely to generate a substantial number of objections from congressional Republicans. There will undoubtedly be efforts in the Congress to amend various appropriations bills and other legislation to reverse the NIH ruling on the use of stem cells in biomedical research, and biomedical organizations that favor the ruling will have to try to generate support from other policy leaders in the scientific community and from the attentive public for biomedical policy to oppose these amendments. It will be important, however, to examine the strategies and the success rate of biomedical communications groups in fostering positive attitudes toward this research among the attentive public for biomedical policy and in converting some of those attitudes into overt policy contacting behaviors.

The assessment of policy communication efforts is not only expensive, but it is sometimes difficult because it involves asking individuals about their personal policy preferences and political activities. But, nonetheless, we will acquire a solid understanding of the processes that produce successful biomedical policy communications only when we have a solid base of empirical assessments of these communications programs and efforts.

THE ESTIMATION OF POLICY COMMUNICATION IMPACT

The general model of biomedical policy communications displayed in Figure 11-1 and the series of questions above suggest a basic approach to estimating the impact of a policy communications program or campaign. For illustrative purposes, assume that we wish to design a communications program to increase support for the use of stem calls in biomedical research among adults attentive to biomedical policy and to encourage these attentive citizens to contact a senator from their state to oppose all amendments seeking to reverse the NIH decision on this matter. Using the form shown in Figure 11-2, we can walk though the process of estimating the likely impact of a specific communications effort on achieving this objective.

The first step is to define the target population, and we think that it is

Line	Instruction	Estimated Number
1	Define the target audience and enter the estimated number of individuals included in this audience in the next column.	30,400,000
2	Estimate the proportion of the target audience that will hear, view, or read the medium (or media) through which you expect this message to be delivered. Enter this proportion (less than 1.0) in the next column.	.42
3	Multiply the number on line 1 by the proportion on line 2 and enter the result on line 3.	12,768,000
4	Estimate the proportion of the target audience that reads the selected media who will read the specific story or information. Enter this proportion on line 4.	.70
5	Multiply the number on line 3 by the proportion on line 4 and enter the result on line 5.	8,937,600
6	Estimate the proportion of the targeted audience that heard, viewed, or read the message that will accept or believe the message and retain it for possible future use. Enter this proportion on line 6.	.60
7	Multiply the number on line 5 by the proportion on line 6 and enter the result on line 7.	5,362,560
8	Estimate the proportion of the target audience that received and accepted the message that will take the desired action within a defined time period. Enter this proportion on line 8.	.05
9	Multiply the number of line 7 by the proportion on line 8 and enter the result on line 9.	268,128
10	Divide the number on line 9 by the number on line 1 and multiply the result by 100. Enter the result on line 10. This is your estimate of the percentage of the target audience that your message will reach and lead to take the desired action.	1 %

Figure 11-2 A worksheet to compute the estimated impact of a message or campaign.

important to try to reach all adults who are attentive to biomedical policy. From our most recent national study in 1999, we determine that 16 percent of adults were attentive to biomedical policy issues, or approximately 30,400,000 individual citizens (see Chapter 7 for a discussion of the definition and composition of this attentive public). In this example, we enter the total target population of 30,4000,000 on line 1.

For our hypothetical policy communications campaign, we decide to use a combination of freelance articles, paid advertisements, and direct mail. We select a group of news, science, and health magazines[2] that are read frequently by adults attentive to biomedical policy issues, and we seek to place freelance articles in those magazines. We buy paid advertising in the same magazines. Slightly later, we rent the circulation lists for those magazines and send a personal letter advocating the use of stem cells in biomedical research and indicating that various pending amendments would reverse the recent NIH ruling that allows this research. From our 1999 database, we determine that approximately 42 percent of the attentive public for biomedical policy would read one of these magazines most months. Enter this proportion on line 2 and multiply line 1 by this proportion. The resulting estimate (see line 3) is that the proposed policy information program using a selected set of magazines would provide potential message exposure to approximately 12.8 million citizens who are attentive to biomedical policy.

We know that even attentive citizens do not read all of the available stories in every magazine that they read, but tend to scan the article titles and front pages and read only selected articles in greater depth. This practice is a reflection of the application of an individual's policy schemas, including their biomedical policy schema(s). We do not have good empirical evidence about the reading rate for biomedical stories among attentive citizens, so we need to make an informed guess. Because the individual who is attentive to biomedical policy already has a high level of interest in the subject and may be a regular reader of the magazines included in this communications program, we think that an estimate of about 70 percent would be reasonable. The important point is that 100 percent of even attentive citizens will not read every article about any biomedical issue, and communicators need to think explicitly about how to determine what the real rate is and how they might seek to increase this reading rate. In this example, we enter .70 on line 4 and multiply the population on line 3 by this proportion. We enter the result on line 5, which indicates that about 8.9 million adults who are attentive to biomedical policy might be expected to read the articles or advertisements in at least one of the selected magazines.

Getting an individual to read an article does not mean that he or she will accept its message and incorporate the new information into their biomedical policy schema(s). This may be especially true for citizens attentive to biomedical policy, because most of these citizens will bring a reasonably well-developed set of biomedical policy schema(s) to the assessment of the message. It is sometimes possible to gain some insights into the acceptance rate through the use of focus groups and small pilot studies, but it is essential to recognize that the artificiality of these groups tends to increase the observed interest in and retention of any kind of information over the rate that we

---

[2]For the purpose of this example, assume that the information campaign would focus on *Time, Newsweek, US News and World Report, Scientific American, National Geographic,* and a small set of health magazines such as *Prevention.*

would expect to observe without the recruitment and rewards associated with the focus group. For illustrative purposes, we estimate that 60 percent of attentive citizens would read and accept a message about the importance of stem cell research. We enter .60 on line 6, multiply the population on line 5 by this proportion, and enter the result on line 7. Following the logic of our assumptions so far, we would estimate that our hypothetical information campaign would produce about 5.3 million adults who have been updated on the importance of allowing biomedical researchers to use stem cells in their work.

Finally, we know that information alone does not lead to overt actions. Rosenau (1974) and others have shown that the process of mobilization to make a policy-related contact is difficult, although we have argued previously that new information technologies are making this process easier. In this example, we apply the estimates obtained by Rosenau in regard to contacting on a nuclear weapons testing treaty and estimate that about 5 percent of those attentive citizens who have received the message and accepted it would contact a senator on the stem cell issue. We enter .05 on line 8, multiply the population on line 7 by this proportion, and enter the result on line 9. We now estimate that our hypothetical information campaign would produce approximately 268,000 contacts with senators in support of stem cell research, urging each senator contacted to vigorously oppose all amendments designed to reverse the NIH ruling on this matter.

The critical point of this exercise for biomedical policy communicators is that we need to be aware of the steps in the communication process and the probabilities of success at each step in the process. More important, by understanding these steps and the associated probabilities, the opportunities to improve the impact of the program by increasing some of the proportions becomes obvious. Let's reexamine the decisions and estimates and think about some of the points of possible intervention to improve the productivity of the process.

First, the hypothetical information campaign focused on a set of national magazines for the information program that other evidence indicated were read by significant numbers of citizens who are attentive to biomedical policy issues. Using survey data collected previously by the authors, we determined the proportion of our target audience reached by these media. We could compute the proportion for other magazines or for other media, such as newspapers or television, and reestimate the reach of the selected media. By being more rigorous and empirical in our definition of the target audience, we are able to select media that are used by this audience and increase our proportion of coverage. It is possible that we could increase this proportion further by utilizing some of the intermediary groups that are trusted by citizens attentive to biomedical policy—major universities, research centers, professional groups and societies, and selected leadership spokespersons. It is unlikely that prominent figures from sports or entertainment activities would appeal to attentive citizens, in contrast to consumer biomedical communications. The analysis of information acquisition patterns in Chapter 8 may be helpful in thinking about the selection of specific media for reaching citizens attentive to biomedical policy issues.

Second, the proportion of our attentive group who examine a particular story carefully is an important part of the equation. Although carefully selected pictures or graphics are helpful for all audiences, the major factor in the reading rate may be the nature of the publication itself. If an attentive citizen has a high level of confidence in the science section of the *New York Times,* he or she may be much more likely to read a story in that paper than a comparable story in their local newspaper (assuming that it is not the *Times*). We need more research on the current reading habits of issue attentives and on their use of new information technologies to gain access to traditional sources such as the *New York Times* on-line as well as new sources—on-line access to the *New England Journal of Medicine* or *Nature* or the Mayo Clinic Web site.

Third, the rate of acceptance of messages by the attentive public for biomedical policy issues may differ substantially by the content of the message. Generally, intermediaries and interpreters may be less important in increasing or decreasing the acceptance rate among attentives than they are among consumers because of the larger and more developed biomedical policy schema(s) already held by attentives, but there is some marginal gain that can be obtained by intermediaries. Biomedical communicators need to understand more about the dynamics of this process. Although the evidence is thin, it appears that the citizens attentive to biomedical policy issues are more likely to be influenced by interpretations and argument by respected institutions than by personal acquaintances. But, substantially more research is needed on this process.

Finally, the conversion of attitudes and information—integrated into one or more biomedical policy schemas—into overt contacting or other policy influencing actions is a critical and essential step in the policy communication process. In our stem cell example, we estimated a mobilization rate of 5 percent, based largely on the earlier work of Rosenau (1974). Although there is an urgent need to improve our estimates about actual mobilization rates and the factors that influence them, the point is not the accuracy of this estimated rate, but the importance of this rate in determining the ultimate effectiveness of a biomedical policy communication campaign. If this rate could be increased to 20 percent, for example, the hypothetical stem cell communications campaign would have produced over a million contacts with senators for the same investment in time and resources. The mobilization rate is a critical factor in policy communications campaigns, and it is rarely recognized and less often understood.

BIOMEDICAL COMMUNICATION POLICIES FOR THE 21ST CENTURY

12
....

POLICIES TO IMPROVE BIOMEDICAL COMMUNICATIONS

....

The preceding chapters have attempted to provide a sound empirical description of the processes of communicating personal health information to consumers and biomedical policy information to citizens. We began this book with an examination of biomedical literacy in the United States, and we now conclude with a discussion of the problems found in the preceding analyses of biomedical communications and make some recommendation for policies and programs to improve the practice, reach, and effectiveness of biomedical communications.

Our summary discussions and recommendations will focus on (1) educational policies to advance biomedical literacy, (2) policies to support informed decision making by consumers, and (3) citizenship and the formulation of biomedical policy. There is an underlying logic to these recommendations. Improved levels of biomedical literacy depend heavily on improvements in the educational achievement of precollege students in the United States. The first result of improved educational efforts to assure that all high school graduates are biomedically literate should be reflected in better consumer judgments and more informed consumer decision making. The second, and longer term, result should produce a broader and better informed public discourse on biomedical policy for the twenty-first century. We have woven these strands together in this chapter because effective solutions to the underlying issues will require substantial achievements in all three areas.

EDUCATIONAL POLICIES TO
ADVANCE BIOMEDICAL LITERACY

Throughout our analysis, we have found that biomedical literacy provides a foundation for consumer understanding and for effective policy communications, but the evidence indicates that only one in five American adults have a level of biomedical literacy sufficient to read a news story in the Science Times section of the *New York Times* or a comparable article in *Prevention* or other health-oriented magazines. This level of biomedical literacy is too low under any condition, but it is dangerously low as we enter a new century of genomic medicine. It is imperative that the biomedical community, the broader scientific community, and federal and state governments join in a sustained effort to significantly increase the level of scientific and biomedical literacy in the United States.

Universal Biomedical Literacy among High School Graduates

The first objective must be universal biomedical literacy for all high school graduates in the United States. It is entirely reasonable to expect that all high school graduates in the twenty-first century should understand the basic concepts of cell biology, including the role of genes and chromosomes in the development of all forms of life. These basic ideas are the vocabulary for understanding the direction of modern medicine and for decoding the numerous public policy disputes that will accompany the development of genomic medicine in the twenty-first century. As simple as this objective may sound, it is clear that a large majority of current high school graduates (and high school teachers) do not qualify as biomedically literate. And, there is evidence that the situation may be eroding rather than improving.

Although the substance of biomedical literacy for adults was discussed in Chapter 2, there are excellent and broadly supported descriptions of the specific biological and scientific concepts that students should understand prior to high school graduation. The American Association for the Advancement of Science's *Science for All Americans* (Rutherford and Ahlgren, 1990) and the National Academy of Science's *National Education Science Standards* (National Research Council, 1996) provide comprehensive descriptions of the central concepts that must be included to obtain biomedical literacy, as well as scientific literacy. There is broad consensus among scientists, educators, and mainstream political leaders on the need for improved science education in the United States and the general substance of scientific literacy for high school graduates. A small segment of the religious right wing of American politics continues to resist the concepts of evolution and natural selection—in contrast to every other major nation in the world—but this opposition should not significantly delay a renewed national effort to improve the quality of elementary and secondary science and mathematics education in the United States.

The evidence from three decades of good national testing of student achievement in science and mathematics indicates that the highest achieving American students are competitive with students anywhere else in the world and that our lowest achieving students rank lower than the average student in some developing nations (Beaton *et al.,* 1996a,b; Schmidt *et al.,* 1998; Mullis *et al.,* 1998). The evidence also indicates that the relative competitiveness of U.S. students—compared to students in other nations—declines as students move through the American school system. It is important to understand these points.

The Third International Mathematics and Science Study (TIMSS) included more than 45 nations, ranging from modern industrial and science-oriented nations such an the United States, Canada, and major western European nations to economically developing nations such as Greece and Columbia. Following the general pattern of the First International Mathematics and Science Study in the 1970s and the Second International Study of Mathematics and Science in the 1980s, TIMSS used international committees of educators and scholars to design achievement tests in science and mathematics and international teams of sampling experts to monitor and supervise the selection of students and the administration of the tests. The tests are achievement tests—how well does a student understand selected concepts and how skillful is a student in defining and solving selected problems—but they are not measures of potential or some innate ability. The results are useful in comparing the level of student achievement in science and mathematics at selected age or grade levels.

In broad terms, the mean score on both science and mathematics for U.S. students in the fourth grade was slightly higher than the mean for fourth-grade students from all 45 nations included in TIMSS. The mean score in both science and mathematics for U.S. eighth-grade students was slightly lower than the mean for eighth-grade students in all 45 countries, but the mean science and mathematics scores for American students in grade 12 was lower than virtually any other major industrial nation in the world (Beaton *et al.,* 1996a,b; Schmidt *et al.,* 1998; Mullis *et al.,* 1998). The inference from these results is clear. American students have a small advantage in science and mathematics achievement in the elementary school years, reflecting the influence of their parent's education and the strong cultural interest in and commitment to science and technology in the United States. This early international advantage, however, is lost before the beginning of high school, and the margin of difference by grade 12 is substantial.

The factors responsible for this relatively uncompetitive level of student performance are equally clear. Both parents and school administrators are ambivalent about the ability of students to attain a solid understanding of science or mathematics. There is a pervasive feeling that these subjects are only for the best and brightest of students, and that average students can only be expected to develop some appreciation of the nature of science or its central concepts. This feeling originates in large part from a misguided effort to identify gifted and talented students in the elementary years and to provide special educational advantages for these students. Reflecting a congressionally imposed rule that only 5 percent of students in a school system can be identified as gifted and talented for federal funding purposes, many school systems introduce rigid tracking systems in the early elementary school years—often organized around reading groups—that segregate the best prepared students from other students and convey a message to at least 80 percent of students that they are not gifted and talented and are average at best. In this context, it would be surprising if most students felt highly motivated to strive for academic excellence.

In practice, this perverse system conveys only minor advantages to the few students selected as gifted and talented, but just enough to persuade the parents of these students that the school system has recognized the potential of their student and to not scrutinize school programs or policies too carefully. For the majority of the students, the tracking system results in lowered expectations, reduced challenges, and lower standards for grading and graduation.

This system is reenforced by a secondary school philosophy that seeks to maximize student happiness over achievement. Too many high school counselors advise students to take easier (lower track) courses to improve their grade point average, reflecting a profound misunderstanding of college admission procedures and the life-cycle consequences of an inferior education. School boards and school administrators have found that extensive athletic programs channel student and parent energies into satisfying activities that reduce concern about low levels of academic achievement. Most high school principals and school boards would happily trade a conference championship in football for 10 additional National Merit Finalists. Unfortunately, that may be exactly the choice that they face in the context of limited financial resources and a declining proportion of voters with children of school age.

The structural problems of the system are compounded by too many science and mathematics teachers with limited or outdated understanding of their subject, too few resources for adequate laboratory or computer resources, too few student hours in substantive classes, and too many days of summer and holiday leave. A full discussion of the systemic problems of the American educational system is beyond the scope of this book or this chapter, but it is essential to recognize that the goal of universal biomedical literacy by the end of high school will require more than a minor tweaking of a few courses.

A few first steps merit a brief discussion. First, it is important to understand that students do not learn science and mathematics by simply being in the same building in which these subjects are taught, but rather that students must actually take and pass the courses. We should expect all high school graduates to have at least 3 years of mathematics and 3 years of science, excluding fraudulent substitutes such as personal finance (in place of algebra) and landscaping (in place of biology). Most nations require students expecting to enter a university to have completed biology, chemistry, physics, and advanced mathematics, and the United States must expect no less from its students.

Second, state legislatures need to learn to say no to interest groups demanding that another special course be mandated for all public schools. Until some of these mandates are folded into core subjects, school boards and school administrators should seek to turn these mandates into opportunities. For example, a personal health course might be redesigned to provide a strong science-based understanding of the biological basis of addiction and the biological consequences of tobacco use or extensive alcohol use. "Just Say No" may be a convenient curriculum, but "Knowing the Consequences" may be a more effective course and may even enhance the biomedical literacy of students.

Third, the extensive national effort to wire every school and to provide expanded student exposure to personal computers and the Internet is meritorious in its own right, but it also offers an opportunity to introduce students to personal health sites that may become a resource throughout their adult years. Undoubtedly the sites will change, but once a student develops the skills needed to locate and bookmark health-relevant sites, it is reasonable to expect that many students will continue to use this kind of resource for current health information. By introducing sites such as the National Library of Medicine's PubMed, the National Institutes of Health (NIH) and nongovernmental sites on specific diseases, and general health information providers, students may learn how to select and evaluate on-line health information, and it is likely that this is a skill that will be useful in the decades ahead.

Improved Informal Science
and Biomedical Education

Although formal schooling must provide a basic understanding of a core of scientific and biomedical constructs for young adults, it is clear that the task of increasing biomedical literacy must include student groups and extracurricular groups focused on specific issues and problems. Four specific examples may illustrate both the need for informal education activities and some of the ways in which this approach has worked in recent years.

First, tobacco use is perhaps the single most serious threat to the health of adolescents and young adults in the United States, and strictly curriculum-based interventions have had limited success. The use of student-based groups in Florida (combined with a general media campaign) appears to have reduced student smoking by at least 30 percent in the initial year and even more in subsequent years.

Second, the combination of student-based groups (Students Against Drunk Driving) and parents (Mothers Against Drunk Driving) over the last decade has reduced the teenage death rate from alcohol-related traffic accidents. Many of these programs have been integrated into school programming and have been able to use school facilities and resources. The combination of student and adult programming is a very useful model, and the jointly signed contracts concerning parent provision of transportation without accusations or punishments in exchange for the student's promise to call for help rather than driving after drinking illustrate the potential for student/parent agreements in influencing both the development of understanding about a health problem and the adoption of appropriate behaviors. It is important to study the factors associated with successful behavioral outcomes from this kind of experience and the factors associated with unsuccessful programs, but even without additional research, it is clear that this general model offers a promising framework for programmatic efforts to increase adolescent and young adult biomedical literacy.

Third, the growth of student-based DARE groups in many schools illustrate another approach to the use of informal extracurricular activities to supplement and enhance curriculum information about the consequences of drug use and abuse. Although the first comparative studies do not find a significant difference in drug use or attitudes between students who participate in DARE and students who do (Lynam *et al.*, 1999; Becker *et al.*, 1992), these programs remain popular with students and parents and provide a useful model for student and parent involvement in learning and thinking about drug use and its consequences.

Finally, intramural and club sports provide a useful source of exercise and fitness experiences for many students who are not participating in interscholastic sports. Although the growth of multiple levels of sports teams within the interscholastic framework has reduced the reach of intramural sports in many schools, this kind of activity offers an important opportunity to link fitness awareness to intramural participation, and to build linkages between health classes, intramural leagues, and club sports. By involving parent and community groups, it would be possible to build programs that would cover both the school year and the summer vacation period. Given the increasing levels of obesity reported in school-aged populations and among American adults, it is important to examine the existing opportunities to build communication and educational programs within the framework of existing institutions and programs.

Web Education for the Life Cycle

In the context of the current information technology revolution, the school years provide an important opportunity to provide students with the skills needed to locate and use Web sites for personal health information. Although the Web includes a number of sites that offer inaccurate health information and outright quackery, it also includes a large number of sites that provide excellent information resources for learning about personal health, prescription drugs, patient support groups for a wide array of diseases, and the location and quality of health care facilities. While specific health-related sites will come and go over the years, it is important for students to learn about appropriate search strategies and about the criteria for discerning between responsible medical information and fraudulent information. Because most adolescents and young adults have little interest in diseases associated with older adults, it may not be possible to promote a strong interest in visiting the sites for the American Heart Association or the American Cancer Society (unless a parent or grandparent has the disease), but it is possible to introduce general health sites such as the Mayo Clinic site, U.S. Centers for Disease Control and Prevention (CDC) sites on communicable diseases and accidents, and Planned Parenthood and selected sites on reproductive health questions. In the context of the genomic revolution in medicine, an introduction to the site for the National Human Genome Research Institute and related institutes at major universities might serve to provide some answers to emerging questions about the relative influence of genetic and environmental factors in various diseases, traits, and behaviors.

This is not a comprehensive agenda for health-related or biomedical Web education, but it does suggest some important possibilities for encouraging students to learn about the information technologies that will become the major conduit for information in their lifetime and to provide some exposure to relevant health and biomedical sites. Even if this experience does not produce immediate increases in biomedical knowledge or in health-related attitudes and behaviors, many students might retain some understanding of how and where to find responsible information when it is needed and in a manner that provides some sense of confidentiality about the inquiry itself.

POLICIES TO SUPPORT INFORMED DECISION MAKING BY CONSUMERS

Although policies to produce biomedically literate high school graduates would—if successfully implemented—provide a long-term foundation for improving biomedical communications, the reality is that most of today's adults are unlikely to return to formal instruction to become biomedically literate. Yet, they will continue to make health-related decisions for themselves, their children, and, in some cases, their parents. They will operate with some level of biomedical understanding, and they will have a personal health schema that includes some collection of information, expectations, attitudes, and experiences. The question is not whether most adults will be able to make health-related decisions, but whether or not they will make those decisions on the basis of an accurate and reasonably comprehensive understanding of biomedical science and the full range of possibilities available at any given time.

There are several policies and programs that might increase the number of adults who have a sufficient personal health schema, including an adequate level of biomedical literacy, to make good personal and family health decisions. We will, in this section, quickly outline some policies that we think would enhance the quality of health decision-making by consumers.

Multiple Messages for Multiple Audiences

It is essential to recognize the wide range of understanding and personal health competence among adults in the United States and to construct messages and information campaigns that produce messages tailored to different levels of biomedical literacy among consumers. We argued for this position in several chapters, and we repeat the imperative for biomedical communicators to abandon the single-message syndrome and begin to think, write, and produce a range of information and messages targeted to different levels of consumer understanding and background.

How can multiple messages be transmitted without insulting the less sophisticated consumer? This is an important question since it would be undesirable to reduce the likelihood of messages being received and accepted by less well educated adults by creating a demeaning tone or impression. Although it is essential to begin with and maintain a high level of sensitivity to this issue, we offer some suggestions about how multiple-level messages might be constructed and disseminated.

First, many announcements and information campaigns provide press packets to journalists, frequently mailing or e-mailing the material to individual journalists at selected publications and outlets. This provides an opportunity to make reasonable differentiations. A basic press kit might be produced that includes the basic information about the event, discovery, or publication. Additional materials might be prepared that provide a more sophisticated discussion of the biomedical science involved in the event or announcement, at a level similar to that found in the *New York Times'* Science Times or a magazine such as *Prevention.* A more advanced package might be constructed for publications such as the *New York Times,* the *Wall Street Journal, Science News,* or *Chemical and Engineering News* that would include reprints of journal articles and related materials to allow the writer to explore the background of the announcement or event without having to engage in library research. It is likely that the published stories that come from this kind of multilevel announcement process would be written at different levels and would be useful to consumers with different levels of biomedical understanding.

Second, Web sites and other on-line information sources (kiosks and information screens in public areas) can be programmed to provide several layers of explanation and information. For example, an excellent exhibit on the evolution of the human brain at the American Museum of Natural History in New York City includes a simple one or two sentence explanation about a topic or screen, and then offers the viewer (who is using a touch-screen surface) a choice of a basic explanation, an advanced explanation, or an expert explanation. Most viewers begin with a basic explanation, then at least look at the advanced explanation to see how much of it they understand. If that explanation is generally comprehensible, the viewer may go to the advanced screen. This basic approach could be used on Web sites, information kiosks, and in a variety of automated information settings. It could also be used by hospitals and medical facilities to allow patients, families, and friends to learn more about personal health information while they are waiting for one purpose or the other.

Third, many organizations write brochures or reports that they print and disseminate to the public, often using purchased mailing lists. This type of information campaign is ideally suited to some differentiation among publications. For example, if an organization wanted to increase public awareness of a particular disease for the purpose of increasing early detection and diagnosis, it might write a simple brochure describing the symptoms of the disease, the early diagnosis procedures, and the eventual impact of the disease if not identified and treated. It would include toll-free telephone numbers and Web addresses for more information or help, and it might include a card to request a full report, which might be written at a more advanced level and would provide additional explanation of the biomedical basis of the disease and some of the current efforts to develop diagnostic procedures or pharmaceutical products to control or cure the disease. It might also include a pitch for contributions to support research in this area, as well as an expanded listing of Web and print resources for readers who would like to obtain additional information. At the most advanced level, the organization might develop a Patient and Family Handbook that would provide more detailed discussions of the causes, symptoms, and current and prospective treatments for the disease. The Handbook would reflect the higher level of information needs of individuals who are experiencing the disease, or who have a family member who is experiencing the disease. The net result of this kind of communications campaign would be a general increase in awareness at virtually all strata of the public, but with differential levels of comprehension and understanding by different strata of the public, reflecting their individual needs and backgrounds.

Fourth, some information campaigns use advertising and seek to deliver their message by selecting publications and outlets that are used by their targeted audiences. This process also allows some differentiation in message sophistication, but care must be taken to avoid the perception that race or ethnicity is being used as a surrogate marker for differential levels of background or ability. But, we know a good deal about the audiences for various publications and broadcasts, and useful differentiations can be made. The general profile of readers for *Parade* magazine, for example, is less sophisticated than the readership of the *Washington Post* or *Smithsonian* magazine. If an organization was seeking to buy advertising space in these publications, it would be possible to differentiate the level and sophistication of the message without offending the readers of any of the publications.

Promote Adult Literacy and Numeracy

Too often, biomedical communicators and their institutions focus on crafting an effective message and ignore the reality that millions of American adults have limited basic literacy and numeracy skills. The long-term effectiveness of communication campaigns, especially campaigns designed to reach older and less well educated adults, depend on the literacy skills of those consumers. Each focused group and organization—a hospital, a health agency, a group practice, a newspaper, a magazine—acknowledge that illiteracy and innumeracy among adults is a serious problem, but insist that it is not their problem. It is too general! It should be handled by the schools or by the public library! It is everyone's problem and no one's problem at the same time.

Although the responsibility for reducing adult illiteracy and innumeracy does not rest with the biomedical community alone, we need to support basic literacy programs and recognize that we can contribute to reducing the problem through creative programming to advance biomedical literacy. Some clinics and community hospitals offer reading materials about pregnancy and reading instruction to mothers as a part of prenatal care. Other hospitals and public libraries have joined forces to provide books to new mothers and to encourage them to bring their young children into library story reading programs—a precursor to early reading programs. New parents are almost universally eager to do whatever they can to help their current or soon-to-arrive children, and parents with low reading skills are often willing to engage in reading and literacy classes or tutoring. It is essential to recognize that most low literacy adults are embarrassed by their situation and may seek to mask it, but there are good model programs of adult literacy that have been successful in communities throughout the nation.

Build Community and Organizational Partnerships

Efforts to communicate about biomedical topics can be made more effective through creative and effective partnerships with various organizations, institutions, and community groups. In the model of biomedical communications to consumers in Chapter 6, we pointed to the role of selected groups as interpreters and mobilizers. It is important to incorporate these groups into a biomedical communications plan. Some examples may be helpful.

First, campaigns to increase awareness of diseases and their early warning symptoms can make effective use of joint mailings and communications from employers, unions, and membership groups with newsletters or Web sites. This kind of partnership may reduce the communication cost by sharing an existing vehicle, and it may significantly enhance the acceptability or credibility of the message itself. In some cases, a program of periodic health information alerts may build a level of confidence among recipients that will increase their willingness to donate to local (or national) biomedical fundraising programs in subsequent requests.

Second, these same organizations may also be willing to sponsor on-site programs for actual screening activities or for the scheduling of screening tests at a local clinic or hospital. For example, the Cancer Research Foundation of America (CRFA) operates a mobile mammogram facility (essentially a refitted bus) that goes to the meetings of community groups and provides on-site services in communities that are underserved by traditional medical service organizations. The CRFA also recently operated an information kiosk at both the Republican and Democratic National Conventions and offered on-site mammograms to delegates and other attendees, providing some additional screening services and increasing the awareness of the importance of early and regular checkups. The range of possible joint alliances is extraordinary and is used too infrequently by biomedical communicators.

Third, public libraries and community colleges are important potential partners with common programmatic interests and substantial resources that are often overlooked by biomedical communicators. As noted in Chapter 5, a majority of American adults visit a public library at least once each year and report moderate levels of use of library resources. Some libraries do provide special exhibits for Cancer Awareness Week or other special events, but it appears that most of the initiative for this kind of programming comes from libraries and librarians rather than from biomedical communicators. Libraries have a high level of credibility among Americans, and they have substantial resources for the purchase of materials, professional staff, good meeting facilities with parking, and longer operating hours than most community-based organizations. They usually have a steady local tax base and are good partners for long-term programs.

Community colleges are organizations with a mission to improve adult education through a wide range of formal and informal—credit and non-credit—programs and activities. Like libraries, these institutions usually have a steady local tax base, professional staff, good meeting facilities with parking, a library of their own, and a good computing facility with extensive Web access. In recent years, many community colleges have struggled to maintain their enrollments and are eager to build joint programming with community organizations. Many community colleges sponsor lectures, have noncredit classes in recreational subjects, and offer evening and weekend programming, including user-friendly opportunities to learn how to use a personal computer and access the Web. Biomedical communicators need to think creatively about how they can work with these institutions to build effective communication programming on biomedical subjects.

Fourth, millions of Americans visit a science center or museum, a natural history museum, or similar facility each year, and many of these institutions are ready partners for the communication of biomedical information. Apart from major exhibitions (which can cost millions of dollars), museums and related institutions have membership lists, hold public lectures, send out newsletters, have a Web site, and have good meeting facilities with parking. Many also operate a food service, including catering for special events. They are usually more interesting and more economical than a hotel, and they offer the prospect for long-term partnerships in activities from newsletter articles to Web site links to information kiosks within the facility. Some museums do some programming on biomedical subjects, but this is usually generated by their own staff and less often by the overtures of biomedical communicators from other organizations.

Finally, there are numerous youth organizations that could be productive partners in biomedical communications efforts. Girl Scouts, Boy Scouts, girls clubs, boys clubs, and 4-H clubs are all examples of groups that already incorporate some health-related information into their programs and could be partners in more extensive efforts to improve youth understanding of biomedical subjects or programs to disseminate information to adult populations. Youth athletic clubs could also be useful partners in tobacco control programming—for themselves and for their parents and friends.

These suggestions do not exhaust the range of possible partnerships, but they hopefully illustrate some of the kinds of partnerships and alliances that could be built into a biomedical communications program. Recalling the general model of biomedical communications to consumers at the end of Chapter 6, this kind of collaborative programming should be seen as a part of a more general communications effort designed to interpret and amplify information and mobilize individual consumers to actions or behaviors.

Recognize the Long-Term Importance of the Web

Although the time frame for the extension of the Web and its electronic successors into the information backbone for the United States can be debated, there is little doubt that this is the direction in which communications are moving. It is unlikely, in our view, that electronic communications will lead to the complete elimination of print materials; we expect a strong convergence of media. Already, most newspapers and many magazines have on-line editions that are widely used. The growth of electronic communications and on-line editions have grown even more rapidly within the trade press. Some of these new electronic ventures will fail, but others will start and many will grow.

It is essential that biomedical communicators recognize now the extraordinary impact that broadband transmission technologies will have on communications in the United States (and most European countries) within the next decade. The Web will be an important channel for communicating with both consumers and citizens who are attentive to biomedical policy, although the sites that they visit and the information that they take in and retain as a part of their schemas will undoubtedly differ. Biomedical communicators need to begin to think now about strategies to use and stay current in the continuing information technology revolution.

For individuals who lead or administer information offices and programs in biomedical institutions and firms, it is important to begin building infrastructure now. It will be important to have staff expertise in video streaming, graphics, and server management. Major centers will need to monitor the acquisition of high-speed receiving equipment by the media and other outlets through which they seek to communicate. Some firms and organizations will find it feasible to build this expertise internally, whereas other firms and groups may find that outsourcing this service is more cost-effective. Regardless of the solution, now is the time to begin serious thinking and planning for acquiring these capabilities.

For journalists and biomedical writers, it is essential to build strong Internet and Web skills. Biomedical journalists and writers need to stay abreast of the emerging technologies and try to maintain their ability to read and use new text, graphical, and audio software. In practical terms, the useful lifetime of most desktop and notebook computers will be no longer than 3 years. It is likely, however, that the price of hardware will continue to decline, although the initial cost of new high definition television screens and office or home servers will be significantly higher than similar equipment in the past. For example, the price of digital cameras was initially high, but the price is declining as the quality increases—reflecting the price/quality pattern for personal computers.

In a broader social context, it is important to encourage and support the expansion of access to personal computing and Web resources. By the end of the twentieth century, a majority of Americans lived in households that had at least one personal computer, and more than 90 percent of college graduates had access to a computer at home or at work. This pattern of personal computer and Web access reflects the distribution pattern for all major technologies in the twentieth century, from automobiles to color television sets. In the case of computer and Web access, the pattern reflects a combination of economic resources and educational resources. Although continued economic growth will alleviate some of these distributional problems in the United States, biomedical institutions interested in advancing biomedical literacy should seek to expand Web access through collaborative programs with public libraries, community colleges, and other partners. In some cases, it may be therapeutically beneficial and cost-effective to provide an inexpensive personal computer and Web training to patients to monitor a posthospital recovery or a therapy that continues over the period of months or years. This may be especially beneficial for patients that have difficulty traveling.

It is also important for biomedical communicators to recognize that the extraordinary growth of the Web—now adding an estimated 5 million pages of information each day—has made the early search engine technology obsolete and that there is a growing and compelling need to build credible points of expert reference. Many hospitals and health plans operate Web sites that include some linkages to other sources of information (the *Physician's Desk Reference* or other prescription drug listings are favorites). This referral function is an important responsibility for biomedical communicators. A senior officer of the National Library of Medicine (NLM) recently pointed out the large staff commitment that the NLM makes to reviewing all of the citations that appear in PubMed (www.ncbi.nlm.nih.gov/PubMed) to eliminate older documents that have been superceded by newer studies and information. Although our democratic instincts argue against a single source of certification of biomedical Web sites, we believe that consumers will increasingly look to authoritative sources for referrals to Web sites relevant to specific health questions and concerns. The same principle applies to respected journalists and biomedical writers, who are beginning to include Web references in their articles, but who may not fully realize the influence of their recommendation on consumers. The inclusion of a Web biomedical reference includes the responsibility to look at that site carefully and to explore its linkages, because less well-informed consumers may logically conclude that a linkage from a recommended site is also recommended by the journalist, writer, or institution.

In short, the Web is here to stay as a major player in biomedical communications, and both individual biomedical communicators and biomedical institutions should begin to think about the implications of these technologies and plan for the effective use of these resources. Even more, leaders in biomedical communications must step forward and play a leadership role in shaping the structure and uses of these technologies.

CITIZENSHIP AND THE FORMULATION OF BIOMEDICAL POLICY

The revolution in genomic biology and medicine will undoubtedly raise important new public policy issues and disputes. We described recent and current patterns of citizen involvement in the formulation of biomedical policy in the United States in Chapters 7 through 11 and suggested some issues and objectives for the future. This section will recommend some general policies to enhance the level of biomedical literacy among adults in the United States and to improve the quality of public policy discourse on these issues.

The Growth of Biomedical Literacy

It is essential to continue to increase the proportion of American adults who are biomedically literate to expand the scope of citizen participation in the discussion of relevant public policy issues. We cannot, however, take the growth of biomedical literacy for granted, assuming that the flow of new students from colleges and universities will provide a sufficient pool of biomedically literate citizens. Given the extraordinary growth of genomic biology research and its likely impact on the practice of medicine over the next several decades, the pace of new knowledge and new concepts that adults will need to understand will outstrip the generational patterns of formal schooling, essentially requiring adults to make overt efforts to keep up with new developments in this area. Most of the pressure to keep up will come from the needs of individuals to make decisions about their own health, but the importance of public policy matters involving biomedical science will increase significantly also.

In the context of the preceding discussion of issue specialization, it will be particularly important to assure the continued biomedical literacy of a large proportion of the attentive public for biomedical policy and of biomedical policy leaders. We have said relatively little about the level of biomedical literacy required by biomedical policy leaders, and it is reasonable to assume that most biomedical policy leaders already have at least a moderately good level of understanding of basic biomedical concepts. It is not clear that insurance company executives, hospital administrators, benefits managers for companies and unions, and the executive staff of professional societies—many of whom would be classified as biomedical policy leaders—are biomedically literate or are in a position to stay current with the substance and implications of the genomic biomedical revolution. We need research to better define biomedical policy leaders and to examine the levels of biomedical understanding that they currently hold.

Similarly, many adults who are attentive to biomedical policy still retain a general understanding of basic biological concepts from their formal schooling and some informal reading about these topics, but may not understand the shifting basis of medicine and the likely affect of genomic-based medical science for diagnosis or therapy. As outlined in Chapters 7 and 8, we know some of the general information acquisition patterns for these attentive citizens, but we need to monitor their utilization of the Internet and Web-based information sources in the years ahead.

Biomedical communicators must recognize the importance of enhancing biomedical literacy and seek to advance that cause through their writing, productions, professional societies, and school programs. Many biomedical communicators have developed an extraordinary skill in understanding and translating biomedical science to lay audiences and display that skill in their daily work in a newspaper, magazine, television show, or other outlet. Some biomedical communicators have undertaken book projects to open a window of understanding to broader audiences. Boyce Rensberger's (1996) *Life Itself: Exploring the Realm of the Living Cell* is a good example. Other biomedical communicators have worked with professional societies and voluntary groups to write brochures, handbooks, and policy papers for members and leaders that broaden their understanding of a disease, a therapy, or a policy proposal. In all of this work, it is important to continue to write good sidebars and appendices—or Web sites—that explain basic concepts such as bacterium, virus, gene, chromosome, immunity, and resistance.

Biomedical institutions must recognize that they bear a major responsibility for communicating to policy leaders on biomedical matters. It is important to seek to enhance the biomedical literacy of executives, board members, donors, and vendors about the forthcoming changes in biomedical science and its impact on the medicines and therapies of the future. Biomedical institutions can sponsor lectures and talks, create and distribute educational materials, provide forums for policy-oriented discussions, and partner with other institutions—universities, libraries, and private associations—to enhance biomedical literacy among their respective clienteles. Most biomedical institutions operate Web sites that can facilitate these objectives.

Regardless of the approaches or methods employed, it is important for biomedical communicators and their institutions to recognize the importance of increasing the proportion of adolescents and adults who are biomedically literate, especially among the attentive public for biomedical policy and biomedical policy leaders.

The Role of Interest Groups

It is important for biomedical communicators and their institutions to recognize the potential role that interest groups can play in enhancing biomedical literacy and in fostering specific attitudes on biomedical policy issues. Although many biomedical communicators recognize the potential role of professional associations and societies in advancing biomedical literacy and specific policy agendas, some are wary of working with groups that are actively involved in lobbying the Congress or who may have an economic interest in health or medical affairs, such as employers, unions, insurance companies, and pharmaceutical companies. We pointed to the important roles of these groups in both consumer communications (Chapter 6) and policy communications (Chapter 11) in the distribution of information, its acceptance, and its influence on subsequent behaviors. Recognizing that different groups have different policy objectives, it may be possible to find common ground in the enhancement of biomedical literacy and in the development of educational and communications programs for that purpose.

We use the term interest groups rather than voluntary groups to emphasize that most groups do have some interests in the outcomes of biomedical policy deliberations. This is not a serious problem—virtually all groups and firms do have some interests or they would not have been formed in the first place. By understanding the interests of all potential partners in programs or communications, it is likely that each of the partners will find the process and the results to be more satisfactory. Many interest groups have built effective organizations to collect and disseminate information about policy matters, and many of these same resources may be utilized to improve the level of biomedical literacy among biomedical policy attentives and leaders.

Some examples may be helpful. Consider the issue of the growing number of antibiotic resistant strains of bacterial diseases in the world. To understand the origins of this problem and the array of feasible policy options available to the United States and similar countries, it would be helpful for an attentive citizen or a biomedical policy leader to understand the difference between a bacterium and a virus, the bacterial basis of a disease such as tuberculosis, the ways in which antibiotic resistance or immunity can develop for a particular bacterium, and the implications of antibiotic resistance on individual and public health. It may also be helpful to know something about the procedures that various countries use to control the distribution of antibiotics and the implications of self-diagnosis and self-medication (using antibiotics) on the development of antibiotic resistance.

If the objective is to increase the level of understanding of the basic biological constructs associated with the identification and treatment of bacterial-based disease among citizens attentive to biomedical policy, several of the following approaches might be employed:

- Persuade major professional societies and interest groups to include information about the growth of antibiotic-resistant bacteria in their journals, magazines, and newsletters, including some explanation of the biological processes that create this kind of resistance.

- Persuade the same groups to utilize their Web sites to include information and explanations about this problem.

- Include panels and symposia into the annual meetings of selected societies and interest groups, and encourage leaders of those groups to participate in these sessions.

- Pool resources among several interest groups to develop materials, print and broadcast, that provide accurate explanations of the biological processes and some of the policy options.

- Encourage joint meetings, workshops, and seminars for members and/ or leaders of cooperating interest groups to enhance their understanding of the issue and its biological basis.

The essential point is that many interest groups can play an important and constructive role in enhancing biomedical literacy among citizens who are attentive to biomedical policy and among biomedical policy leaders, and biomedical communicators need to build creative partnerships with those interest groups whose general objectives are compatible with the objectives of the communicator and his or her organization.

Provide Forums for Leadership Discussions of Biomedical Policy Issues

In addition to improving biomedical literacy and providing information about biomedical issues, it is important to provide forums for leadership discussions of biomedical issues and trends. It is likely that the number and complexity of biomedical policy issues will grow in the decades ahead, and leadership discussions and debates are one of the best methods to inform the attentive public for biomedical policy about the relevant issues and options.

To illustrate the role of leadership discussions on the formulation of public policy, consider the example of foreign policy. For nearly 50 years, a Council on Foreign Relations—with minor variations in name—has operated in most major cities in the United States. The leadership of these foreign relations councils are usually individuals who may have a policy leadership role in foreign policy, and virtually all of their members would qualify as being attentive to foreign policy. These groups provide a forum for invited speakers on current and emergent foreign policy issues. When divisive issues arise— such as the Vietnam War—these councils frequently provide a debate forum for directly opposing views. In less contentious times, these groups provide in-depth understanding of major areas of the world, introduce leaders from other nations to leaders of major interest groups in the United States, sponsor foreign travel for interested and attentive Americans to visit other countries and talk with some of their leaders, and organize informal social activities to encourage the maintenance of foreign language skills. Foreign Relations Councils have become an important part of the infrastructure of foreign policy discourse in the United States.

Whereas these formal organizations are limited to a few major cities, similar foreign policy leadership forums have emerged in the form of narrow-audience broadcasting. *Meet the Press* and similar Sunday morning television interview shows have served this purpose for several decades, serving many policy arenas beyond foreign policy. The growth of cable-based broadcasting has produced a small number of serious news discussion shows, but virtually no programming focused on scientific or biomedical issues. C-Span covers some congressional committee hearings on scientific and biomedical topics, and the C-Span2 weekend book programming covers some histories and popularizations of science, medicine, and health. The biomedical community—including biomedical communicators—should work with C-Span and similar narrow-casting media to sponsor leadership discussion forums on issues ranging from stem cell research to global warming to infectious diseases.

In the longer term, the growth of broadband communications will allow thousands of groups and institutions to use video streaming and its successor technologies to Web-cast to narrow audiences on specific topics. Until those technologies are operational, however, biomedical communicators should explore opportunities to create and disseminate leadership discussions of major biomedical issues.

Recognize and Prepare for Religious Conflict

Most biomedical organizations and biomedical communicators have had limited experience with the politics of conflict and confrontation. The evolution controversy that continued through most of the twentieth century, however, is a precursor to the kind of controversy that genomic biology is likely to provoke in the United States. Although the United States has been unique in the nature and depth of the rejection of biological evolution by religious fundamentalists, Europe is experiencing a Green-led rejection of agricultural genomics and the rise of an environmental fundamentalism that seeks to freeze and preserve nature in its present form. Undoubtedly, genomic research will provide a detailed and persuasive description of the development of life from its microbial beginnings to our current biological diversity and will offer the possibility for numerous interventions to cure specific diseases and modify genomes of both plants and animals, including humans. Whereas some of the issues involving the nature and extent of genomic intervention merit serious public policy discussion, the emergence of these issues will give rise to fundamentalist resistance to the basic science itself.

Although we are optimistic that the accuracy, elegance, and utility of the science will prevail, it is important for the biomedical community to recognize that this passage will not occur without turbulence. It is imperative that the biomedical and scientific communities endure the controversy and engage in accurate and thoughtful discourse about the nature and benefits of genomic biology and related sciences. Confrontation is never fun, as many biomedical researchers and communicators have discovered through the continuing confrontation by People for the Ethical Treatment of Animals (PETA), but the price of acquiescence is far greater than the discomfort of the conflict.

RESEARCH AND
BIOMEDICAL COMMUNICATIONS

We started this book with a discussion of the value of a research-based approach to biomedical communications, and we will end it with a discussion of research that is needed to advance our understanding of biomedical communications. We have tried in the preceding analyses to draw conclusions when the data supported a conclusion, but to point to the unresolved nature of various questions when the data did not allow a good empirical determination. From this experience, we would offer these suggestions to improve the understanding of biomedical communications.

First, it is essential to continue to monitor what the public—at all levels—knows and think about biomedical subjects and issues. Although the National Science Foundation has sponsored a 20-year time series on general scientific literacy, a comparable time series has not been supported by either major federal agencies or major nongovernmental foundations with a strong commitment to biomedical research. Although some of the data reported in the preceding analysis provide some interesting and useful data for what might be called the pre-genetic-revolution period, or perhaps the early genetic revolution period, it is critical to build good monitoring programs now to describe and understand the public reaction to and utilization of the tidal wave of new genomic information that will become available in the decades ahead.

Second, it is important to encourage similar monitoring programs in all of the major industrial nations of the world and to begin to explore the possibility of selective sampling in the developing world. Microbes have no nationality. The careless use of antibiotics over the last 50 years has created a growing number of antibiotic-resistant strains of major diseases. Tuberculosis was once thought to be near eradication, but its new antibiotic-resistant form is now one of the world's major causes of death. The solution to this and similar events requires sound public health policies and a sufficient level of understanding of basic biomedical science by both medical providers and patients to use available medications carefully and wisely. The global community has a need to know about biomedical literacy, attitudes, and behaviors that can effect the health of every nation.

Third, it is important to initiate adult panel studies that measure biomedical literacy, attitudes, and behaviors of the same individuals over a long period of time—at least several years. Virtually all of our current data on biomedical literacy, attitudes, behaviors, and the effectiveness of communications is based on cross-sectional studies. We can ask background questions and build statistical models to predict current knowledge, attitudes, and behaviors, but we know from educational research that longitudinal studies of children, adolescents, and young adults have provided invaluable insights into the learning process that were unavailable from cross-sectional data sets. Longitudinal panel studies are expensive, but there is no substitute for the data and insights that they provide.

Fourth, we need to design studies to understand the interaction of formal schooling, changes in life circumstances, and the influence of biomedical communications. We can see from our cross-sectional analyses that access to information, trust in the source of that information, and the size of an individual's personal health schema interact to influence current decisions and behaviors. We could obtain some useful insights from the panel studies described above, but we need to explore the use of experiments and related studies to examine the influence of various kinds of messages and arguments on individual decision making. Currently, we know far more about the factors that influence an individual to buy an automobile than the factors that lead to tobacco use.

Finally, we need to study how adolescents and adults integrate information about genomic research into their more general schemas about life, illness, disease, and health. The new genetics-based biology will be able to describe the web of life that links plants, animals, and humans, and many adults will come to understand some of the universal building blocks on which all life is based. It is important to understand how adolescents and adults incorporate this information into their mental models of their origins and their prospects for the future. In the worst scenario, we might see a resurgence of eugenics, reflecting a novice's understanding of the new biology. In the best scenario, adolescents and adults might develop a deeper and more profound understanding of the biological basis of all life and its interactions with its environment. We can do more than just hope for the best—we can try to use our communications skills to improve the level of biomedical understanding in our society.

The analyses presented in this book rely on data from three primary sources: the 1993 Study of Biomedical Literacy, the 1998 U.S. Biotechnology Study, and the *Science and Engineering Indicators* studies. The questionnaire used in each of these studies is provided in this appendix.

The 1993 Study of Biomedical Literacy was conducted by the Public Opinion Laboratory (POL) located at Northern Illinois University, under the direction of Jon Miller. The study was funded by the National Institutes of Health, and asked a national sample of adults a wide range of knowledge, behavior, and attitude questions about health and biomedical matters. The study was designed to disproportionately sample African-Americans, Hispanic-Americans, and Other Americans—including an oversample of college-educated African-Americans and Hispanic-Americans—to allow for reliable estimates based on race and ethnicity. The majority of telephone interviews conducted by the study were completed by the POL, using a random-digit sample of telephone numbers. Screening interviews to obtain oversamples of African-Americans and Hispanic-Americans, as well as the interviews of college-educated African-Americans and Hispanic-Americans, were conducted by the Market Facts telephone facility in Evanston, Illinois. A total of 3111 interviews were completed between February and August of 1993. The study had a response rate of 70 percent.

The 1998 U.S. Biotechnology Study was conducted by the International Center for the Advancement of Scientific Literacy (ICASL) of the Chicago Academy of Sciences, under the direction of Jon Miller. The study was funded by the National Science Foundation and was designed to (1) repeat selected sets of items from a 1996 Eurobarometer (46.1) and (2) measure public understanding of and attitudes toward biotechnology in the United States. The study measured knowledge and attitudes about biotechnology through a combination of general questions and a set of examples of genetic modification. The interview also obtained extensive information about relative interest levels in selected issues, attentiveness to issues, and various forms of political participation. Telephone interviews were conducted between November 11, 1997, and February 14, 1998, by Market Facts. One important aspect of this study was the incorporation of a large number of open-ended questions that were collected verbatim using .WAV digital recording. The study obtained a high rate (95+ percent) from respondents for the recording of the responses, but the awareness of the recording appears to have encouraged respondents to give longer responses. The sample for the study should be viewed as a quota sample. The original design was for a probability sample with approximately 1500 cases, but the introduction of the .WAV recording technology led to a major increase in the average length of interview. Rather than trying to reduce the length of the interview schedule after approximately 500 completions, the total size of the sample was reduced to approximately 1100 respondents.

The 1999 Science and Engineering Indicators Study was conducted by the ICASL of the Chicago Academy of Sciences for the National Science Foundation. The 1999 study is the most recent in a series of studies sponsored by the National Science Foundation since 1979 for inclusion in the chapter on public attitudes in *Science and Engineering Indicators.* Telephone interviews for the 1999 study were conducted by the National Opinion Research Center (NORC) interviewing facility in Downer's Grove, Illinois, using a random-digit sample of telephone numbers. A total of 1882 interviews were conducted between March 29, 1999, and August 7, 1999. For the 1999 study, the response rate was 66 percent. The 1999 and 1997 studies used virtually identical questionnaires. The questionnaire used in the 1999 study is included in this appendix.

QUESTIONNAIRE FOR THE 1993 STUDY OF BIOMEDICAL LITERACY

Question: 0
Hello, my name is [   ]. I'm calling long distance from the Public Opinion Laboratory. We are conducting a national survey of people's opinions about current issues and your telephone number has been selected. Have you ever been interviewed for a national opinion survey before? WAIT FOR RESPONSE. As you may know, we are a university group and we have no products to sell. We are interested in your opinions on some current topics and we will treat your answers with strict confidence. IF THE RESPONDENT

WANTS MORE INFORMATION, TELL THEM THAT THEY CAN WRITE TO OFFICE OF MANAGEMENT AND BUDGET, Paperwork Reduction Project #3145–0033, Washington, DC 20503. IF RESPONDENT ASKS, TELL THEM INTERVIEW WILL LAST BETWEEN 15–25 MINUTES DEPENDING ON THEIR INTERESTS.

Question: 1
Hello, my name is [   ]. I'm calling long distance from the Public Opinion Laboratory. We are conducting a national survey of people's opinions about current issues and your telephone number has been selected. Have you ever been interviewed for a national opinion survey before? WAIT FOR RESPONSE. As you may know, we are a university group and we have no products to sell. We are interested in your opinions on some current topics and we will treat your answers with strict confidence. IF THE RESPONDENT WANTS MORE INFORMATION, TELL THEM THAT THEY CAN WRITE TO OFFICE OF MANAGEMENT AND BUDGET, Paperwork Reduction Project #3145–0033, Washington, DC 20503. IF RESPONDENT ASKS, TELL THEM INTERVIEW WILL LAST 15–25 MINUTES DEPENDING ON THEIR INTERESTS.

Question: 3
Now, to assure a cross-section of people, I need to talk to just one person who lives at this number and I need your help in selecting that person. I would like to speak to the person aged 18 or over who had the most recent birthday? What is that person's first name? ENTER NAME.

Question: 4
IF SPEAKING TO R: May we begin now? PRESS ENTER TO BEGIN. IF R IS NOT AVAILABLE, ASK: What would be the best time to call back and reach R? AND MAKE AN APPOINTMENT.

Question: 5
IF R HAS NOT HEARD INTRODUCTION: Hello, my name is [   ]. I'm calling long distance from the Public Opinion Laboratory. We are conducting a national survey of people's opinions about current issues and your telephone number has been selected. Have you ever been interviewed for a national opinion survey before? WAIT FOR RESPONSE. As you may know, we are a university group and we have no products to sell. We are interested in your opinions on some current topics and we will treat your answers with strict confidence. IF RESPONDENT WANTS MORE INFORMATION, TELL THEM THAT THEY CAN WRITE TO OFFICE OF MANAGEMENT AND BUDGET, Paperwork Reduction Project #3145–0033 Washington, DC 20503. IF RESPONDENT ASKS, TELL THEM INTERVIEW WILL LAST 15–25 MINUTES DEPENDING ON THEIR INTERESTS.

Question: 9

We need to make sure we have a representative cross-section of households in the United States, so I need to begin by asking you a few questions about yourself. First, What is the highest level of education you completed? DO NOT READ OPTIONS!

0> Grade 6 or less

1> Grade 7 through 9

2> Grade 10 or 11

3> High school diploma/GED

4> Vocational less than 2 years

5> Associate (AA, AS)

6> Baccalaureate (BA, BS)

7> Masters (MA, MS)

8> Doctorate (Ph.D., Ed.D.)

9> Professional (medical, dental, legal)

10> Other

Question: 10 Ask if Q9 > 4

In what field was the degree? ENTER EXACT RESPONSE.

Question: 11

Are you currently married, widowed, divorced, separated, or have you never been married?

1> married

2> widowed

3> divorced

4> separated

5> never married

Question: 12 Ask if Q11 ≠ 5

Do you have any children? IF YES, ASK: How many? (MAX = 20) OR ZERO FOR NONE. ENTER NUMBER OF CHILDREN

Question: 13 Ask if Q11 ≠ 5 AND Q12 > 0

Do you have any children under age 18 who currently live with you? IF YES, ASK: How many? ENTER NUMBER OF CHILDREN (MAX = 20) OR ZERO FOR NONE.

Question: 14

Are you of Spanish origin or descent?

1> yes

2> no

Question: 15 Ask if Q14 = 1
To which Hispanic group do you belong? USE FOLLOWING CODES, BUT DO NOT READ LIST.
1> Mexican, Mexican-American, Chicano
2> Puerto Rican
3> Cuban
4> Central American
5> South American
6> Other Hispanic origin

Question: 16 Ask if Q14 = 2
What race do you consider yourself? ENTER EXACT RESPONSE. IF R IS UNSURE, OR SAYS "AMERICAN," OR "HUMAN" ASK: WHICH OF THE FOL-LOWING CENSUS CATEGORIES DO YOU CONSIDER YOURSELF: BLACK, HISPANIC, WHITE/CAUCASIAN, ASIAN, OR OTHER? ENTER EXACT RE-SPONSE.

Question: 20
Let me start by asking how interested you are in current news events. Would you say that you are very interested, moderately interested, or not at all in-terested in current news events?
1> very interested
2> moderately interested
3> not at all interested

Question: 21
There are a lot of issues in the news and it is hard to keep up with every area. I'm going to read you a short list of issues and for each one—after I read it— I would like you to tell me if you are very interested, moderately interested, or not at all interested. First, local school issues. Are you very interested, moderately interested, or not at all interested?
1> very interested
2> moderately interested
3> not at all interested

Question: 22
Information about health. Are you very interested, moderately interested, or not at all interested?
1> very interested
2> moderately interested
3> not at all interested

Question: 23
Issues about new scientific discoveries. Are you very interested, moderately interested, or not at all interested?
1> very interested
2> moderately interested
3> not at all interested

Question: 24
Economic issues and business conditions. Are you very interested, moderately interested, or not at all interested?
1> very interested
2> moderately interested
3> not at all interested

Question: 25
Issues about the use of new inventions and technologies. Are you very interested, moderately interested, or not at all interested?
1> very interested
2> moderately interested
3> not at all interested

Question: 26
Issues about new medical discoveries. Are you very interested, moderately interested, or not at all interested?
1> very interested
2> moderately interested
3> not at all interested

Question: 28
Issues about environmental pollution. Are you very interested, moderately interested, or not at all interested?
1> very interested
2> moderately interested
3> not at all interested

Question: 30
Now, I'd like to go through this list with you again and for each issue I'd like you to tell me if you are very well informed, moderately well informed, or poorly informed. First, local school issues. Are you very well informed, moderately well informed, or poorly informed?
1> very well informed
2> moderately well informed
3> poorly informed

Question: 32
Information about health. Are you very well informed, moderately well informed, or poorly informed?
1> very well informed
2> moderately well informed
3> poorly informed

Question: 33
Issues about new scientific discoveries. Are you very well informed, moderately well informed, or poorly informed?
1> very well informed
2> moderately well informed
3> poorly informed

Question: 34
Economic issues and business conditions. Are you very well informed, moderately well informed, or poorly informed?
1> very well informed
2> moderately well informed
3> poorly informed

Question: 35
Issues about the use of new inventions and technologies. Are you very well informed, moderately well informed, or poorly informed?
1> very well informed
2> moderately well informed
3> poorly informed

Question: 36
Issues about new medical discoveries. Are you very well informed, moderately well informed, or poorly informed?
1> very well informed
2> moderately well informed
3> poorly informed

Question: 37
Issues about environmental pollution. Are you very well informed, moderately well informed, or poorly informed?
1> very well informed
2> moderately well informed
3> poorly informed

Question: 41
Now let me change the topic slightly and ask you how you get information. First, how often do you read a newspaper: every day, a few times a week, once a week, or less than once a week?
1> every day
2> a few times a week
3> once a week
4> less than once a week

Question: 43
Are there any magazines that you read regularly; that is, most of the time? What magazine would that be? ENTER MAGAZINE NAME.

Question: 44
IF R NAMED A MAGAZINE ON THE PREVIOUS SCREEN, ASK: Is there another magazine that you read regularly? What magazine would that be? ENTER MAGAZINE NAME. PRESS F3 IF NO MAGAZINE.

Question: 48
Do you ever read any *health* magazines? What magazine would that be? ENTER MAGAZINE NAME.

Question: 49
IF R NAMED A MAGAZINE ON THE PREVIOUS SCREEN, ASK: Do you read any other *health* magazines? What magazine would that be? PRESS F3 IF NO MAGAZINE. ENTER MAGAZINE NAME.

Question: 56
Altogether, on an average day, about how many hours would you say that you watch television? ENTER NUMBER OF HOURS (ROUND TO NEAREST WHOLE HOUR; ENTER ZERO FOR NONE; ENTER .5 FOR 30 MINUTES, ENTER .2 FOR 15 MINUTES; ENTER ZERO FOR LESS THAN 15 MINUTES)

Question: 57 Ask if Q56 > 0
About how many of those hours are news reports or news shows? ENTER NUMBER OF HOURS (ROUND TO NEAREST WHOLE HOUR; ENTER ZERO FOR NONE; ENTER .5 FOR 30 MINUTES. ENTER .2 FOR 15 MINUTES; ENTER ZERO FOR LESS THAN 15 MINUTES).

Question: 58
Altogether, on an average day, about how many hours would you say that you listen to the radio? ENTER NUMBER OF HOURS (ROUND TO NEAREST WHOLE HOUR. ENTER ZERO FOR NONE; ENTER .5 FOR 30 MINUTES;

ENTER .2 FOR 15 MINUTES; ENTER ZERO FOR LESS THAN 15 MIN-
UTES).

Question: 59 Ask if Q58 > 0
About how many of those hours are news reports or news shows? ENTER
NUMBER OF HOURS (ROUND TO NEAREST WHOLE HOUR; ENTER
ZERO FOR NONE; ENTER .5 FOR 30 MINUTES; ENTER .2 FOR 15 MIN-
UTES; ENTER ZERO FOR LESS THAN 15 MINUTES).

Question: 60
Now, let me ask you to think about news or information about health and
medicine. What is your most important source of information about health
and medicine? INTERVIEWERS: ENTER THE CODE USING THE FOL-
LOWING POSSIBILITIES, A SPACE, AND THEN THE EXACT RESPONSE.
PROBE IF R IS UNSURE: THINK OF A HEALTH PROBLEM, IF YOU WANT-
ED TO GET MORE INFORMATION, HOW WOULD YOU GET IT?
10> radio
11> television
12> newspapers
13> magazines
14> books
15> talking to other people
16> health clinics
17> social workers
18> doctors
19> nurses
20> other sources

Question: 62
What is the most important health or science information you have heard in
the last two months? ENTER EXACT RESPONSE (MAXIMUM 74 CHAR-
ACTERS).

Question: 63
How did you come to know about this information? ENTER EXACT RE-
SPONSE (MAXIMUM 74 CHARACTERS).

Question: 70
Now, let me turn to a slightly different type of question. When you read news
stories, you see certain sets of words and terms. We are interested in how
many people recognize certain kinds of terms and I would like to ask you a
few brief questions in that regard. First, some articles refer to the results of
a *scientific study*. When you read or hear the term *scientific study* do

you have a clear understanding of what it means, a general sense of what it means, or little understanding of what it means?
1> clear understanding
2> general sense
3> little understanding

Question: 71 Ask if Q70 = 1 OR Q70 = 2
In your own words, could you tell me what it means to study something *scientifically*? ENTER EXACT RESPONSE: TWO ADDITIONAL SCREENS IF NEEDED.

Question: 72 Ask if Q70 = 1 OR Q70 = 2
FIRST ADDITIONAL SCREEN IF NEEDED. ENTER F3 IF NOT NEEDED.

Question: 73 Ask if Q70 = 1 OR Q70 = 2
SECOND ADDITIONAL SCREEN IF NEEDED. ENTER F3 IF NOT NEEDED.

Question: 78
Next, in articles and on television news shows, the term DNA has been used. When you hear the term DNA, do you have a clear understanding of what it means, a general sense of what it means, or little understanding of what it means?
1> clear understanding
2> general sense
3> little understanding

Question: 79 Ask if Q78 = 1 OR Q78 = 2
Please tell me—in your own words—what is *DNA*? ENTER EXACT RESPONSE BELOW. TWO ADDITIONAL SCREENS IF NEEDED.

Question: 80 Ask if Q78 = 1 OR Q78 = 2
FIRST ADDITIONAL SCREEN IF NEEDED. ENTER F3 IF NOT NEEDED.

Question: 81 Ask if Q78 = 1 OR Q78 = 2
SECOND ADDITIONAL SCREEN IF NEEDED. ENTER F3 IF NOT NEEDED.

Question: 84
Next, *bacteria*. When you read or hear the term *bacteria*, do you have a clear understanding of what it means, a general sense of what it means, or little understanding of what it means?
1> clear understanding

2> general sense
3> little understanding

Question: 85 Ask if Q84 = 1 OR Q84 = 2
Please tell me—in your own words—what are *bacteria*? ENTER EXACT RESPONSE BELOW. TWO ADDITIONAL SCREENS IF NEEDED.

Question: 86 Ask if Q84 = 1 OR Q84 = 2
FIRST ADDITIONAL SCREEN IF NEEDED. ENTER F3 IF NOT NEEDED.

Question: 87 Ask if Q84 = 1 OR Q84 = 2
SECOND ADDITIONAL SCREEN IF NEEDED. ENTER F3 IF NOT NEEDED.

There was a split ballot on the confidence in information battery. Version A included the phrase "heart disease" Version B included the phrase "losing weight."

Confidence in Information Battery Version A

Question: 90
Earlier we talked about the sources from which you get your information about various issues. Now, I would like to ask you to tell me how much confidence or trust you would have in various kinds of information about *heart disease.* Let me read you a short list of news sources that might include some information about *heart disease,* and, for each one, I would like you to tell me if you have a high level of confidence in information from that source, a moderate level of confidence, or a low level of confidence. OK? PRESS RETURN TO GET QUESTION.

Question: 91
First, a story in your local newspaper. Would you have a high, moderate, or low level of confidence in information about heart disease from it?
1> high confidence
2> moderate confidence
3> low confidence

Question: 92
An article in *Time* or *Newsweek.* Would you have a high, moderate, or low level of confidence in information about heart disease from it?
1> high confidence
2> moderate confidence
3> low confidence

Question: 93
A story on the evening television news. Would you have a high, moderate, or low level of confidence in information about heart disease from it?
1> high confidence
2> moderate confidence
3> low confidence

Question: 95
A television talk show like the *Oprah Winfrey Show* or the *Phil Donahue Show*. Would you have a high, moderate, or low level of confidence in information about heart disease from it?
1> high confidence
2> moderate confidence
3> low confidence

Question: 96
A conversation with your physician? Would you have a high, moderate, or low level of confidence in information about heart disease from it?
1> high confidence
2> moderate confidence
3> low confidence

Question: 97
An article by a scientist? Would you have a high, moderate, or low level of confidence in information about heart disease from it?
1> high confidence
2> moderate confidence
3> low confidence

Question: 98
A report from the National Institutes of Health? Would you have a high, moderate, or low level of confidence in information about heart disease from it?
1> high confidence
2> moderate confidence
3> low confidence

Confidence in Information Battery Version B

Question: 99
Earlier we talked about the sources from which you get your information about various issues. Now, I would like to ask you to tell me how much confidence or trust you would have in various kinds of information about *losing weight.* Let me read you a short list of news sources that might include

some information about *losing weight,* and, for each one, I would like you to tell me if you have a high level of confidence in information from that source, a moderate level of confidence, or a low level of confidence. OK? PRESS RETURN TO GET QUESTION.

Question: 100
First, a story in your local newspaper. Would you have a high, moderate, or low level of confidence in information about losing weight from it?
1> high confidence
2> moderate confidence
3> low confidence

Question: 101
An article in *Time* or *Newsweek.* Would you have a high, moderate, or low level of confidence in information about losing weight from it?
1> high confidence
2> moderate confidence
3> low confidence

Question: 102
A story on the evening television news. Would you have a high, moderate, or low level of confidence in information about losing weight from it?
1> high confidence
2> moderate confidence
3> low confidence

Question: 103
A television talk show like the *Oprah Winfrey Show* or the *Phil Donahue Show.* Would you have a high, moderate, or low level of confidence in information about losing weight from it?
1> high confidence
2> moderate confidence
3> low confidence

Question: 104
A conversation with your physician? Would you have a high, moderate, or low level of confidence in information about losing weight from it?
1> high confidence
2> moderate confidence
3> low confidence

Question: 105
An article by a scientist? Would you have a high, moderate, or low level of confidence in information about losing weight from it?

1> high confidence
2> moderate confidence
3> low confidence

Question: 106
A report from the National Institutes of Health? Would you have a high, moderate, or low level of confidence in information about losing weight from it?
1> high confidence
2> moderate confidence
3> low confidence

Question: 110
Now, I would like to read you some statements. For each statement, please tell me if you generally agree or generally disagree. If you feel especially strongly about a statement, please tell me that you *strongly agree* or *strongly disagree*. OK? PRESS ENTER.

Question: 111
First, science and technology are making our lives healthier, easier, and more comfortable. Do you strongly agree, agree, disagree, or strongly disagree?
1> strongly agree
2> agree
3> disagree
4> strongly disagree

Question: 112
The fact that scientists repeat and check each other's work, effectively prevents fraud or cheating by scientists. Do you strongly agree, agree, disagree, or strongly disagree?
1> strongly agree
2> agree
3> disagree
4> strongly disagree

Question: 115
We depend too much on science and not enough on faith. Do you strongly agree, agree, disagree, or strongly disagree?
1> strongly agree
2> agree
3> disagree
4> strongly disagree

Question: 116
Even if it brings no immediate benefits, scientific research which advances the frontiers of knowledge is necessary and should be supported by the federal government. Do you strongly agree, agree, disagree, or strongly disagree?
1> strongly agree
2> agree
3> disagree
4> strongly disagree

Question: 118
Scientists should be allowed to do research that causes pain and injury to animals like dogs and chimpanzees *if* it produces new information about human health problems. Do you strongly agree, agree, disagree, or strongly disagree?
1> strongly agree
2> agree
3> disagree
4> strongly disagree

Question: 119
It is not important for me to know about science in my daily life. Do you strongly agree, agree, disagree, or strongly disagree?
1> strongly agree
2> agree
3> disagree
4> strongly disagree

Question: 120
Some numbers are especially lucky for some people. Do you strongly agree, agree, disagree, or strongly disagree?
1> strongly agree
2> agree
3> disagree
4> strongly disagree

Question: 121
Science makes our way of life change too fast. Do you strongly agree, agree, disagree, or strongly disagree?
1> strongly agree
2> agree
3> disagree
4> strongly disagree

Question: 125
Many scientists make up or falsify research results to advance their careers
or make money. Do you strongly agree, agree, disagree, or strongly disagree?
1> strongly agree
2> agree
3> disagree
4> strongly disagree

Question: 129
New inventions will always be found to counteract any harmful consequences of technological development. Do you strongly agree, agree, disagree, or strongly disagree?
1> strongly agree
2> agree
3> disagree
4> strongly disagree

Question: 130
Most scientists want to work on things that will make life better for the average person. Do you strongly agree, agree, disagree, or strongly disagree?
1> strongly agree
2> agree
3> disagree
4> strongly disagree

Question: 134
Of all the people who are alcoholic in the United States, the greatest number come from among those who are *both* poor and unemployed. Do you
strongly agree, agree, disagree, or strongly disagree?
1> strongly agree
2> agree
3> disagree
4> strongly disagree

Question: 138
Now, for a different type of question. People have frequently noted that scientific research has produced both beneficial and harmful consequences.
Would you say that, on balance, the benefits of scientific research have outweighed the harmful results, *or* have the harmful results of scientific research been greater than its benefits?
1> beneficial results greater
2> about equal
3> harmful results greater

Question: 139 Ask if Q138 = 1
Would you say that the balance has been strongly in favor of beneficial results, or only slightly?
1> strongly
2> only slightly

Question: 140 Ask if Q138 = 3
Would you say that the balance has been strongly in favor of harmful results,
or only slightly?
1> strongly
2> only slightly

Question: 141
Thinking back over the last 10 years—that is, since 1983—what do you think
was the most important medical discovery or achievement in the United
States? ENTER EXACT RESPONSE BELOW.

Question: 152
Now, please think about this situation. Two scientists want to know if a certain drug is effective against high blood pressure. The first scientist wants to
give the drug to 1000 people with high blood pressure and see how many of
them experience lower blood pressure levels. The second scientist wants to
give the drug to 500 people with high blood pressure, and not give the drug
to another 500 people with high blood pressure, and see how many in both
groups experience lower blood pressure levels. Which is the better way to
test this drug?
1> First scientist—all 1000 get drug
2> Second scientist—500 get drug, 500 don't get drug

Question: 153
Why is it better to test the drug this way? ENTER EXACT RESPONSE (CON-
TINUE ON NEXT TWO SCREENS IF NECESSARY).

Question: 154
RESPONSE CONTINUES (PRESS ENTER IF SCREEN NOT NEEDED).

Question: 155
RESPONSE CONTINUES (PRESS ENTER IF SCREEN NOT NEEDED).

Question: 170
Now, let me ask you to think about the long-term future. I am going to read
you a list of possible results and ask you how likely you think it is that each
of these results will occur in the next 25 years or so. First, *the accidental

release of a dangerous man-made organism that could contaminate the environment?* Do you think that it is very likely, possible but not too likely, or not at all likely that this result will occur within the next 25 years?
1> very likely
2> possible but not too likely
3> not at all likely

Question: 171
Next, the development of medical technologies that will extend the average age of Americans to approximately 90 years. Do you think it is very likely, possible but not too likely, or not at all likely that this result will occur within the next 25 years?
1> very likely
2> possible but not too likely
3> not at all likely

Question: 172
A major nuclear power plant accident? Do you think it is very likely, possible but not too likely, or not at all likely that this result will occur within the next 25 years?
1> very likely
2> possible but not too likely
3> not at all likely

Question: 173
A cure for the common forms of cancer. Do you think it is very likely, possible but not too likely, or not at all likely that this result will occur within the next 25 years?
1> very likely
2> possible but not too likely
3> not at all likely

Question: 176
A vaccine for the disease AIDS. Do you think it is very likely, possible but not too likely, or not at all likely that this result will occur within the next 25 years?
1> very likely
2> possible but not too likely
3> not at all likely

Question: 177
A significant deterioration in the quality of our environment. Do you think that it is very likely, possible but not too likely, or not at all likely that this result will occur within the next 25 years?

1> very likely
2> possible but not too likely
3> not at all likely

Question: 183
Now, I would like to ask you a few short quiz-type questions like you might see on a television game show. For each statement that I read, please tell me if it is true or false. If you don't know or aren't sure, just tell me so and we will skip to the next question. Remember: true, false, or don't know.

Question: 185
The oxygen we breathe comes from plants. Is that true or false?
1> true
2> false

Question: 186
DNA regulates inherited characteristics for all plants and animals. Is that true or false?
1> true
2> false

Question: 187
Human beings can survive on almost any combination of foods, provided that the total diet includes enough calories. Is that true or false?
1> true
2> false

Question: 188
The body's immune system protects us from bacteria as well as viruses. Is that true or false?
1> true
2> false

Question: 189
Senility is inevitable as the brain ages and loses tissue. Is that true or false?
1> true
2> false

Question: 190
Brain damage may occur in persons with AIDS. Is that true or false?
1> true
2> false

Question: 191
All bacteria are harmful to humans. Is that true or false?
1> true
2> false

Question: 192
Chemical addiction to a substance, like drugs or alcohol, is a sign of personal *moral failure*, rather than a disease. Is that true or false?
1> true
2> false

Question: 195
Having several alcoholic drinks within 30 minutes makes you act strange because the alcohol reduces the ability of your blood to carry oxygen to your brain. Is that true or false?
1 > true
2> false

Question: 196
In general, to be effective, a vaccine must be administered before an infection occurs. Is that true or false?
1> true
2> false

Question: 204
Human beings, as we know them today, developed from earlier species of animals. Is that true or false?
1> true
2> false

Question: 205
Intelligence *in humans* is related to the size of the brain. Is that true or false?
1> true
2> false

Question: 208
The human immune system has no defense against viruses. Is that true or false?
1> true
2> false

Question: 209
The process of evolution is continuing today. Is that true or false?

1> true
2> false

There was a split ballot on the probability battery to test for question-order effects.

Probability Battery—Version A

Question: 212
Now, think about this situation. A doctor tells a couple that their *genetic makeup* means that they've got *one in four chances* of having a child with an inherited illness. Does this mean that each of the couple's children will have the same risk of suffering from the illness?
1> yes
2> no

Question: 213
Does this mean that if their first child has the illness, the next three will not?
1> yes
2> no

Question: 214
Does this mean that if their first three children are healthy, the fourth will have the illness?
1> yes
2> no

Question: 215
Does this mean that if they only have three children, none will have the illness?
1> yes
2> no

Probability Battery—Version B

Question: 216
Now, think about this situation. A doctor tells a couple that their *genetic makeup* means that they've got *one in four chances* of having a child with an inherited illness. Does this mean that if their first three children are healthy, the fourth will have the illness?
1> yes
2> no

Question: 217
Does this mean that if their first child has the illness, the next three will not?
1> yes
2> no

Question: 218
Does this mean that each of the couple's children will have the same risk of suffering from the illness?
1> yes
2> no

Question: 219
Does this mean that if they have only three children, none will have the illness?
1> yes
2> no

Question: 220
Would you say that astrology is very scientific, sort of scientific, or not at all scientific?
1> Very scientific
2> Sort of scientific
3> Not at all scientific

Question: 243 Ask if Q9 > 1
Now, let me ask you to think about some of the courses you took in high school. What was the highest level of math that you completed in high school? DO NOT READ OPTIONS!
0> no math in HS; didn't go to HS
1> general math, business or vocational math
2> pre-algebra
3> one year of algebra
4> two years of algebra
5> geometry (plane or solid or both)
6> trigonometry/linear programming/analysis
7> pre-calculus
8> calculus
9> statistics/probability
10> Other

Question: 244 Ask if Q243 = 10
ENTER OTHER MATH CLASS HERE. PROBE FOR SUBJECT MATTER IF NECESSARY.

Question: 245 Ask if Q9 > 1
Did you take a high school biology course?
1> yes
2> no

Question: 246 Ask if Q9 > 1
Did you take a high school chemistry course?
1> yes
2> no

Question: 247 Ask if Q9 > 1
Did you take a high school physics course?
1> yes
2> no

Question: 248 Ask if Q9 > 2
Have you ever taken any college-level science courses? IF YES: How many?
ENTER NUMBER OF COURSES OR ZERO FOR NONE. MAXIMUM 50.

Question: 250
Last week, were you working full-time, working part-time, going to school or
what? IF R SAYS GOING TO SCHOOL AND WORKING, PROBE FOR WHICH
ONE R THINKS IS MOST IMPORTANT.
1> working full-time
2> working part-time
3> has job, but on vacation or strike
4> retired
5> unemployed, laid off, or looking for work
6> in school (full-time)
7> keeping house
8> other, disabled, not looking for work

Question: 251 Ask if Q250 > 0 AND Q250 < 5
What kind of work do/did you normally do? What is/was your job called? DE-
SCRIBE OCCUPATION BELOW (40 chars max). PROBE FOR FUNCTIONS
AND DUTIES.

Question: 252 Ask if Q250 > 0 AND Q250 < 4
Are you employed by a unit of government, a private corporation, or are you
self-employed?
1> a unit of government
2> a private corporation
3> self-employed
4> other

Question: 255 Ask if Q250 > 0 AND Q250 < 5
Does/did the organization or firm for which you work conduct or sponsor any scientific or technological research?
1> yes
2> no

Question: 258
Are you currently enrolled in school?
1> yes
2> no

Question: 259 Ask if Q258 = 1
What program are you enrolled in? PROBE IF NECESSARY: WHAT DEGREE OR CERTIFICATE DO YOU EXPECT TO EARN? ENTER EXACT RESPONSE (MAXIMUM 74 CHARS).

Question: 265
Do you have any chronic or continuing illness?
1> yes
2> no

Question: 266 Ask if Q11 = 1
Does your husband/wife have any chronic or continuing illness?
1> yes
2> no

Question: 267 Ask if Q13 > 0
Do any of your children *who live at home* have a chronic or continuing illness?
1> yes
2> no

Question: 268
Now, please think about your own health. Using a thermometer, if 10 stands for perfect health and zero stands for very poor health, how would you rate your own health? ENTER NUMBER BETWEEN ZERO AND 10.

Question: 269 Ask if Q11 = 1
How would you rate your husband's/wife's health? ENTER NUMBER BETWEEN ZERO AND TEN.

Question: 270 Ask if Q13 > 0
Using the same thermometer, how would you rate the overall health of your children *who live at home*? ENTER NUMBER BETWEEN ZERO AND TEN.

Question: 274
What is the ZIP code of your residence? ENTER ZIP CODE BELOW (5 DIG-ITS ONLY). IF R ASKS WHY WE WANT TO KNOW EXPLAIN WE WILL NOT ASK FOR THEIR EXACT STREET ADDRESS, WE ARE JUST LOOKING FOR SOME GENERAL INFORMATION ABOUT THE TYPE OF AREA THEY LIVE IN.

Question: 275
Do you live in a city, town, or village, or do you live in an *unincorporated* area?
1> city, town, or village
2> unincorporated area

Question: 276 Ask if Q275 = 1
What is the name of your city, town, or village? ASK FOR SPELLING IF UN-CERTAIN. ENTER NAME (40 CHARS MAX).

Question: 277
How many adults 18 years of age or older regularly live in your home? EN-TER NUMBER OF ADULTS.

Question: 278
In what year were you born? ENTER ALL FOUR DIGITS OF BIRTH YEAR. IF R WON'T GIVE EXACT YEAR, ASK FOR DECADE, AND ENTER MID-POINT. EXAMPLE: 1940s IS ENTERED AS 1945.

Question: 279 Ask if Q14 = 1
What race do you consider yourself? ENTER EXACT RESPONSE. IF R IS UNSURE, OR SAYS "AMERICAN", ASK: WHICH OF THE FOLLOWING CEN-SUS CATEGORIES DO YOU CONSIDER YOURSELF: BLACK, HISPANIC, WHITE/CAUCASIAN, ASIAN, OR OTHER? ENTER EXACT RESPONSE.

Question: 280
In what country were you born? ENTER EXACT RESPONSE (40 CHARS MAX). IF R WAS BORN IN THIS COUNTRY ENTER USA.

Question: 281
IF RESPONDENT WAS BORN IN UNITED STATES ASK THIS QUESTION, OTHERWISE PRESS F3: About how many miles would you say that you cur-rently live from the place that you were born? ENTER NUMBER OF MILES. IF RESPONDENT SAYS THEY LIVE IN THE SAME LOCATION, ENTER ZERO.

Question: 282
IF RESPONDENT WAS BORN OUTSIDE THE UNITED STATES ASK THIS
QUESTION, OTHERWISE PRESS F3: At what age did you come to the United States? ENTER AGE.

Question: 284
This completes our interview. Thank you for taking the time to talk with me.
Have a good day/evening. CODE RESPONDENT GENDER. ASK ONLY IF
UNSURE. "I HAVE TO READ EVERY QUESTION ON MY SCREEN AND
NOW MY COMPUTER WANTS ME TO ASK IF YOU ARE MALE OR FE-
MALE."
1> Male
2> Female

QUESTIONNAIRE FOR THE 1998
U.S. BIOTECHNOLOGY STUDY

Hello, my name is _____. I'm calling long distance for the Chicago Academy
of Sciences. We are conducting a national survey of people's opinions about
some current issues in the news, and your telephone number has been selected. Have you ever been interviewed for a national opinion survey before?
WAIT FOR RESPONSE.

**(LISTED SAMPLE ONLY SAY: Do you recall receiving a letter in the
past few days from the Chicago Academy of Sciences describing this
study?)**

We are interested in learning more about the attitudes of citizens on several important issues and we have no products to sell. We would like to talk to
one person in this household. We will treat your answers with strict confidence.

Now, I would like to speak to the person aged 18 or over who had the most
recent birthday. What is that person's first name? ENTER NAME.

May I speak to NAME? IF NAME IS NOT AVAILABLE, ASK: What would be
the best time to call back and reach [NAME]? AND MAKE AN APPOINT-
MENT.

IF R HAS NOT HEARD INTRODUCTION: Hello, my name is _____. I'm calling long distance for the Chicago Academy of Sciences. We are conducting a
national survey of people's opinions about some current issues in the news,

and your telephone number has been selected. We are interested in learning more about the attitudes of citizens on several important issues and we have no products to sell. Have you ever been interviewed for a national opinion survey before? WAIT FOR RESPONSE.

We will treat your answers with strict confidence. This interview will take between 15 and 25 minutes, depending largely on your answers. May we begin now? MAKE APPOINTMENT IF NECESSARY.

Question: 6
Let me start by asking how interested you are in current news events. Would you say that you are very interested, moderately interested, or not at all interested in current news events?
1> very interested
2> moderately interested
3> not at all interested

Question: 7
There are a lot of issues in the news, and it is hard to keep up with every area. I'm going to read you a short list of issues, and for each one—as I read it—I would like you to tell me if you are very interested, moderately interested, or not at all interested. First, agricultural and farm issues. Are you very interested, moderately interested, or not at all interested?
1> very interested
2> moderately interested
3> not at all interested

Question: 8
Economic issues and business conditions. Are you very interested, moderately interested, or not at all interested?
1> very interested
2> moderately interested
3> not at all interested

Question: 9
Issues about new scientific discoveries. Are you very interested, moderately interested, or not at all interested?
1> very interested
2> moderately interested
3> not at all interested

Question: 10
Issues about the use of new inventions and technologies. Are you very interested, moderately interested, or not at all interested?

1> very interested
2> moderately interested
3> not at all interested

Question: 11
Issues about new medical discoveries. Are you very interested, moderately interested, or not at all interested?
1> very interested
2> moderately interested
3> not at all interested

Question: 12
Issues about environmental pollution. Are you very interested, moderately interested, or not at all interested?
1> very interested
2> moderately interested
3> not at all interested

Question: 13
Issues about the quality and cost of health care services. Are you very interested, moderately interested, or not at all interested?
1> very interested
2> moderately interested
3> not at all interested

Question: 14
Now, I'd like to go through this list with you again, and for each issue I'd like you to tell me if you are very well informed, moderately well informed, or poorly informed. First, agricultural and farm issues. Are you very well informed, moderately well informed, or poorly informed?
1> very well informed
2> moderately well informed
3> poorly informed

Question: 15
Economic issues and business conditions. Are you very well informed, moderately well informed, or poorly informed?
1> very well informed
2> moderately well informed
3> poorly informed

Question: 16
Issues about new scientific discoveries. Are you very well informed, moderately well informed, or poorly informed?

1> very well informed
2> moderately well informed
3> poorly informed

Question: 17
Issues about the use of new inventions and technologies. Are you very well informed, moderately well informed, or poorly informed?
1> very well informed
2> moderately well informed
3> poorly informed

Question: 18
Issues about new medical discoveries. Are you very well informed, moderately well informed, or poorly informed?
1> very well informed
2> moderately well informed
3> poorly informed

Question: 19
Issues about environmental pollution. Are you very well informed, moderately well informed, or poorly informed?
1> very well informed
2> moderately well informed
3> poorly informed

Question: 20
Issues about the quality and cost of health care services. Are you very well informed, moderately well informed, or poorly informed?
1> very well informed
2> moderately well informed
3> poorly informed

Question: 21
Now let me change the topic slightly and ask you how you get information. First, how often do you read a newspaper: every day, a few times a week, once a week, or less than once a week? IF THE RESPONDENT ASKS IF IT COUNTS IF THEY READ THE NEWSPAPER ON THE WEB, SAY "YES"
1> every day
2> a few times a week
3> once a week
4> less than once a week (ENTER IF R SAYS THEY NEVER READ THE NEWSPAPER)

Question: 22

Are there any magazines that you read regularly, that is, most of the time? What magazine would that be? ENTER MAGAZINE NAME. IF THE RESPONDENT ASKS IF IT COUNTS IF THEY READ A MAGAZINE ON THE WEB, SAY "YES."

Question: 23

IF R NAMED A MAGAZINE ON THE PREVIOUS SCREEN, ASK: Is there another magazine that you read regularly? What magazine would that be? ENTER MAGAZINE NAME. IF THE RESPONDENT ASKS IF IT COUNTS IF THEY READ A MAGAZINE ON THE WEB, SAY "YES."

Question: 24

IF R NAMED A MAGAZINE ON THE PREVIOUS SCREEN, ASK: Is there another magazine that you read regularly? What magazine would that be? ENTER MAGAZINE NAME. IF THE RESPONDENT ASKS IF IT COUNTS IF THEY READ A MAGAZINE ON THE WEB, SAY "YES."

Question: 25

Are there any health or science magazines that you read regularly, that is most of the time? What magazine would that be? ENTER MAGAZINE NAME. IF THE RESPONDENT ASKS IF IT COUNTS IF THEY READ A MAGAZINE ON THE WEB, SAY "YES." IF A RESPONDENT SAYS "I JUST TOLD YOU A HEALTH OR SCIENCE MAGAZINE" JUST TYPE IN "SEE EARLIER RESPONSE" AND GO TO THE NEXT QUESTION.

Question: 26

IF R NAMED A MAGAZINE ON THE PREVIOUS SCREEN, ASK: Is there another health or science magazine that you read regularly? What magazine would that be? ENTER MAGAZINE NAME IF THE RESPONDENT ASKS IF IT COUNTS IF THEY READ A MAGAZINE ON THE WEB, SAY "YES."

Question: 27

IF R NAMED A MAGAZINE ON THE PREVIOUS SCREEN, ASK: Is there another health or science magazine that you read regularly? What magazine would that be? ENTER MAGAZINE NAME. IF THE RESPONDENT ASKS IF IT COUNTS IF THEY READ A MAGAZINE ON THE WEB, SAY "YES."

Question: 28

Do you subscribe to any health newsletters? IF YES: Which health newsletter is that? ENTER NEWSLETTER NAME.

Question: 45

Now, let me ask you a different kind of question. Science and technology change the way we live. I am going to read out a list of areas in which new technologies are currently developing. For each of these areas, do you think it will improve our way of life in the next 20 years, it will have no effect, or it will make things worse? First, solar energy. Do you think solar energy will improve our way of life in the next 20 years, have no effect, or make things worse?

1> Improve our way of life
2> Have no effect
3> Make things worse

Question: 46

Do you think computers and information technology will improve our way of life in the next 20 years, have no effect, or make things worse?

1> Improve our way of life
2> Have no effect
3> Make things worse

There was a split ballot on question 47. Half of the sample was asked about "biotechnology," while the other half was asked about "genetic engineering."

Question: 47

Do you think biotechnology [genetic engineering] will improve our way of life in the next 20 years, have no effect, or make things worse?

1> Improve our way of life
2> Have no effect
3> Make things worse

Question: 48

Do you think telecommunications will improve our way of life in the next 20 years, have no effect, or make things worse?

1> Improve our way of life
2> Have no effect
3> Make things worse

Question: 49

Do you think space exploration will improve our way of life in the next 20 years, have no effect, or make things worse?

1> Improve our way of life
2> Have no effect
3> Make things worse

Question: 50
You've just indicated to what degree you think various new technologies will change the way we live. Now, I would like to ask you what comes to mind when you think about modern biotechnology in a broad sense, that is including genetic engineering. Before you answer, let me ask you if I might use my computer to record your exact answer, rather than having me try to type it as you speak. Since my typing is a lot slower than your speaking, this will allow me to capture your answer more accurately. It is all right to record this answer?
1> Yes [**activate Wave recording**]
2> No

Question: 51
Now, let me ask you again what comes to mind when you think about modern biotechnology in a broad sense, that is including genetic engineering. INTERVIEWER: PROMPT "ANYTHING ELSE?" AFTER EACH PHRASE; WRITE VERBATIMS IN FULL IF NOT RECORDING.
INTERVIEWER: AFTER COMPLETION OF RESPONSE TO Q51, TELL RESPONDENT: For the rest of this survey, we are using the term modern biotechnology in a broad sense to include genetic engineering.

Question: 52
Over the last three months, have you heard or read anything about issues involving modern biotechnology?
1> Yes
3> No

Question: 53 Ask if Q52 = 1
What did you hear or read about modern biotechnology? ENTER EXACT RESPONSE.

Question: 54 Ask if Q52 = 1
How did you come to know about this information? ENTER THE FIRST RESPONSE.
01 library
02 newspaper
03 magazine
04 book, other printed (includes encyclopedias)
05 television or radio
06 government agency
07 family member

08 friend or colleague
09 Internet or World Wide Web
10 Computer CD-ROM
11 Computer in general
12 College or other school
13 Museum
14 Other

Question: 55 Ask if Q52 = 1
If you wanted to learn more about this topic, how would you get more information? ENTER THE FIRST RESPONSE.
01 library
02 newspaper
03 magazine
04 book, other printed (includes encyclopedias)
05 television or radio
06 government agency
07 family member
08 friend or colleague
09 Internet or World Wide Web
10 computer CD-ROM
11 computer in general
12 college or other school
13 museum
14 other

Question: 56 Ask if didn't mention Dolly in above questions
Have you heard or read about the cloning of a sheep named Dolly in Scotland?
1> Yes
2> No

Question: 57
Now, let me turn to a slightly different type of question. When you read news stories, you see certain sets of words and terms. We are interested in how many people recognize certain kinds of terms, and I would like to ask you a few brief questions in that regard. In articles and on television news shows, the term DNA has been used. When you hear the term DNA, do you have a clear understanding of what it means, a general sense of what it means, or little understanding of what it means?
1> clear understanding
2> general sense
3> little understanding

Question: 58a Ask if Q57 = 1 or Q57 = 2
Now, I'm going to ask you to tell me, in your own words, what is DNA? Before you begin, I need to ask you if the computer can record your exact response to this question, and to similar questions that would require me to type your exact response. This recording will be used to allow our data editors to classify your response, and your confidentiality is assured. May I use my computer's digital recorder for this and similar open-ended responses?
1> Yes
2> No

Question: 58b **[Use Wave recording if Q58a = 1]**
Now, please tell me, in your own words, what is DNA?
ENTER EXACT RESPONSE. DO NOT PROBE FOR ADDITIONAL INFORMATION

Question: 59
Next, when you read or hear the term molecule, do you have a clear understanding of what it means, a general sense of what it means, or little understanding of what it means?
1> clear understanding
2> general sense
3> little understanding

Question: 60a Ask if Q57 = 3 and (Q59 is 1 or 2)
Now, I'm going to ask you to tell me, in your own words, what is a molecule? Before you begin, I need to ask you if the computer can record your exact response to this question, and to similar questions that would require me to type your exact response. This recording will be used to allow our data editors to classify your response, and your confidentiality is assured. May I use my computer's digital recorder for this and similar open-ended responses?
1> Yes
2> No

Question: 60b Ask if Q59 = 1 or Q59 = 2 **[Use Wave recording if Q58a = 1 or Q60A 5 1]**
Please tell me, in your own words, what is a molecule?
ENTER EXACT RESPONSE. DO NOT PROBE FOR ADDITIONAL INFORMATION.

Question: 68
Now I am going to read you a list of applications which may come out of modern biotechnology. For each one, please tell me whether you have heard of

the application, then let me know whether you definitely agree, tend to agree, tend to disagree, or definitely disagree with the questions that follow. First, have you heard of using modern biotechnology in the production of food and drinks, for example, to make them higher in protein, keep longer, or taste better?
1> Yes
2> No

Question: 69
The use of modern biotechnology in the production of food and drinks is useful for society. Do you definitely agree, tend to agree, tend to disagree, or definitely disagree?
1> Definitely agree
2> Tend to agree
3> Tend to disagree
4> Definitely disagree

Question: 70
The use of modern biotechnology in the production of food and drinks is risky for society. Do you definitely agree, tend to agree, tend to disagree, or definitely disagree?
1> Definitely agree
2> Tend to agree
3> Tend to disagree
4> Definitely disagree

Question: 71
The use of modern biotechnology in the production of food and drinks is morally acceptable for society. Do you definitely agree, tend to agree, tend to disagree, or definitely disagree?
1> Definitely agree
2> Tend to agree
3> Tend to disagree
4> Definitely disagree

Question: 72
All in all, the use of modern biotechnology in the production of food and drinks should be encouraged. Do you definitely agree, tend to agree, tend to disagree, or definitely disagree?
1> Definitely agree
2> Tend to agree
3> Tend to disagree
4> Definitely disagree

Question: 73
Next, have you heard of using biotechnology to insert genes from one plant into a crop plant to make it more resistant to insect pests?
1> Yes
2> No

Question: 74
Using biotechnology to insert genes from one plant into a crop plant is useful for society. Do you definitely agree, tend to agree, tend to disagree, or definitely disagree?
1> Definitely agree
2> Tend to agree
3> Tend to disagree
4> Definitely disagree

Question: 75
Using biotechnology to insert genes from one plant into a crop plant is risky for society. Do you definitely agree, tend to agree, tend to disagree, or definitely disagree?
1> Definitely agree
2> Tend to agree
3> Tend to disagree
4> Definitely disagree

Question: 76
Using biotechnology to insert genes from one plant into a crop plant is morally acceptable for society. Do you definitely agree, tend to agree, tend to disagree, or definitely disagree?
1> Definitely agree
2> Tend to agree
3> Tend to disagree
4> Definitely disagree

Question: 77
All in all, using biotechnology to insert genes from one plant into a crop plant should be encouraged. Do you definitely agree, tend to agree, tend to disagree, or definitely disagree?
1> Definitely agree
2> Tend to agree
3> Tend to disagree
4> Definitely disagree

Question: 78
Next, have you heard of using biotechnology to introduce human genes into bacteria to produce medicines and vaccines, for example, the production of insulin for people with diabetes?
1> Yes
2> No

Question: 79
Using biotechnology to introduce human genes into bacteria to produce medicines and vaccines is useful for society. Do you definitely agree, tend to agree, tend to disagree, or definitely disagree?
1> Definitely agree
2> Tend to agree
3> Tend to disagree
4> Definitely disagree

Question: 80
Using biotechnology to introduce human genes into bacteria to produce medicines and vaccines is risky for society. Do you definitely agree, tend to agree, tend to disagree, or definitely disagree?
1> Definitely agree
2> Tend to agree
3> Tend to disagree
4> Definitely disagree

Question: 81
Using biotechnology to introduce human genes into bacteria to produce medicines and vaccines is morally acceptable for society. Do you definitely agree, tend to agree, tend to disagree, or definitely disagree?
1> Definitely agree
2> Tend to agree
3> Tend to disagree
4> Definitely disagree

Question: 82
All in all, using biotechnology to introduce human genes into bacteria to produce medicines and vaccines should be encouraged. Do you definitely agree, tend to agree, tend to disagree, or definitely disagree?
1> Definitely agree
2> Tend to agree
3> Tend to disagree
4> Definitely disagree

Question: 88
Next, have you heard of using biotechnology to introduce human genes into animals to produce organs for human transplants, such as pigs for human hearts?
1> Yes
2> No

Question: 89
Using biotechnology to introduce human genes into animals to produce organs for human transplants is useful for society. Do you definitely agree, tend to agree, tend to disagree, or definitely disagree?
1> Definitely agree
2> Tend to agree
3> Tend to disagree
4> Definitely disagree

Question: 90
Using biotechnology to introduce human genes into animals to produce organs for human transplants is risky for society. Do you definitely agree, tend to agree, tend to disagree, or definitely disagree?
1> Definitely agree
2> Tend to agree
3> Tend to disagree
4> Definitely disagree

Question: 91
Using biotechnology to introduce human genes into animals to produce organs for human transplants is morally acceptable for society. Do you definitely agree, tend to agree, tend to disagree, or definitely disagree?
1> Definitely agree
2> Tend to agree
3> Tend to disagree
4> Definitely disagree

Question: 92
All in all, using biotechnology to introduce human genes into animals to produce organs for human transplants should be encouraged. Do you definitely agree, tend to agree, tend to disagree, or definitely disagree?
1> Definitely agree
2> Tend to agree
3> Tend to disagree
4> Definitely disagree

Question: 93
Next, have you heard of using genetic testing to determine whether an unborn child has a genetic predisposition for a serious disease such as cystic fibrosis?
1> Yes
2> No

Question: 94
Using genetic testing to determine whether an unborn child has a genetic predisposition for a serious disease is useful for society. Do you definitely agree, tend to agree, tend to disagree, or definitely disagree?
1> Definitely agree
2> Tend to agree
3> Tend to disagree
4> Definitely disagree

Question: 95
Using genetic testing to determine whether an unborn child has a genetic predisposition for a serious disease is risky for society. Do you definitely agree, tend to agree, tend to disagree, or definitely disagree?
1> Definitely agree
2> Tend to agree
3> Tend to disagree
4> Definitely disagree

Question: 96
Using genetic testing to determine whether an unborn child has a genetic predisposition for a serious disease is morally acceptable for society. Do you definitely agree, tend to agree, tend to disagree, or definitely disagree?
1> Definitely agree
2> Tend to agree
3> Tend to disagree
4> Definitely disagree

Question: 97
All in all, using genetic testing to determine whether an unborn child has a genetic predisposition for a serious disease should be encouraged. Do you definitely agree, tend to agree, tend to disagree, or definitely disagree?
1> Definitely agree
2> Tend to agree
3> Tend to disagree
4> Definitely disagree

Question:103
Now I am going to read you a list of groups. For each of these groups, if they made a public statement about the safety of biotechnology, would you have a lot, some, or no trust in the statement about biotechnology. First, the American Medical Association. Would you have a lot of trust, some trust, or no trust in a statement made by the American Medical Association about biotechnology?
1> lot of trust
2> some trust
3> no trust

Question: 104
The federal Food and Drug Administration. Would you have a lot of trust, some trust, or no trust in a statement made by the Food and Drug Administration about biotechnology?
1> lot of trust
2> some trust
3> no trust

Question: 105
Scientists from a university. Would you have a lot of trust, some trust, or no trust in a statement made by scientists from a university in your own state about biotechnology?
1> lot of trust
2> some trust
3> no trust

Question: 106
Food manufacturers. Would you have a lot of trust, some trust, or no trust in a statement made by food manufacturers about biotechnology?
1> lot of trust
2> some trust
3> no trust

Question: 107
The National Institutes of Health. Would you have a lot of trust, some trust, or no trust in a statement made by the National Institutes of health about biotechnology?
1> lot of trust
2> some trust
3> no trust

Question: 108
Reporters on a television news show like *60 Minutes*. Would you have a lot of trust, some trust, or no trust in a statement made by reporters on a television news show like *60 Minutes* about biotechnology?
1> lot of trust
2> some trust
3> no trust

Question: 109
The U.S. Department of Agriculture. Would you have a lot of trust, some trust, or no trust in a statement made by the Department of Agriculture in your own state about biotechnology?
1> lot of trust
2> some trust
3> no trust

Question: 110
An article in *Time* or *Newsweek*. Would you have a lot of trust, some trust, or no trust in a statement made by an article in *Time* or *Newsweek?*
1> lot of trust
2> some trust
3> no trust

Question: 111
An article in *Consumer Reports* magazine. Would you have a lot of trust, some trust, or no trust in a statement made by an article in *Consumer Reports* magazine?
1> lot of trust
2> some trust
3> no trust

Question: 112
Now I'm going to read to you some statements such as those you might find in a newspaper or magazine article. For each statement, please tell me if you *generally agree* or *generally disagree*. If you feel especially strongly about a statement, please tell me that you *strongly agree* or *strongly disagree*. OK?

First, the interested and informed citizen can often have some influence on government policies toward science and technology if he or she is willing to make the effort. Do you strongly agree, agree, disagree, or strongly disagree?
1> strongly agree
2> agree
3> disagree
4> strongly disagree

Question: 113
Even if it brings no immediate benefits, scientific research which advances
the frontiers of knowledge is necessary and should be supported by the federal government. Do you strongly agree, agree, disagree, or strongly disagree?
1> strongly agree
2> agree
3> disagree
4> strongly disagree

Question: 114
Scientists should be allowed to do research that causes pain and injury to animals like dogs and chimpanzees if it produces new information about human
health problems. Do you strongly agree, agree, disagree, or strongly disagree?
1> strongly agree
2> agree
3> disagree
4> strongly disagree

Question: 115
Current regulations are sufficient to protect people from any risks linked to
modern biotechnology. Do you strongly agree, agree, disagree, or strongly
disagree?
1> strongly agree
2> agree
3> disagree
4> strongly disagree

Question: 116
Biotechnology will personally benefit people like me in the next five years.
Do you strongly agree, agree, disagree, or strongly disagree?
1> strongly agree
2> agree
3> disagree
4> strongly disagree

Question: 117
My family and I have already benefited from biotechnology. Do you strongly
agree, agree, disagree, or strongly disagree?
1> strongly agree
2> agree

3> disagree
4> strongly disagree

Question: 118
The Bible is the actual word of God and is to be taken literally. Do you strongly agree, agree, disagree, or strongly disagree?
1> strongly agree
2> agree
3> disagree
4> strongly disagree

Question: 119
Plants and animals exist primarily to be used by humans. Do you strongly agree, agree, disagree, or strongly disagree?
1> strongly agree
2> agree
3> disagree
4> strongly disagree

Question: 120
The regulation of biotechnology should be left mainly to industry. Do you strongly agree, agree, disagree, or strongly disagree?
1> strongly agree
2> agree
3> disagree
4> strongly disagree

Question: 121
Modern biotechnology is so complex that public involvement in the policy process is a waste of time. Do you strongly agree, agree, disagree, or strongly disagree?
1> strongly agree
2> agree
3> disagree
4> strongly disagree

Question: 122
There is a personal God who hears the prayers of individual men and women. Do you strongly agree, agree, disagree, or strongly disagree?
1>strongly agree
2>agree
3>disagree
4>strongly disagree

Question: 124
It is not worth putting special labels on genetically modified foods. Do you
strongly agree, agree, disagree, or strongly disagree?
1> strongly agree
2> agree
3> disagree
4> strongly disagree

Question: 125
Animals have rights that people should not violate. Do you strongly agree,
agree, disagree or strongly disagree.
1> strongly agree
2> agree
3> disagree
4> strongly disagree

Question: 126
Now, please tell me whether you support or oppose the use of biotechnology in agriculture and food production?
1> Support
2> Oppose

Question: 126b Ask if (Q57 = 3 and Q59 = 3) and (Q126 = 1)
Now, I'm going to ask you to tell me why you support the use of biotechnology in agriculture and food production. Before you begin, I need to ask you
if the computer can record your exact response to this question, and to one
other similar question that would require me to type your exact response.
This recording will be used to allow our data editors to classify your response,
and your confidentiality is assured. May I use my computer's digital recorder
for this and similar open-ended responses?
1> Yes
2> No

Question: 127A Ask if Q126 = 1 [**Use Wave Recording if Q126b = 1 OR
Q58A = 1 OR Q60A = 1**]
Please tell me why you support the use of biotechnology in agriculture and
food production?
DO NOT PROMPT FOR ADDITIONAL INFORMATION.

Question: 127C Ask if Q126 = 2 [**Use Wave Recording if Q58A = 1 OR
Q60A = 1**]
Please tell me why you oppose the use of biotechnology in agriculture and
food production?
DO NOT PROMPT FOR ADDITIONAL INFORMATION.

Question: 128
Do you support or oppose the use of biotechnology to develop new medicines to treat human disease?
1> Support
2> Oppose

Question: 129A Ask if Q128 = 1 [**Use Wave Recording if Q58A = 1 OR Q60A = 1 OR Q126B = 1 OR Q127B = 1**]
Please tell me why you support the use of biotechnology to develop new medicines to treat human disease. DO NOT PROMPT FOR ADDITIONAL INFORMATION.

Question: 129B Ask if Q128 = 2 [**Use Wave Recording if Q58a = 1 OR Q60A = 1 OR Q126B = 1 OR Q127B = 1**]
Please tell me why you oppose the use of biotechnology to develop new medicines to treat human disease. DO NOT PROMPT FOR ADDITIONAL INFORMATION.

Question: 130
There are differing views about whether people inherit particular characteristics, that is whether people are born with these characteristics, or whether they acquire them mainly from their upbringing, or the conditions in which they lived. I am going to read you a list of characteristics, and I would like you to tell me, for each one, whether you think it is mainly inherited or mainly the result of upbringing and living conditions. First, eye color. Is eye color mainly inherited or mainly the result of upbringing and living conditions?
1> mainly inherited
2> mainly the result of upbringing and living conditions

Question: 131
Next, intelligence. Is intelligence mainly inherited or mainly the result of upbringing and living conditions?
1> mainly inherited
2> mainly the result of upbringing and living conditions

Question: 132
A tendency to be happy. Is a tendency to be happy mainly inherited or mainly the result of upbringing and living conditions?
1> mainly inherited
2> mainly the result of upbringing and living conditions

Question: 133
Athletic abilities. Are athletic abilities mainly inherited or mainly the result of upbringing and living conditions?

1> mainly inherited
2> mainly the result of upbringing and living conditions

Question: 134
A person's attitude toward work. Is a person's attitude toward work mainly inherited or mainly the result of upbringing and living conditions?
1> mainly inherited
2> mainly the result of upbringing and living conditions

Question: 135
Finally, musical abilities. Are musical abilities mainly inherited or mainly the result of upbringing and living conditions?
1> mainly inherited
2> mainly the result of upbringing and living conditions

Question: 136
Now I am going to read you a list of things that might happen within the next 20 years as a result of modern biotechnology. For each one, please say whether you think it is likely or unlikely to happen within the next 20 years. First, substantially reducing environmental pollution. Is this likely or unlikely to happen within the next 20 years?
1> likely
2> unlikely

Question: 137
Next, creating dangerous new diseases. Is this likely or unlikely to happen within the next 20 years?
1> likely
2> unlikely

Question: 138
Substantially reducing world hunger. Is this likely or unlikely to happen within the next 20 years?
1> likely
2> unlikely

Question: 139
Reducing the range of fruits and vegetables we can get. Is this likely or unlikely to happen within the next 20 years?
1> likely
2> unlikely

Question: 140
Curing most genetic diseases. Is this likely or unlikely to happen within the next 20 years?
1> likely
2> unlikely

Question: 141
Getting more out of natural resources in Third World countries. Is this likely or unlikely to happen within the next 20 years?
1> likely
2> unlikely

Question: 142
Producing designer babies. Is this likely or unlikely to happen within the next 20 years?
1> likely
2> unlikely

Question: 143
Replacing most existing food products with new varieties. Is this likely or unlikely to happen within the next 20 years?
1> likely
2> unlikely

Question: 144
Now, let me return to a question about words and terms you may read or hear in the news. Some articles refer to the results of a **scientific study**. When you read or hear the term scientific study do you have a clear understanding of what it means, a general sense of what it means, or little understanding of what it means?
1> clear understanding
2> general sense
3> little understanding

Question: 145 Ask if Q144 = 1 or Q144 = 2 [**Use Wave Recording if Q58a = 1 OR Q60A = 1 OR Q126B = 1 OR Q127B = 1**]
In your own words, could you tell me what it means to study something scientifically?
ENTER EXACT RESPONSE. DO NOT PROBE FOR ADDITIONAL INFORMATION!

Question: 146
Now, please think about this situation. Two scientists want to know if a certain drug is effective against high blood pressure. The first scientist wants to

give the drug to a 1000 people with high blood pressure and see how many of them experience lower blood pressure levels. The second scientist wants to give the drug to 500 people with high blood pressure, and not give the drug to another 500 people with high blood pressure, and see how many in both groups experience lower blood pressure levels. Which is the better way to test this drug?

1> All 1000 get the drug
2> 500 get the drug; 500 don't

> NOTE: IF THE RESPONDENT ASKS WHETHER OR NOT A PLACEBO WAS GIVEN, SAY "IN THIS CASE, NO PLACEBO WAS GIVEN."

Question: 147 [Use Wave Recording if Q58a = 1 OR Q60A = 1 OR Q126B = 1 OR Q127B]

Why is it better to test the drug this way?
ENTER EXACT RESPONSE. DO NOT PROBE FOR ADDITIONAL INFORMATION!

Question: 148

Now, I would like to ask you a few short quiz-type questions such as you might see on a television game show. For each statement that I read, please tell me if it is true or false. If you don't know or aren't sure, just tell me so and we will skip to the next question. Remember: true, false, or don't know. First, DNA regulates inherited characteristics in all plants, animals, and humans. Is that true or false?

1> true
2> false

Question: 149

All bacteria are harmful to humans. Is that true or false?
1> true
2> false

Question: 150

Antibiotics kill viruses as well as bacteria. Is that true or false?
1> true
2> false

Question: 151

Senility is inevitable as the brain ages and loses tissue. Is that true or false?
1> true
2> false

Question: 152
Given today's biotechnology, scientists can now create new genes that never existed in nature. Is that true or false?
1> true
2> false

Question: 153
More than half of human genes are identical to those with chimpanzees. Is that true or false?
1> true
2> false

Question: 154
Viruses can be contaminated by bacteria. Is that true or false?
1> true
2> false

Question: 155
Human beings, as we know them today, developed from earlier species of animals. Is that true or false?
1> true
2> false

Question: 156
The cloning of living things produces exactly identical offspring. Is that true or false?
1> true
2> false

Question: 157
Yeast for brewing beer consists of living organisms. Is that true or false?
1> true
2> false

Question: 158
Human beings can survive on almost any combination of foods, provided that the total diet includes enough calories. Is that true or false?
1> true
2> false

Question: 159
The human immune system has no defense against viruses. Is that true or false?

1> true
2> false

Question: 160
Ordinary tomatoes do not contain genes while genetically modified tomatoes do. Is that true or false?
1> true
2> false

Question: 161
It is possible to find out in the first few months of pregnancy whether or not an unborn child will have Down's Syndrome. Is that true or false?
1> true
2> false

Question: 162
By eating a genetically modified fruit, a person's genes could also become modified. Is that true or false?
1> true
2> false

Question: 163
It is impossible to transfer animal genes into plants. Is that true or false?
1> true
2> false

Question: 164
Intelligence in humans is related to the size of the brain. Is that true or false?
1> true
2> false

Question: 165
Genetically modified animals are always bigger than ordinary ones. Is that true or false?
1> true
2> false

Question: 166
Now, think about this situation. A doctor tells a couple that their *genetic makeup* means that they've got *one in four chances* of having a child with an inherited illness. Does this mean that if their first three children are healthy, the fourth will have the illness?
1> yes
2> no

Question: 167
Does this mean that if their first child has the illness, the next three will not?
1> yes
2> no

Question: 168
Does this mean that each of the couple's children will have the same risk of suffering from the illness?
1> yes
2> no

Question: 169
Does this mean that if they have only three children, none will have the illness?
1> yes
2> no

Question: 170
We've been discussing several issues to do with modern biotechnology. Some people think these issues are very important while others don't think so. On a scale from zero to ten where zero is not at all important and ten is extremely important, how important are these issues for you personally? ENTER NUMBER.

Question: 171
Now, using the same scale, how well informed would you say you are about biotechnology, if zero means you are not at all informed about biotechnology and ten means you are very well informed about biotechnology. ENTER NUMBER.

Question: 172
Before today, had you ever talked about modern biotechnology with someone? IF YES: Had you talked about it frequently, occasionally, or only once or twice?
1> no, never
2> yes, frequently
3> yes, occasionally
4> yes, only once or twice

Question: 173
Now, let me change the subject. During the last year, have you written or spoken to any public official or legislator about any *political issue or problem?*
1> yes
2> no

Question: 174 Ask if Q173 = 1
Can you recall an issue that you made a contact about? ENTER EXACT RE-
SPONSE. IF R MENTIONS A PIECE OF LEGISLATION BY NUMBER,
PROBE FOR CONTENT OF BILL.

Question: 175   Ask if named issue on Q174
IF R NAMED AN ISSUE ON THE PREVIOUS SCREEN, ASK: Can you recall
another issue that you made a contact about? ENTER EXACT RESPONSE.

Question: 176 Ask if named issue on Q175
IF R NAMED AN ISSUE ON THE PREVIOUS SCREEN, ASK: Can you recall
another issue that you made a contact about? ENTER EXACT RESPONSE.

Question: 177
Politically speaking, would you call yourself a Democrat, a Republican, or an
independent?
1> Democrat
2> Independent
3> Republican

Question: 178 Ask if Q177 = 1
Would you call yourself a strong Democrat or not so strong?
1> strong
2> not so strong

Question: 179 Ask if Q177 = 3
Would you call yourself a strong Republican or not so strong?
1> strong
2> not so strong

Question: 180 Ask if Q177 = 2
Would you say that you lean toward the Democrats, lean toward the Republicans, or that you do not lean toward either party?
1> lean toward Democrats
2> lean toward Republicans
3> do not lean toward either

Question 181:
Are you currently registered to vote?
1> yes
2> no

Question: 182
Did you vote in the 1996 presidential election?

1> yes
2> no

Question: 183 Ask if Q182 = 1
Did you vote for Mr. Clinton, Mr. Dole, Mr. Perot, or someone else?
1> Clinton
2> Dole
3> Perot
4> Other

Question: 184
Are you currently a member of the American Association of Retired Persons, that is, the AARP?
1> Yes
2> No

Question: 185
During the last 12 months, about how many times have you attended religious services. ENTER EXACT NUMBER. IF R SAYS "NEVER" ENTER ZERO. IF R SAYS "ONCE A WEEK" ENTER 52.

Question: 186
What is your religious preference or denomination? Is it Protestant, Catholic, Jewish, some other religion, or no religion?
1> Protestant
2> Catholic
3> Jewish
4> Other
5> None

Question: 187 Ask if 186 = 1
What specific denomination is that, if any? ENTER EXACT RESPONSE.

Question: 188
Thinking of a scale from zero to ten where ten is very religious and zero is not at all religious, how religious would you say that you are? ENTER NUMBER.

Question: 189
Now, let me ask you a few brief questions about yourself. First, are you currently married, widowed, divorced, separated, or have you never been married?
1> married

2> widowed
3> divorced
4> separated
5> never married

Question: 190
How many adults 18 years of age or older regularly live in your home?
ENTER NUMBER OF ADULTS. IF THE RESPONDENT REFUSES TO IN-
DICATE HOW MANY ADULTS LIVE IN THE HOUSEHOLD READ ANY POR-
TION OF THE FOLLOWING TEXT NECESSARY TO GET A RESPONSE: I
can certainly understand your hesitation in answering this question. When
we gather information it is important to know if people of various ages, races,
levels of education, and so forth have different needs. When we run our statistics with this information they will have more meaning. I assure you that
protecting your privacy is a major concern and when the results are published they are reported as statistics and it is impossible to associate the answers directly with anyone we've talked to.

Question: 191
Do you have any children?
IF YES, ASK: How many? ENTER NUMBER OF CHILDREN OR ZERO FOR
NONE.

Question: 192 Ask if Q191 > 0
Do you have any children under age 18 who currently live with you?
IF YES, ASK: How many? ENTER NUMBER OF CHILDREN OR ZERO FOR
NONE.

Question: 193
What is the highest level of education you completed? DO NOT READ OP-
TIONS!
0> Grade 6 or less
1> Grade 7 through 9
2> Grade 10 or 11
3> High school diploma/GED
4> Vocational less than 2 years
5> Associate (AA, AS)
6> Baccalaureate (BA, BS)
7> Masters (MA, MS)
8> Doctorate (Ph.D., Ed.D.)
9> Professional (medical, dental, legal)
10> Other

IF RESPONDENT REFUSES TO GIVE HIGHEST LEVEL OF EDUCATION READ AS MUCH OF THE FOLLOWING AS POSSIBLE TO GET AN ANSWER: I can certainly understand your hesitation in answering this question. When we gather information it is important to know if people of various ages, races, levels of education, and so forth have different needs. When we run our statistics with this information they will have more meaning. I assure you that protecting your privacy is a major concern and when the results are published they are reported as statistics and it is impossible to associate the answers directly with anyone we've talked to. Into which of these groups could we categorize your responses? Would you say less than a high school diploma, you received a high school diploma/GED, or you have a baccalaureate degree or higher?

Question: 195   Ask if Q193 > 4 and not = 10
In what field was the degree? ENTER EXACT RESPONSE.

Question: 196   Ask if Q193 > 2
Have you ever taken any college-level science courses? IF YES: How many? ENTER NUMBER OF COURSES OR ZERO FOR NONE.

Question: 197   Ask if Q193 > 1
Now, let me ask you to think about the courses you took in high school. What was the highest level of math that you completed in high school? DO NOT READ OPTIONS!
0> no math in HS; didn't go to HS
1> general math, business or vocational math
2> pre-algebra
3> one year of algebra
4> two years of algebra—Algebra 2
5> geometry (plane or solid or both)
6> trigonometry/linear programming/analysis
7> pre-calculus
8> calculus
9> statistics/probability
10> Other

IF A RESPONDENT SAYS "SENIOR MATH" "MATH 2," "MATH 100," OR SOME OTHER GENERAL COURSE PLEASE ASK THEM: Would that be algebra, algebra two, geometry, trigonometry, pre-calculus, calculus, or general math?

Question: 199   Ask if Q193 > 1
Did you take a high school biology course?

1> yes
2> no

Question: 200   Ask if Q193 > 1
Did you take a high school chemistry course?
1> yes
2> no

Question: 201   Ask if Q193 > 1
Did you take a high school physics course?
1> yes
2> no

Question: 202
Are you currently enrolled in school?
1> yes
2> no

Question: 203   Ask if Q202 = 1
What program are you enrolled in? IF R JUST NAMES A SUBJECT SUCH AS
"ENGLISH" OR "MATH" ASK IF THEY EXPECT TO EARN A DEGREE, AND
IF SO, WHAT DEGREE.
1> High school diploma/GED
2> Vocational/Technical Program/Certificate
3> Associate Degree
4> Academic subject, no degree
5> Bachelor's degree
6> Master's degree
7> PhD/MD/JD
8> Personal enjoyment
9> Other

Question: 204
Last week, were you working full-time, working part-time, going to school,
or something else? IF R SAYS GOING TO SCHOOL AND WORKING, ASK
HOW MANY HOURS OF WORK PER WEEK AND CODE AS FULL-TIME (35
HOURS OR MORE) OR PART-TIME WORK.
1> working full-time
2> working part-time
3> has job, but on vacation or strike
4> retired
5> unemployed, laid off, or looking for work
6> in school (full-time)

7> keeping house
8> other, disabled, not looking for work

Question: 205   Ask if Q204 > 0 and Q204 < 5
What kind of work do/did you normally do? What is/was your job called?
DESCRIBE OCCUPATION. PROBE FOR FUNCTIONS AND DUTIES. IF THE
RESPONDENT SAYS THEY ARE "SELF-EMPLOYED" PROBE FOR FUNC-
TIONS AND DUTIES. IF THE RESPONDENT SIMPLY GIVES THE NAME
OF A COMPANY THEY WORK FOR (FOR EXAMPLE, "I WORK AT BUR
GER KING," "I WORK FOR FORD") PROBE FOR FUNCTIONS AND DU-
TIES.

Question: 206 Ask if Q204 > 0 and Q204 < 5
Are/were you employed by a unit of government, a private corporation, or
are you self-employed?
1> a unit of government
2> a private corporation
3> self-employed
4> other

Question: 207   Ask if Q204 > 0 and Q204 < 5
Does/did the organization or firm for which you work conduct or sponsor any
scientific or technological research?
1> yes
2> no

Question: 208   Ask if Q204 > 0 and Q204 < 4
Do you use a computer in your work?
1> yes
2> no

Question: 209
Do you have any pets?
1> yes
2> no

Question: 210
What is the primary language spoken in you home?
1> English
2> Spanish
3> Vietnamese
4> Chinese
5> Japanese

6> Polish
7> Other

Question: 211
Do you presently have a home computer in your household?
1> yes
2> no

Question: 212
Do you have access to the World Wide Web at home or work?
1> yes
2> no

Question: 213 Ask if Q212 = 1
During the last month, about how many hours have you spent on the Web?
ENTER NUMBER OF HOURS.

Question 216 Ask if Q212 = 1
Have you ever looked for information about health or medicine on the Internet or the World Wide Web?
1> yes
2> no

Question: 219
Do you smoke?
1> yes
2> no

Question: 220   Ask if Q219 = 1
On an average day, about how many cigarettes, cigars, or pipes do you smoke?
ENTER NUMBER. THERE ARE 20 CIGARETTES IN A PACK. IF A RESPONDENT SAYS THEY SMOKE "ONE PACK A DAY" ENTER "20." IF THEY SAY THEY SMOKE "HALF A PACK" ENTER "10."

Question: 221
What is the ZIP code of your residence? ENTER ZIP CODE BELOW (5 DIGITS ONLY).

Question: 222
Do you live in a city, town, or village, or do you live in an unincorporated area?
1> city, town, or village
2> unincorporated area

Question: 223   Ask if Q222 = 1
What is the name of your city, town, or village? ENTER NAME. ASK FOR SPELLING IF UNCERTAIN.

Question: 224
What race do you consider yourself? IF R IS UNSURE, OR SAYS "AMERI-CAN," ASK: Which of the following Census categories do you consider yourself: African American, Hispanic American, White/Caucasian, Asian or Pacific Islander, or American Indian or Alaskan Native?
1> African American
2> Hispanic American
3> White/Caucasian
3> Asian or Pacific Islander
4> American Indian/Native American
5> Alaskan Native

IF THE RESPONDENT REFUSES TO ANSWER THIS QUESTION, READ ANY PORTION OF THE FOLLOWING TEXT NECESSARY TO GET A RE-SPONSE.

I can certainly understand your hesitation in answering this question. When we gather information it is important to know if people of various ages, races, levels of education, and so forth have different needs. When we run our statistics with this information they will have more meaning. I assure you that protecting your privacy is a major concern and when the results are published they are reported as statistics and it is impossible to associate the answers directly with anyone we've talked to. Into which of these groups could we categorize your responses, African American, Hispanic American, or all other groups?

Question: 225 Ask if Q224 is not 2
Are you of Hispanic origin or descent?
1> yes
2> no

Question: 226
In what year were you born? ENTER ALL FOUR DIGITS OF BIRTH YEAR. IF R WON'T GIVE EXACT YEAR, ASK FOR DECADE, AND ENTER MID-POINT. EXAMPLE: 1940s IS ENTERED AS 1945.

IF R REFUSES TO GIVE A YEAR OF BIRTH, READ ANY PORTION OF THE FOLLOWING TEXT NECESSARY TO OBTAIN A RESPONSE:

I can certainly understand your hesitation in answering this question. When we gather information it is important to know if people of various ages, races, levels of education, and so forth have different needs. When we run our statistics with this information they will have more meaning. I assure you that protecting your privacy is a major concern and when the results are published they are reported as statistics and it is impossible to associate the answers directly with anyone we've talked to. Into which of these groups could we categorize your response? Either 18–24, 25–34, 35–44, 45–64, or 65 years of age and older?

Question: 227
This completes our interview. Thank you for taking the time to talk with me. Have a good day/evening.

CODE RESPONDENT GENDER. IF UNSURE, ASK: "I have to read every question on my screen and now my computer wants me to ask if you are male or female."
1> male
2> female

QUESTIONNAIRE FOR THE 1999 U.S. SCIENCE AND ENGINEERING INDICATORS STUDY

Question: 1
Hello, my name is _____. I'm calling for the National Science Foundation. We are a university conducting a national survey of people's opinions about some current issues in the news, and your telephone number has been selected. We have no products to sell. [IF LETTER RESPONDENT: You may recall receiving a letter from us about this study.] IF RESPONDENT REQUESTS A MAILING OR REMAIL OF THE ADVANCE LETTER:

I would like to confirm your name and address so that we can mail the letter to you. OR IF NOT AN ORIGINAL LETTER RESPONDENT: In order to mail the letter to you, I'll need your name and address.

INTERVIEWER: CONFIRM ADDRESS OR COLLECT ADDRESS IF NO ADDRESS INFORMATION IS PRESENT. IF NECESSARY BACKSPACE OVER EXISTING DATA AND ENTER CORRECTIONS. ASSUME R WILL CONTINUE WITH THE INTERVIEW. IF R WILL NOT CONTINUE, MAKE AN APPOINTMENT TO TAKE THE INTERVIEW ONE WEEK FROM TODAY.

Have you ever been interviewed for a national opinion survey before? WAIT FOR RESPONSE.

As you may know, the National Science Foundation is a part of the federal government and is responsible for supporting scientific and engineering research. We are interested in learning more about the attitudes of citizens on several important issues and we would like to talk to one person in this household. We will treat your answers with strict confidence.

IF THE RESPONDENT WANTS MORE INFORMATION, TELL THEM THAT THEY CAN WRITE TO Suzanne H. Plimpton, Division of Administrative Services, National Science Foundation, 4201 Wilson Boulevard, Arlington, VA 22230.

Question: 3
Now, I would like to speak to the person aged 18 or older who had the most recent birthday. What is that person's first name? ENTER NAME.

Question: 4
IS THIS PERSON CURRENTLY ON THE PHONE? IF NOT: May I speak to NAME? IF NAME IS NOT AVAILABLE, ASK: What would be the best time to call back and reach [NAME]? AND MAKE AN APPOINTMENT.

Question: 5 Ask if Q2 > 1
IF R HAS NOT HEARD INTRODUCTION: Hello, my name is _____. I'm calling long distance for the National Science Foundation. We are a university conducting a national survey of people's opinions about some current issues in the news, and your telephone number has been selected. We have no products to sell. [IF LETTER RESPONDENT: You may recall receiving a letter from us about this study.] Have you ever been interviewed for a national opinion survey before? WAIT FOR RESPONSE.

As you may know, the National Science Foundation is a part of the federal government and is responsible for supporting scientific and engineering research. We will treat your answers with strict confidence.

IF THE RESPONDENT WANTS MORE INFORMATION, TELL THEM THAT THEY CAN WRITE TO OFFICE OF MANAGEMENT AND BUDGET, Paperwork Reduction Project, Washington, DC 20503.

Question: 6   Ask if Q2 = 1
This interview will take between 15 and 30 minutes, depending largely on your answers. Let's begin now?

MAKE APPOINTMENT IF NECESSARY. MAKE AN APPOINTMENT TO TAKE THE INTERVIEW AS SOON AS IT IS CONVENIENT FOR THE RESPONDENT. REMIND THE RESPONDENT THAT WE CAN TAKE THE INTERVIEW IN MULTIPLE SITTINGS, THAT WE ARE OPEN FROM 9 AM TIL 10 PM, AND THAT WE CAN CALL ON THE WEEKEND. EXECUTE <CTRL><END>, UPDATE CALL NOTES AND SELECT THE APPROPRIATE OUTCOME. CONFIRM APPOINTMENT TIME AND <CTRL><END> TO SUSPEND CASE.

Question: 7
Let me start by asking how interested you are in current news events. Would you say that you are very interested, moderately interested, or not at all interested in current news events?
1> very interested
2> moderately interested
3> not at all interested

Question: 8
There are a lot of issues in the news, and it is hard to keep up with every area. I'm going to read you a short list of issues, and for each one—as I read it—I would like you to tell me if you are very interested, moderately interested, or not at all interested. First, international and foreign policy issues. Are you very interested, moderately interested, or not at all interested?
1> very interested
2> moderately interested
3> not at all interested

Question: 9
Agricultural and farm issues. Are you very interested, moderately interested, or not at all interested?
1> very interested
2> moderately interested
3> not at all interested

Question: 10
Local school issues. Are you very interested, moderately interested, or not at all interested?
1> very interested
2> moderately interested
3> not at all interested

Question: 11
Issues about new scientific discoveries. Are you very interested, moderately interested, or not at all interested?

1> very interested
2> moderately interested
3> not at all interested

Question: 12
Economic issues and business conditions. Are you very interested, moderately interested, or not at all interested?
1> very interested
2> moderately interested
3> not at all interested

Question: 13
Issues about the use of new inventions and technologies. Are you very interested, moderately interested, or not at all interested?
1> very interested
2> moderately interested
3> not at all interested

Question: 14
Issues about the use of nuclear energy to generate electricity. Are you very interested, moderately interested, or not at all interested?
1> very interested
2> moderately interested
3> not at all interested

Question: 15
Issues about new medical discoveries. Are you very interested, moderately interested, or not at all interested?
1> very interested
2> moderately interested
3> not at all interested

Question: 16
Issues about space exploration. Are you very interested, moderately interested, or not at all interested?
1> very interested
2> moderately interested
3> not at all interested

Question: 17
Issues about environmental pollution. Are you very interested, moderately interested, or not at all interested?
1> very interested

2> moderately interested
3> not at all interested

Question: 18
Issues about military and defense policy. Are you very interested, moderately interested, or not at all interested?
1> very interested
2> moderately interested
3> not at all interested

Question: 19
Now, I'd like to go through this list with you again, and for each issue I'd like you to tell me if you are very well informed, moderately well informed, or poorly informed. First, international and foreign policy issues. Are you very well informed, moderately well informed, or poorly informed?
1> very well informed
2> moderately well informed
3> poorly informed

Question: 20
Agricultural and farm issues. Are you very well informed, moderately well informed, or poorly informed?
1> very well informed
2> moderately well informed
3> poorly informed

Question: 21
Local school issues. Are you very well informed, moderately well informed, or poorly informed?
1> very well informed
2> moderately well informed
3> poorly informed

Question: 22
Issues about new scientific discoveries. Are you very well informed, moderately well informed, or poorly informed?
1> very well informed
2> moderately well informed
3> poorly informed

Question: 23
Economic issues and business conditions. Are you very well informed, moderately well informed, or poorly informed?

1> very well informed
2> moderately well informed
3> poorly informed

Question: 24
Issues about the use of new inventions and technologies. Are you very well informed, moderately well informed, or poorly informed?
1> very well informed
2> moderately well informed
3> poorly informed

Question: 25
Issues about the use of nuclear power to generate electricity. Are you very well informed, moderately well informed, or poorly informed?
1> very well informed
2> moderately well informed
3> poorly informed

Question: 26
Issues about new medical discoveries. Are you very well informed, moderately well informed, or poorly informed?
1> very well informed
2> moderately well informed
3> poorly informed

Question: 27
Issues about space exploration. Are you very well informed, moderately well informed, or poorly informed?
1> very well informed
2> moderately well informed
3> poorly informed

Question: 28
Issues about environmental pollution. Are you very well informed, moderately well informed, or poorly informed?
1> very well informed
2> moderately well informed
3> poorly informed

Question: 29
Issues about military and defense policy. Are you very well informed, moderately well informed, or poorly informed?
1> very well informed

2> moderately well informed

3> poorly informed

Question: 30

Now let me change the topic slightly and ask you how you get information. First, how often do you read a newspaper: every day, a few times a week, once a week, or less than once a week? IF RESPONDENT ASKS IF IT COUNTS IF THEY READ THE NEWSPAPER ON THE WEB, SAY YES.

1> every day

2> a few times a week

3> once a week

4> less than once a week

Question: 31

Are there any magazines that you read regularly, that is, most of the time? IF YES: What magazine would that be? ENTER MAGAZINE NAME. IF RESPONDENT ASKS IF IT COUNTS IF THEY READ A MAGAZINE ON THE WEB, SAY YES.

Question: 32

IF R NAMED A MAGAZINE ON THE PREVIOUS SCREEN, ASK: Is there another magazine that you read regularly? IF YES: What magazine would that be? ENTER MAGAZINE NAME. IF RESPONDENT ASKS IF IT COUNTS IF THEY READ A MAGAZINE ON THE WEB, SAY YES.

Question: 33

IF R NAMED A MAGAZINE ON THE PREVIOUS SCREEN, ASK: Is there another magazine that you read regularly? IF YES: What magazine would that be? ENTER MAGAZINE NAME. IF RESPONDENT ASKS IF IT COUNTS IF THEY READ A MAGAZINE ON THE WEB, SAY YES.

Question: 34

IF R NAMED A MAGAZINE ON THE PREVIOUS SCREEN, ASK: Is there another magazine that you read regularly? IF YES: What magazine would that be? ENTER MAGAZINE NAME. IF RESPONDENT ASKS IF IT COUNTS IF THEY READ A MAGAZINE ON THE WEB, SAY YES.

Question: 35

IF R NAMED A MAGAZINE ON THE PREVIOUS SCREEN, ASK: Is there another magazine that you read regularly? IF YES: What magazine would that be? ENTER MAGAZINE NAME. IF RESPONDENT ASKS IF IT COUNTS IF THEY READ A MAGAZINE ON THE WEB, SAY YES.

Question: 36
Do you ever read any science magazines? IF YES: What magazine would that be? ENTER MAGAZINE NAME. IF THE RESPONDENT ASKS IF IT COUNTS IF THEY READ A MAGAZINE ON THE WEB, SAY YES.

Question: 37
IF R NAMED A MAGAZINE ON THE PREVIOUS SCREEN, ASK: Do you read any other science magazines? IF YES: What magazine would that be? ENTER MAGAZINE NAME. IF RESPONDENT ASKS IF IT COUNTS IF THEY READ A MAGAZINE ON THE WEB, SAY YES.

Question: 38
IF R NAMED A MAGAZINE ON THE PREVIOUS SCREEN, ASK: Do you read any other science magazines? IF YES: What magazine would that be? ENTER MAGAZINE NAME. IF RESPONDENT ASKS IF IT COUNTS IF THEY READ A MAGAZINE ON THE WEB, SAY YES.

Question: 39
Altogether, on an average day, about how many hours would you say that you watch television? ENTER ZERO FOR NONE OR LESS THAN 15 MINUTES. ENTER HOURS. ENTER MINUTES.

Question: 40 Ask if Q39 > 0
About how many of those hours are news reports or news shows? ENTER ZERO FOR NONE OR LESS THAN 15 MINUTES. ENTER HOURS. ENTER MINUTES.

Question: 41
Do you have cable or satellite television service in your home?
1> yes
2> no
3> satellite TV

Question: 43
Do you watch any television shows that focus primarily on science or nature?
1> yes
2> no

Question: 44   Ask if Q43 = 1
Which science or nature show do you watch most often? ENTER EXACT RESPONSE. IF "DISCOVERY," OR "DISCOVERY CHANNEL" PROBE FOR SPECIFIC SHOW. IF R SAYS "CHANNEL 8" OR "CHANNEL 13" TRY AND PROBE FOR THE NAME OF A SPECIFIC SHOW OR TYPE OF CHANNEL.

Question: 45   Ask if Q43 = 1

About how many times a month do you watch this show? ENTER NUMBER OR ZERO IF R CAN'T NAME A SPECIFIC SHOW, OR IF R WATCHES LESS THAN ONCE A MONTH.

Question: 46   Ask if Q45 GT 0

Is there another science or nature show that you watch sometimes?
1> yes
2> no

Question: 47   Ask if Q46 = 1

What is the name of that show? ENTER EXACT RESPONSE. IF "DISCOV-ERY," OR "DISCOVERY CHANNEL" PROBE FOR SPECIFIC SHOW. IF R SAYS "CHANNEL 8" OR "CHANNEL 13" TRY AND PROBE FOR THE NAME OF A SPECIFIC SHOW OR TYPE OF CHANNEL.

Question: 48   Ask if Q46 = 1

About how many times a month do you watch this show? ENTER NUMBER OR ZERO IF R CAN'T NAME A SPECIFIC SHOW, OR IF R WATCHES LESS THAN ONCE A MONTH.

Question: 49   Ask if Q48 GT 0

Is there another science or nature show that you watch sometimes?
1> yes
2> no

Question: 50   Ask if Q49 = 1

What is the name of that show? ENTER EXACT RESPONSE. IF "DISCOV-ERY," OR "DISCOVERY CHANNEL" PROBE FOR SPECIFIC SHOW. IF R SAYS "CHANNEL 8" OR "CHANNEL 13" TRY AND PROBE FOR THE NAME OF A SPECIFIC SHOW OR TYPE OF CHANNEL.

Question: 51   Ask if Q49 = 1

About how many times a month do you watch this show? ENTER NUMBER OR ZERO IF R CAN'T NAME A SPECIFIC SHOW, OR IF R WATCHES LESS THAN ONCE A MONTH.

Question: 52

On an average day, about how many hours would you say that you listen to a radio? ENTER ZERO FOR NONE OR LESS THAN 15 MINUTES. ENTER HOURS. ENTER MINUTES.

Question: 53   Ask if Q52 > 0
About how many of those hours are news reports or news shows? ENTER ZERO FOR NONE OR FOR LESS THAN 15 MINUTES. ENTER HOURS. ENTER MINUTES.

Question: 54
Now, let me ask you about your use of museums, zoos, and similar institutions. I am going to read you a short list of places and ask you to tell me how many times you visited each type of place during the last year, that is, the last 12 months. If you did not visit any given place, just say none. First, an art museum. How many times did you visit it during the last year? ENTER NUMBER OF VISITS OR ZERO. IF R GIVES A RANGE ANSWER, FOR EXAMPLE, THAT THEY VISITED 2 TO 3 TIMES, TYPE IN THE LOWEST NUMBER. IF R GIVES A RANGE SUCH AS 15 TO 20 TIMES, TYPE IN THE MID-RANGE, FOR EXAMPLE, 17. DO NOT PROBE FOR A MORE SPECIFIC ANSWER.

Question: 55
Next, a natural history museum. How many times did you visit it during the last year? ENTER NUMBER OF VISITS OR ZERO. IF R GIVES A RANGE ANSWER, FOR EXAMPLE, THAT THEY VISITED 2 TO 3 TIMES, TYPE IN THE LOWEST NUMBER. IF R GIVES A RANGE SUCH AS 15 TO 20 TIMES, TYPE IN THE MID-RANGE, FOR EXAMPLE, 17. DO NOT PROBE FOR A MORE SPECIFIC ANSWER.

Question: 56
A zoo or aquarium. How many times did you visit it during the last year? ENTER NUMBER OF VISITS OR ZERO. IF R GIVES A RANGE ANSWER, FOR EXAMPLE, THAT THEY VISITED 2 TO 3 TIMES, TYPE IN THE LOWEST NUMBER. IF R GIVES A RANGE SUCH AS 15 TO 20 TIMES, TYPE IN THE MID-RANGE, FOR EXAMPLE, 17. DO NOT PROBE FOR A MORE SPECIFIC ANSWER.

Question: 57
A science or technology museum. How many times did you visit it during the last year? ENTER NUMBER OF VISITS OR ZERO (maximum number is 95). IF R GIVES A RANGE ANSWER, FOR EXAMPLE, THAT THEY VISITED 2 TO 3 TIMES, TYPE IN THE LOWEST NUMBER. IF R GIVES A RANGE SUCH AS 15 TO 20 TIMES, TYPE IN THE MID-RANGE, FOR EXAMPLE, 17. DO NOT PROBE FOR A MORE SPECIFIC ANSWER.

Question: 58a
A public library. How many times did you visit it during the last year?

ENTER NUMBER OF VISITS OR ZERO. IF R GIVES A RANGE ANSWER, FOR EXAMPLE, THAT THEY VISITED 2 TO 3 TIMES, TYPE IN THE LOWEST NUMBER. IF R GIVES A RANGE SUCH AS 15 TO 20 TIMES, TYPE IN THE MID-RANGE, FOR EXAMPLE, 17. DO NOT PROBE FOR A MORE SPECIFIC ANSWER.

Question: 58b   Ask if Q58a > 0
During the last 12 months, did you borrow any books from the public library?
1> yes
2> no

Question: 58c   Ask if Q58b = 1
About how many books did you borrow during the last year? ENTER NUMBER.

Question: 58d   Ask if Q58a > 0
During the last 12 months, did you borrow any videotapes from the public library? IF YES, ASK: About how many? ENTER NUMBER OR ZERO.

Question: 59a
During the last 12 months, did you buy any books?
1> yes
2> no

Question: 59b   Ask if Q59a = 1
About how many books did you buy during the last year? ENTER NUMBER.

Question: 59c   Ask if Q59a = 1
Were any of those books about science, mathematics, or technology, including computers or computer use? IF YES, ASK: About how many? (IF NECESSARY: of those books, how many were about science, mathematics, or technology, including computers or computer use?) ENTER NUMBER OR ZERO.

Question: 60
Now, for a different type of question. All things considered, would you say that the world is better off, or worse off, because of science?
1> better off
2> about equal (CODE BUT DO NOT OFFER)
3> worse off

Question: 61
Now, let me turn to a slightly different type of question. When you read news

stories, you see certain sets of words and terms. We are interested in how many people recognize certain kinds of terms, and I would like to ask you a few brief questions in that regard. First, some articles refer to the results of a **scientific study**. When you read or hear the term scientific study do you have a clear understanding of what it means, a general sense of what it means, or little understanding of what it means?
1> clear understanding
2> general sense
3> little understanding

Question: 62   Ask if Q61 = 1 or Q61 = 2
In your own words, could you tell me what it means to **study something scientifically**? ENTER EXACT RESPONSE. DO NOT PROBE FOR FUR-THER RESPONSE.

Question: 63
Next, the Internet. When you read or hear the term the Internet, do you have a clear understanding of what it means, a general sense of what it means, or little understanding of what it means?
1> clear understanding
2> general sense
3> little understanding

Question: 64   Ask if Q63 = 1 or Q63 = 2
Please tell me, in your own words, what is the Internet? ENTER EXACT RE-SPONSE. DO NOT PROBE FOR FURTHER RESPONSE.

Question: 65
Next, in articles and on television news shows, the term DNA has been used. When you hear the term DNA, do you have a clear understanding of what it means, a general sense of what it means, or little understanding of what it means?
1> clear understanding
2> general sense
3> little understanding

Question: 66   Ask if Q65 = 1 or Q65 = 2
Please tell me, in your own words, what is DNA? ENTER EXACT RE-SPONSE. DO NOT PROBE FOR FURTHER RESPONSE.

Question: 66a Ask if Q65 = 1 or Q65 = 2
If you wanted to find DNA in the human body, where would you expect to find it? ENTER EXACT RESPONSE. PROBE FOR ADDITIONAL RE-

SPONSES. WHEN THE RESPONDENT NAMES ONE LOCATION, SAY "ANYWHERE ELSE?"

Question: 67
Next, when you read or hear the term molecule, do you have a clear understanding of what it means, a general sense of what it means, or little understanding of what it means?
1> clear understanding
2> general sense
3> little understanding

Question: 68   Ask if Q67 = 1 or Q67 = 2
Please tell me, in your own words, what is a molecule? ENTER EXACT RESPONSE. DO NOT PROBE FOR FURTHER RESPONSE.

Question: 69
Next, when you read or hear the term radiation, do you have a clear understanding of what it means, a general sense of what it means, or little understanding of what it means?
1> clear understanding
2> general sense
3> little understanding

Question: 70   Ask if Q69 = 1 or Q69 = 2
Please tell me, in your own words, what is radiation? ENTER EXACT RESPONSE. DO NOT PROBE FOR FURTHER RESPONSE.

Question: 79
Now, please think about this situation. Two scientists want to know if a certain drug is effective against high blood pressure. The first scientist wants to give the drug to 1000 people with high blood pressure and see how many of them experience lower blood pressure levels. The second scientist wants to give the drug to 500 people with high blood pressure, and not give the drug to another 500 people with high blood pressure, and see how many in both groups experience lower blood pressure levels. Which is the better way to test this drug? IF R ASKS WHETHER OR NOT A PLACEBO WAS GIVEN, INDICATE THAT "IN THIS CASE THERE WAS NO PLACEBO GIVEN."
1> All 1000 get the drug
2> 500 get the drug; 500 don't

Question: 80
Why is it better to test the drug this way? ENTER EXACT RESPONSE. DO NOT PROBE FOR FURTHER RESPONSE.

Question: 82
I'm going to read to you some statements such as those you might find in a newspaper or magazine article. For each statement, please tell me if you *generally agree* or *generally disagree*. If you feel especially strongly about a statement, please tell me that you *strongly agree* or *strongly disagree*. OK? First, science and technology are making our lives healthier, easier, and more comfortable. Do you strongly agree, agree, disagree, or strongly disagree?
1> strongly agree
2> agree
3> disagree
4> strongly disagree

Question: 83
The quality of science and mathematics education in American schools is inadequate. Do you strongly agree, agree, disagree, or strongly disagree?
1> strongly agree
2> agree
3> disagree
4> strongly disagree

Question: 84
In general, computers and factory automation will create more jobs than they will eliminate. Do you strongly agree, agree, disagree, or strongly disagree?
1> strongly agree
2> agree
3> disagree
4> strongly disagree

Question: 85
We depend too much on science and not enough on faith. Do you strongly agree, agree, disagree, or strongly disagree?
1> strongly agree
2> agree
3> disagree
4> strongly disagree

Question: 86
Even if it brings no immediate benefits, scientific research which advances the frontiers of knowledge is necessary and should be supported by the federal government. Do you strongly agree, agree, disagree, or strongly disagree?
1> strongly agree
2> agree

3> disagree
4> strongly disagree

There was a split ballot regarding the order of questions 87 and 96b. Version A asked about "dogs and chimpanzees" in question 87 and about "mice" in question 96b. Version B asked about "mice" in question 87 and "dogs and chimpanzees" in question 96b.

Question: 87
Scientists should be allowed to do research that causes pain and injury to animals like dogs and chimpanzees if it produces new information about human health problems. Do you strongly agree, agree, disagree, or strongly disagree?
1> strongly agree
2> agree
3> disagree
4> strongly disagree

Question: 88
It is not important for me to know about science in my daily life. Do you strongly agree, agree, disagree, or strongly disagree?
1> strongly agree
2> agree
3> disagree
4> strongly disagree

Question: 89
The American space program should build a space station large enough to house scientific and manufacturing experiments. Do you strongly agree, agree, disagree, or strongly disagree?
1> strongly agree
2> agree
3> disagree
4> strongly disagree

Question: 90
Some numbers are especially lucky for some people. Do you strongly agree, agree, disagree, or strongly disagree?
1> strongly agree
2> agree
3> disagree
4> strongly disagree

Question: 91
Science makes our way of life change too fast. Do you strongly agree, agree, disagree, or strongly disagree?
1> strongly agree
2> agree
3> disagree
4> strongly disagree

Question: 92
Most scientists want to work on things that will make life better for the average person. Do you strongly agree, agree, disagree, or strongly disagree?
1> strongly agree
2> agree
3> disagree
4> strongly disagree

Question: 93
Technological discoveries will eventually destroy the earth. Do you strongly agree, agree, disagree, or strongly disagree?
1> strongly agree
2> agree
3> disagree
4> strongly disagree

Question: 94
With the application of science and new technology, work will become more interesting. Do you strongly agree, agree, disagree, or strongly disagree?
1> strongly agree
2> agree
3> disagree
4> strongly disagree

Question: 95
Because of science and technology, there will be more opportunities for the next generation. Do you strongly agree, agree, disagree, or strongly disagree?
1> strongly agree
2> agree
3> disagree
4> strongly disagree

Question: 96
Technological development creates an artificial and inhuman way of living. Do you strongly agree, agree, disagree, or strongly disagree?
1> strongly agree

2> agree
3> disagree
4> strongly disagree

Question: 96b
Scientists should be allowed to do research that causes pain and injury to animals like mice if it produces new information about human health problems. Do you strongly agree, agree, disagree, or strongly disagree?
1> strongly agree
2> agree
3> disagree
4> strongly disagree

Question: 97a
New inventions will always be found to counteract any harmful consequences of technological development. Do you strongly agree, agree, disagree, or strongly disagree?
1> strongly agree
2> agree
3> disagree
4> strongly disagree

Question: 97b
People would do better by living a simpler life without so much technology. Do you strongly agree, agree, disagree, or strongly disagree?
1> strongly agree
2> agree
3> disagree
4> strongly disagree

Question: 98
Now for a different type of question. People have frequently noted that scientific research has produced both beneficial and harmful consequences. Would you say that, on balance, the benefits of scientific research have outweighed the harmful results, or have the harmful results of scientific research been greater than its benefits?
1> beneficial results greater
2> about equal
3> harmful results greater

Question: 99   Ask if Q98 = 1
Would you say that the balance has been strongly in favor of beneficial results, or only slightly?

1> strongly
2> only slightly

Question: 100   Ask if Q98 = 3
Would you say that the balance has been strongly in favor of harmful results,
or only slightly?
1> strongly
2> only slightly

*There was a split ballot on question 101 to examine two alternate forms
of wording. Version A included the words "the creation of new life
forms" and version B included the words "the modification of existing
life forms."*

Question: 101
Some persons have argued that the creation of new life forms [modification
of existing life forms] through genetic engineering research constitutes a serious risk, while other persons have argued that this research may yield major benefits for society. In your opinion, have the benefits of genetic engineering research outweighed the harmful results, or have the harmful results
of genetic engineering research been greater than its benefits?
1> benefits greater
2> about equal
3> harms greater

Question: 102   Ask if Q101 = 1
Would you say that the balance has been strongly in favor of beneficial results, or only slightly?
1> strongly
2> slightly

Question: 103   Ask if Q101 = 3
Would you say that the balance has been strongly in favor of harmful results,
or only slightly?
1> strongly
2> slightly

Question: 104
In the current debate over the use of nuclear reactors to generate electricity, there is broad agreement that there are some risks and some benefits associated with nuclear power. In your opinion, have the benefits associated
with nuclear power outweighed the harmful results, or have the harmful results associated with nuclear power been greater than its benefits?

1> benefits greater
2> about equal
3> harms greater

Question: 105   Ask if Q104 = 1
Would you say that the balance has been strongly in favor of beneficial results, or only slightly?
1> strongly
2> slightly

Question: 106   Ask if Q104 = 3
Would you say that the balance has been strongly in favor of harmful results, or only slightly?
1> strongly
2> slightly

Question: 107
Many current issues in science and technology may be viewed as a judgment of relative costs and benefits. Thinking first about the space program, some persons have argued that the costs of the space program may have exceeded its benefits, while other people have argued that the benefits of space exploration have exceeded its costs. In your opinion, have the costs of space exploration exceeded its benefits, or have the benefits of space exploration exceeded its costs?
1> benefits greater
2> about equal
3> costs greater

Question: 108   Ask if Q107 = 1
Would you say that the benefits have substantially exceeded the costs, or only slightly exceeded the costs?
1> substantially
2> slightly

Question: 109   Ask if Q107 = 3
Would you say that the costs have substantially exceeded the benefits, or only slightly exceeded the benefits?
1> substantially
2> slightly

Question: 110
We are faced with many problems in this country. I'm going to name some of these problems, and for each one, I'd like you to tell me if you think that the

government is spending too little money on it, about the right amount, or too much. First, exploring space. Is the government spending too little, about the right amount, or too much on exploring space?
1> too little
2> about the right amount
3> too much

Question: 111
Next, reducing pollution. Is the government spending too little, about the right amount, or too much on reducing pollution?
1> too little
2> about the right amount
3> too much

Question: 112
Improving health care. Is the government spending too little, about the right amount, or too much on improving health care?
1> too little
2> about the right amount
3> too much

Question: 113
Supporting scientific research. Is the government spending too little, about the right amount, or too much on supporting scientific research?
1> too little
2> about the right amount
3> too much

Question: 114
Improving education. Is the government spending too little, about the right amount, or too much on improving education?
1> too little
2> about the right amount
3> too much

Question: 115
Helping older people. Is the government spending too little, about the right amount, or too much on helping older people?
1> too little
2> about the right amount
3> too much

Question: 116
Improving national defense. Is the government spending too little, about the right amount, or too much on improving national defense?
1> too little
2> about the right amount
3> too much

Question: 117
Helping low-income persons. Is the government spending too little, about the right amount, or too much on helping low-income persons?
1> too little
2> about the right amount
3> too much

Question: 120
Now, I would like to ask you a few short quiz-type questions such as you might see on a television game show. For each statement that I read, please tell me if it is true or false. If you don't know or aren't sure, just tell me so and we will skip to the next question. Remember: true, false, or don't know. First, the center of the Earth is very hot. Is that true or false?
1> true
2> false

Question: 121
All radioactivity is man-made. Is that true or false?
1> true
2> false

Question: 122
The oxygen we breathe comes from plants. Is that true or false?
1> true
2> false

Question: 123
It is the father's gene which decides whether the baby is a boy or a girl. Is that true or false?
1> true
2> false

Question: 124
Lasers work by focusing sound waves. Is that true or false?
1> true
2> false

Question: 125
Electrons are smaller than atoms. Is that true or false?
1> true
2> false

Question: 126
Antibiotics kill viruses as well as bacteria. Is that true or false?
1> true
2> false

Question: 127
The universe began with a huge explosion. Is that true or false?
1> true
2> false

Question: 128
The continents on which we live have been moving their location for millions of years and will continue to move in the future. Is that true or false?
1> true
2> false

Question: 129
Human beings, as we know them today, developed from earlier species of animals. Is that true or false?
1> true
2> false

Question: 130
Cigarette smoking causes lung cancer. Is that true or false?
1> true
2> false

Question: 131
The earliest humans lived at the same time as the dinosaurs. Is that true or false?
1> true
2> false

Question: 132
Radioactive milk can be made safe by boiling it. Is that true or false?
1> true
2> false

Question: 133
Which travels faster: light or sound?
1> light
2> sound
3> both the same

Question: 134
Does the Earth go around the Sun, or does the Sun go around the Earth?
1> Earth goes around Sun
2> Sun goes around Earth

Question: 135   Ask if Q134 = 1
How long does it take for the Earth to go around the Sun: one day, one month, or one year?
1> one day
2> one month
3> one year
4> other time period (CODE BUT DO NOT OFFER)

Question: 136
Now, think about this situation. A doctor tells a couple that their *genetic makeup* means that they've got *one in four chances* of having a child with an inherited illness. Does this mean that if their first three children are healthy, the fourth will have the illness?
1> yes
2> no

Question: 137
Does this mean that if their first child has the illness, the next three will not?
1> yes
2> no

Question: 138
Does this mean that each of the couple's children will have the same risk of suffering from the illness?
1> yes
2> no

Question: 139
Does this mean that if they have only three children, none will have the illness?
1> yes
2> no

Question: 140
Now, a new subject. Do you ever read a horoscope or your personal astrology report?
1> yes
2> no

Question: 141   Ask if Q140 = 1
Do you read an astrology report every day, quite often, just occasionally, or almost never?
1> every day
2> quite often
3> just occasionally
4> almost never

Question: 142
Would you say that astrology is very scientific, sort of scientific, or not at all scientific?
1> very scientific
2> sort of scientific
3> not at all scientific

Question: 143
Now, let me change the subject. During the last year, have you written or spoken to any public official or legislator about any *political issue or problem*?
1> yes
2> no

Question: 144   Ask if Q143 = 1
Can you recall an issue that you made a contact about? ENTER EXACT RESPONSE. IF R MENTIONS A PIECE OF LEGISLATION BY NUMBER, PROBE FOR CONTENT OF BILL.

Question: 145   Ask if Q143 = 1
IF R NAMED AN ISSUE ON THE PREVIOUS SCREEN, ASK: Can you recall another issue that you made a contact about? ENTER EXACT RESPONSE. IF R MENTIONS A PIECE OF LEGISLATION BY NUMBER, PROBE FOR CONTENT OF BILL.

Question: 146
IF R NAMED AN ISSUE ON THE PREVIOUS SCREEN, ASK: Can you recall another issue that you made a contact about? ENTER EXACT RESPONSE. IF R MENTIONS A PIECE OF LEGISLATION BY NUMBER, PROBE FOR CONTENT OF BILL.

Question: 147
Now, let me ask you a few brief questions about yourself. First, are you currently married, widowed, divorced, separated, or have you never been married?
1> married
2> widowed
3> divorced
4> separated
5> never married

Question: 147a
How many adults 18 years of age or older regularly live in your home? ENTER NUMBER OF ADULTS.

READ IF REFUSED: I can certainly understand your hesitation in answering this question. When we gather information it is important to know if people of various ages, races, levels of education, and so forth have different needs. When we run our statistics with this information they will have more meaning. I assure you that protecting your privacy is a major concern and when the results are published they are reported as statistics and it is impossible to associate the answers directly with anyone we've talked to. ATTENTION INTERVIEWER: THIS IS A CRITICAL ITEM.

Question: 148
Do you have any children? IF YES, ASK: How many? ENTER NUMBER OF CHILDREN OR ZERO FOR NONE.

Question: 149   Ask if Q148 > 0
Do you have any children under age 18 who currently live with you? IF YES, ASK: How many? ENTER NUMBER OF CHILDREN OR ZERO FOR NONE.

Question: 150
What is the highest level of education you completed? ATTENTION INTERVIEWER: THIS IS A CRITICAL ITEM!
0> Grade 6 or less
1> Grade 7 through 9
2> Grade 10 or 11
3> High school diploma/GED
4> Vocational less than 2 years
5> Associate (AA, AS)
6> Baccalaureate (BA, BS)
7> Masters (MA, MS)
8> Doctorate (Ph.D., Ed.D.)

9> Professional (medical, dental, legal)

10> Other

READ IF REFUSED: I can certainly understand your hesitation in answering this question. When we gather information it is important to know if people of various ages, races, levels of education, and so forth have different needs. When we run our statistics with this information they will have more meaning. I assure you that protecting your privacy is a major concern and when the results are published they are reported as statistics and it is impossible to associate the answers directly with anyone we've talked to. Into which of these groups could we categorize your response, would you say less than a high school diploma, you received a high school diploma/GED, or you have a baccalaureate degree or higher?

Question: 150a Ask if Q150 = 10
What level would that be? ENTER R DESCRIPTION OF HIGHEST LEVEL OF EDUCATION.

Question: 151 Ask if Q150 > 4 and Q150 ≠ 10
In what field was the degree? ENTER EXACT RESPONSE.

Question: 152 Ask if Q150 > 2
Have you ever taken any college-level science courses? IF YES: How many? ENTER NUMBER OF COURSES OR ZERO FOR NONE.

Question: 153 Ask if Q150>1
Now, let me ask you to think about the courses you took in high school. What was the highest level of math that you completed in high school? IF RESPONDENT SAYS "SENIOR MATH," "MATH 2," "MATH 100," OR SOME OTHER GENERAL COURSE, ASK THEM: Would that be algebra, algebra two, geometry, trigonometry, pre-calculus, calculus, or general math?

1> no math in HS; didn't go to HS

2> general math, business or vocational math

3> pre-algebra

4> one year of algebra

5> two years of algebra

6> geometry (plane or solid or both)

7> trigonometry/linear programming/analysis

8> pre-calculus

9> calculus

10> statistics/probability

11> other, specify

Question: 154   Ask if Q153 = 10
ENTER OTHER MATH CLASS HERE. PROBE FOR SUBJECT MATTER IF
NECESSARY.

Question: 155   Ask if Q150 > 1
Did you take a high school biology course?
1> yes
2> no

Question: 156   Ask if Q150 > 1
Did you take a high school chemistry course?
1> yes
2> no

Question: 157   Ask if Q150 > 1
Did you take a high school physics course?
1> yes
2> no

Question: 158
Are you currently enrolled in school?
1> yes
2> no

Question: 159   Ask if Q158 = 1
What program are you enrolled in? ENTER EXACT RESPONSE. IF RE-
PONDENT GIVES A SUBJECT (BIOLOGY, COMPUTER PROGRAMMING)
ASK: What type of degree or certificate do you expect to earn?

Question: 160
Last week, were you working full-time, working part-time, going to school,
or what? IF R SAYS GOING TO SCHOOL AND WORKING, ASK HOW MANY
HOURS OF WORK PER WEEK AND CODE AS FULL-TIME (35 HOURS OR
MORE) OR PART-TIME WORK.
1> working full-time
2> working part-time
3> has job, but on vacation or strike
4> retired
5> unemployed, laid off, or looking for work
6> in school (full-time)
7> keeping house
8> other, disabled, not looking for work

Question: 161   Ask if Q160 > 0 and Q160 < 5
What kind of work do/did you normally do? What is/was your job called? IF RESPONDENT SAYS THEY ARE SELF-EMPLOYED, PROBE FOR FUNC-TIONS AND DUTIES. IF RESPONDENT SIMPLY GIVES THE NAME OF THE COMPANY THEY WORK FOR (BURGER KING ETC.) PROBE FOR FUNC-TIONS AND DUTIES. ENTER DESCRIPTION.

Question: 162 Ask if Q160 > 0 and Q160 < 5
Are/were you employed by a unit of government, a private corporation, or are you self-employed?
1> a unit of government
2> a private corporation (for profit and not for profit corporations)
3> self-employed
4> other

Question: 163   Ask if Q160 > 0 and Q160 < 5
Does/did the organization or firm for which you work/worked conduct or sponsor any scientific or technological research?
1> yes
2> no

Question: 164   Ask if Q160 > 0 and Q160 < 4
Do you use a computer in your work?
1> yes
2> no

Question: 165a Ask if Q164 = 1
About how many hours do you personally use your work computer in a typ-ical week? ENTER EXACT RESPONSE TO NEAREST WHOLE HOUR.

Question: 165b Ask if Q164 = 1
Do you have an e-mail address for use at work?
1> yes
2> no

Question: 165c Ask if Q164 = 1
Do you have access to the World Wide Web through your work computer?
1> yes
2> no

Question: 165d Ask if Q165c = 1
During the last month, about how many hours have you spent on the Web at work? ENTER NUMBER OF HOURS

Question: 166a
Do you presently have a home computer in your household?
1> yes
2> no

Question: 166b Ask if Q166a = 1
Do you have more than one computer in your household?
1> yes
2> no

Question: 166c Ask if Q166b = 1
How many computers do you have in your household that are in working order? ENTER NUMBER OF COMPUTERS

Question: 167   Ask if Q166 = 1
About how many hours do you personally use your home computer in a typical week? ENTER EXACT RESPONSE TO NEAREST WHOLE HOUR.

Question: 170   Ask if Q166 = 1
Do you have a CD-ROM reader in your home computer?
1> yes
2> no

Question: 171   Ask if Q166 = 1
Do you have a modem in your home computer?
1> yes
2> no

Question: 173   Ask if Q171 = 1
Do you presently subscribe to any network service like Compuserve, Prodigy, America Online, or any other dial-in service?
1> yes
2> no

Question: 174a Ask if Q173 = 1
About how many hours a month do you use a dial-in or network service? EN-
TER EXACT NUMBER TO NEAREST WHOLE HOUR.

Question: 174b Ask if Q165b = 1
Do you have an e-mail address that you use with your home computer, separate from your e-mail address at work?
1> yes
2> no

Question: 174c Ask if Q165b = 2
Do you have an e-mail address that you can use with your home computer?
1> yes
2> no

Question: 174d
Do you have WEB television in your home? That is, do you have access to the World Wide Web through your television?
1> yes
2> no

Question: 175a Ask if Q173 = 1 or Q174d = 1
Do your ever access the World Wide Web through your home computer?
1> yes
2> no

Question: 175b Ask if Q175a = 1
During the last month, about how many hours have you spent on the Web at home? ENTER NUMBER OF HOURS.

Question 175c   Ask if Q175a = 1 or Q165c = 1 or Q174d = 1
Have you ever tried to get information about a specific topic or problem on the Internet or the World Wide Web either at work or home, or do you usually just browse to see what you can find?
1> Have tried to get specific information
2> Usually just browse

Question 175d   Ask if Q175c = 1
Can you recall the most recent topic or problem that you looked for information about on the Internet or the World Wide Web? IF YES: Could you describe that topic or problem to me? ENTER EXACT RESPONSE.

Question 175e Ask if Q175d = YES
Have you ever looked for information about a scientific or technological topic or problem on the Internet or the World Wide Web? IF YES: Could you describe that topic or problem to me? ENTER EXACT RESPONSE.

Question 175f Ask if Q175e = YES
Have you looked for information about another scientific or technological topic or problem on the Internet or the World Wide Web? IF YES: Could you describe that topic or problem to me? ENTER EXACT RESPONSE.

Question 175g Ask if Q175f = YES
Have you looked for information about another scientific or technological topic or problem on the Internet or the World Wide Web? IF YES: Could you describe that topic or problem to me? ENTER EXACT RESPONSE.

Question: 176a
Do you smoke?
1> yes
2> no

Question: 176b Ask if Q16a = 1
On an average day, about how many cigarettes, cigars, or pipes do you smoke?
ENTER NUMBER.

Question: 177a
What is the ZIP code of your residence? [IF MATCHED REPONDENT: I'd like to confirm your zip code. Is it _____?] ENTER ZIP CODE BELOW (5 DIGITS ONLY).

Question: 177b
Do you live in a city, town, or village, or do you live in an unincorporated area?
1> city, town, or village
2> unincorporated area

Question: 177c Ask if Q177b = 1
What is the name of your city, town, or village? ENTER NAME. ASK FOR SPELLING IF UNCERTAIN.

Question: 179
What race do you consider yourself?
ENTER EXACT RESPONSE. IF R IS UNSURE, OR SAYS "AMERICAN", ASK: Which of the following Census categories do you consider yourself: African American, Hispanic American, White/Caucasian, Asian or Pacific Islander, or American Indian or Alaskan Native?

ATTENTION INTERVIEWER: THIS IS A CRITICAL QUESTION. IF REFUSED READ: I can certainly understand your hesitation in answering this question. When we gather information it is important to know if people of various ages, races, levels of education, and so forth have different needs. When we run our statistics with this information they will have more meaning. I assure you that protecting your privacy is a major concern and when the results are published they are reported as statistics and it is impossible to associate the answers directly with anyone we've talked to. Into which of these groups could we categorize your response, either African American, Hispanic, or all other groups?

Question: 180
IF RESPONDENT DID NOT INDICATE THAT THEY WERE HISPANIC IN THE PREVIOUS QUESTION, ASK THIS QUESTION: Are you of Hispanic origin or descent?
1> yes
2> no

Question: 181
In what year were you born? ENTER ALL FOUR DIGITS OF BIRTH YEAR.

ATTENTION INTERVIEWER: THIS IS A CRITICAL QUESTION. IF RE-FUSED READ: I can certainly understand your hesitation in answering this question. When we gather information it is important to know if people of various ages, races, levels of education, and so forth have different needs. When we run our statistics with this information they will have more meaning. I assure you that protecting your privacy is a major concern and when the results are published they are reported as statistics and it is impossible to associate the answers directly with anyone we've talked to. Into which of these groups could we categorize your response, either 18–24, 25–34, 35–44, 45–64, or 65 and older?

Question: 182
This completes our interview. Thank you for taking the time to talk with me. Have a good day/evening.

ATTENTION INTERVIEWER: THIS IS A CRITICAL QUESTION: CODE RE-SPONDENT GENDER. IF UNSURE, ASK: "I have to read every question on my screen and now my computer wants me to ask if you are male or female."
1> male
2> female

B

·········

CONSTRUCTED VARIABLES

················

The analyses presented in this book use a number of variables that were constructed from one or more questions included in the original surveys. This appendix provides a detailed description of how those variables were constructed, organized by the first chapter in which a constructed variable is used.

CHAPTER 2

Index of Biomedical Literacy

Each respondent's level of biomedical literacy is estimated by a five-level ordinal variable. To ensure that all of the knowledge questions measured the same construct, a confirmatory factor analysis was conducted, using LISREL8. Unlike previous studies of civic scientific literacy (Miller, 1983a, 1987a, 1995, 1998; Miller and Pardo, 2000; Miller *et al.*, 1997), the items measuring biomedical vocabulary and the items measuring an understanding of the nature of scientific inquiry loaded on a single factor. Accepting this pattern, biomedical literacy scores were calculated using the Item Response Theory (IRT) method, as reflected in the BILOG-MG program. The resulting IRT scores were an interval-level measure, which was then converted into a zero to 100 index by equating the lowest IRT score to zero and the highest IRT score to 100 and computing the relative value of each IRT score in between. A five-level ordinal measure of biomedical literacy was created from the original scores, using the following categories: (1) scores from 0 to 30;

(2) scores from 31 to 40; (3) scores from 41 to 49; (4) scores from 50 to 64; and (5) scores of 65 or more.

Level of Education

All respondents were asked the question, "What is the highest level of education you completed?" Interviewers coded the responses into the following categories: (1) grade 6 or less, (2) grade 7 through 9, (3) grade 10 or 11, (4) high school diploma/GED, (5) vocational training (less than 2 years), (6) associate degree, (7) baccalaureate degree, (8) masters degree, (9) doctorate, and (10) professional degree (medical, dental, or legal). The coded responses have been collapsed into three different variables that measure the level of education.

- A three-level measure of education categorized respondents as having (1) less than a high school degree, (2) a high school diploma, and (3) a baccalaureate degree or higher. This variable is used in some of the models using data from the 1993 National Institutes of Health (NIH) study and in some figures and bar charts.
- A four-level measure of education categorized respondents as having (1) less than a high school diploma, (2), a high school diploma, (3) a baccalaureate degree, and (4) a graduate or professional degree. This variable is used in several bar charts and descriptive text discussions of respondent education.
- A five-level measure of education categorized respondents as having (1) less than a high school diploma, (2) a high school diploma, (3) an associate degree, (4) a baccalaureate degree, or (5) a graduate or professional degree. This variable was used in virtually all of the structural equation models other than those based on the 1993 NIH study.

All three variables are highly correlated (.90 or more) and provide the same substantive results. The decision was to use a small number of classifications in more descriptive figures and in text discussions. The five-category variable was preferred for model building and testing to maximize the original variance in each model.

College Science Courses

All respondents who had completed at least a tenth grade education were asked, "Have you ever taken any college-level science courses?" Those respondents indicating that they had not taken any courses were coded as zero for college-level science courses. All other respondents were asked how many courses they had completed. The responses to these questions were collapsed to create a three-level ordinal variable: (1) zero courses, (2) one, two, or three courses, and (3) four or more courses.

Age

Respondents were asked, "In what year were you born?" Year of birth was converted into years of age. Several ordinal measures of age were created by collapsing the respondents' actual age. In virtually all of the models, a six-level age variable was used: (1) 18–24 years, (2) 25–34 years, (3) 35–44 years, (4) 45–54 years, (5) 55–64 years, and (6) 65 years or older.

Children at Home

Respondents were asked, "Do you have any children?" If those respondents indicating that they had children were then asked, "Do you have any children under age 18 who currently live with you?" All respondents indicating that they had at least one child under age 18 who currently lived in their home were classified as having children in their home. All other respondents were classified as not having children in their home.

Read News

The variable READ NEWS is a count of four different types of news reading—newspapers, newsmagazines, science magazines, and health magazines—and can range from zero to four. Respondents were asked a series of questions to measure their use of newspapers and magazines. Each respondent was asked, "Now let me change the topic slightly and ask you how you get information. First, how often do you read a newspaper: every day, a few times a week, once a week, or less than once a week?" Respondents were then asked, "Are there any magazines that you read regularly, that is, most of the time?" If they responded yes, they were asked, "What magazine would that be?" and were prompted for additional magazines. In the 1993 Biomedical Literacy Study, respondents were also asked, "Do you ever read any health magazines?" If they responded yes, they were asked, "What magazine would that be?" and were prompted for additional magazines. The answer to each magazine question was coded as to the type of magazine that was read. All those who read a newspaper every day were given one point, while others were given no points. Respondents were given one additional point for reading a newsmagazine, another point if they read a science magazine, and another point if they read a health magazine.

Race/Ethnicity

Respondents in the 1993 Biomedical Literacy Study were asked two questions in order to determine their race/ethnicity. Respondents were first asked, "Are you of Spanish origin or descent?" All respondents were also asked, "What race do you consider yourself?" A three-category measure of race/ethnicity was created based on the two questions. All respondents who indicated that they were African-American, were classified as African-American. All respondents who indicated that they were of Spanish origin or descent, in one of the two questions, but that they were not African-American, were classified as Hispanic-American. All other respondents were classified as Other Americans. The race/ethnicity variable is used in several analyses using the 1993 Biomedical Literacy Study because the sample for the 1993 study was designed to compensate for the lower levels of educational attainment among the current African-Americans and Hispanic-Americans. The variable is not used in any analyses using either the 1998 Biotechnology Study or any of the *Science and Engineering Indicators* studies because those samples were not designed to support the use of a race/ethnicity variable.

Personal Health

A dichotomous variable was created to represent excellent personal health. Two questions were included in the 1993 Biomedical Literacy Study to obtain a self-report on personal health. Respondents were asked, "Do you have any chronic or continuing illness?" and later, "Now, please think about your own health. Using a thermometer, if ten stands for perfect health and zero stands for very poor health, how would you rate your own health?" All respondents who indicated that they did not have any chronic or continuing illness and who rated their health as being eight or higher, were assigned a value of one for personal health status, while all other respondents were assigned a value of zero.

Family Health Problems

A dichotomous variable was created from the 1993 Biomedical Literacy data set to indicate that a spouse or child had chronic health problems. Respondents were asked "Does your husband/wife have any chronic or continuing illness?" and "Do any of your children who live at home have a chronic or continuing illness?" They were later asked, "Using the same thermometer, how would you rate your husband's [or wife's] health?" and "Using the same thermometer, how would you rate the overall health of your children who live at home?"

As a first step, a dichotomous measure of poor children's health status was created. Respondents who both indicated that one or more of their children had a chronic or continuing illness and rated their children's health as being five or less, were assigned a value of one, representing poor health status for their children. Respondents were also assigned a one if they said that their children did not have a chronic or continuing illness, but rated their children's health status as three or lower. All other respondents were assigned a value of zero for children's health status.

Second, a dichotomous measure of poor spouse health was created. Respondents who both indicated that their spouse had a chronic or continuing illness and rated their spouse's health as being five or less, were assigned a value of one, representing poor health status for their spouse. Respondents were also assigned a one if they said that their spouse did not have a chronic or continuing illness, but rated their spouse's health status as three or lower. All other respondents were assigned a value of zero for spouse's health status.

Finally, all respondents assigned a value of one for either spouse health status or children's health status were assigned a value of one for family health problems, indicating that either their spouse or their children suffered from poor personal health. All other respondents were assigned a value of zero for family health problems.

CHAPTER 3

Interest in Health Information

In the 1993 Biomedical Literacy Study, each respondent was asked a series of questions to measure his or her interest in a variety of topics. Each respondent was told, "There are a lot of issues in the news and it is hard to keep up with every area. I'm going to read you a short list of issues and for each one—as I read it—I would like you to tell me if you are very interested, moderately interested, or not at all interested." The interviewers then read a list of topics to the respondents, including, "Information about health." In the structural equation models presented in Chapter 3, interest in health was treated as a dichotomous variable, with those respondents who indicated that they were "very interested" assigned a value of one for interest in health, while all other respondents were assigned a value of zero.

CHAPTER 4

Average Hours of Television Viewing per Year

Each respondent was asked, "Altogether, on an average day, about how many hours would you say that you watch television?" Responses of 12 or more hours were truncated to 12 hours. The resulting number was multiplied by 350 to provide an estimate of the number of hours of television viewed each year.

Average Hours of Radio Listening per Year

Each respondent was asked, "On an average day, about how many hours would you say that you listen to a radio?" Responses of 12 or more hours were truncated to 12 hours of radio listening per day. The resulting number was multiplied by 350 to provide an estimate of the number of hours of radio listening per year.

Newsmagazine Reading

Each respondent in each of the studies used in the preceding analyses were asked, "Are there any magazines that you read regularly, that is, most of the time?" If the respondent said that he or she read a magazine, they were asked, "What magazine would that be?" and were prompted to name additional magazines. Interviewers typed in the exact name of each magazine. These responses were later assigned numeric codes reflecting the type of magazine (e.g., science, news, women's, health, computer) that was read. A dichotomous variable was created indicating whether or not the respondent read any newsmagazines. Respondents were assigned a value of one if they named at least one newsmagazine, and zero if they did not name any newsmagazines.

Science Magazine Reading

A dichotomous variable was created indicating whether or not the respondent read any science magazines, based on the magazine questions included in the studies. Respondents were assigned a value of one if they named at least one science magazine, and zero if they did not name any science magazines.

Women's Magazine Reading

A dichotomous variable was created indicating whether or not the respondent read any women's magazines based on the magazine questions included in the studies. Respondents were assigned a value of one if they named at least one women's magazine, and zero if they did not name any women's magazines.

Health Magazine Reading

A dichotomous variable was created indicating whether or not the respondent read any health magazines based on the magazine questions included in the studies. Respondents were assigned a value of one if they named at least one health magazine, and zero if they did not name any health magazines.

Health Newsletter Reading

In the 1998 Biotechnology Study, Each respondent was asked, "Do you subscribe to any health newsletters?" Respondents were assigned a code of one if they said "yes," and a code of zero if they said "no."

Home Computer Access

Each respondent was asked, "Do you presently have a home computer in your household?" Respondents were assigned a code of one if they said "yes," and a code of zero if they said "no."

Access to the World Wide Web

Three questions were used to create a measure of access to the World Wide Web. Each respondent who indicated that he or she had a home computer with a modem was asked, "Do you presently subscribe to any network service like Compuserve, Prodigy, American Online, or any other dial-in service?" All respondents were also asked, "Do you have WEB television in your home? That is, do you have access to the World Wide Web through your television?"

Each respondent who indicated that he or she used a computer in their work were asked, "Do you have access to the World Wide Web through your work computer?" Respondents who answered "yes" to any of the three questions were coded as having access to the World Wide Web. All other respondents were coded as not having access to the World Wide Web.

Looked for Health Information
on the World Wide Web

Each respondent with access to the World Wide Web either at home or work was asked, "Have you ever tried to get information about a specific topic or problem on the Internet or the World Wide Web either at work or home, or do you usually just browse to see what you can find?" Those respondents who had looked for a specific topic or problem were then asked, "Can you recall the most recent topic or problem that you looked for information about on the Internet or the World Wide Web?" If they said yes, they were asked, "Could you describe that topic or problem to me?" Respondents who were able to name a topic were asked, "Have you ever looked for information about a scientific or technological topic or problem on the Internet or the World Wide Web?" Respondents who replied affirmatively were asked, "Could you describe that topic or problem to me?" and were prompted for up to two additional scientific or technological topics. The verbatim responses to the four questions were assigned numeric codes to represent the type of topic that had been searched for. Respondents were categorized as having looked for health information on the World Wide Web if they named a health or medical topic in any of the four questions.

Public Library Visits per Year

A series of questions were included in the *Science and Engineering Indicators* studies to measure the public's use of libraries, museums, and other institutions. Respondents were first told, "Now let me ask you about your use of museums, zoos, and similar institutions. I am going to read you a short list of places and ask you to tell me how many times you visited each type of place during the last year, that is, the last 12 months. If you did not visit any given place, just say none. Respondents were then read a list of institutions, including, "a public library." Responses of 50 or more visits per year were truncated to 50 visits to calculate the average number of public library visits per year.

On-line Hours per Year

Separate estimates of yearly on-line hours at home and at work were created first. Respondents who subscribed to an on-line service at home were asked, "About how many hours a month do you use a dial-in or network service?" Responses of 60 or more hours were truncated to 60. The resulting number was multiplied by 11 to provide an estimate of yearly home on-line hours. Respondents who used a computer at work were asked, "Do you have access to the World Wide Web through your work computer?" Those responding yes were asked, "During the last month, about how many hours have you spent on the Web at work?" Responses of 60 or more hours were truncated to 60, with the resulting number multiplied by 11 to provide an estimate of yearly work on-line hours. The measures of yearly home and work on-line hours were combined to provide an estimate of the number of on-line hours per year.

Educational Status

In addition to being asked about their highest level of education, respondents were also asked, "Are you currently enrolled in school?" All those indicating that they were currently students were asked, "What program are you enrolled in?" A measure of educational status was created for young adults from these three questions containing the following five categories: (1) high school dropout—less than a high school diploma and not currently a student; (2) high school student—currently working on a GED or high school diploma; (3) high school graduate—not currently a student with the highest level of education being a high school diploma, some vocational training after high school, or an associate degree; (4) college student—currently working on an associate, baccalaureate, or graduate or professional degree; and (5) college graduate—not currently a student with at least a baccalaureate degree.

Parents

Each respondent was asked, "Do you have any children?" Those respondents indicating that they had children were then asked, "Do you have any children under age 18 who currently live with you?" Any respondent indicating that he or she had at least one child under age 18 currently living in their home was classified as being a parent.

Older Adults

A dichotomous measure of age was created to indicate whether or not each respondent was an older adult. Any respondent who was 60 years of age or older was assigned a value of one, while all other respondents were assigned a value of zero (see Age in Chapter 2 above).

CHAPTER 5

Current Health Information Consumers, 1993

Two questions from the 1993 Biomedical Literacy Study were used to construct a dichotomous measure of current health information consumption. Each respondent was asked, "What is the most important health or science information you have heard in the last two months?" All respondents who were able to name at least one piece of information were asked, "How did you come to know about this information?" All respondents who were able to both name a piece of information and recall the source of that information were classified as being current health information consumers, and were assigned a value of one. All other individuals were classified as latent information consumers, and were assigned a value of zero.

Current Health Information Consumers for Heart Disease/Cancer, 1998

A dichotomous measure of current health information consumption for heart disease/cancer was created from two questions included in the 1998 Social and Behavioral Indicators Survey. Respondents were first asked, "Over the last three months, have you heard or read anything about heart disease or cancer?" Those respondents who answered yes were asked, "How did you come to know this information?" Respondents who reported that they had heard or read something about heart disease or cancer and were able to name the source of that information recall were assigned a value of one and categorized as current information consumers for heart disease/cancer. All other respondents were assigned a value of zero and classified as latent information consumers.

Current Health Information Consumers for Mental Health/Alcoholism, 1998

A dichotomous measure of current health information consumption for mental health/alcoholism was created from two questions included in the 1998 Social and Behavioral Indicators Survey. Each respondent was asked, "Over the last three months, have you heard or read anything about alcoholism or serious mental health problems like depression or schizophrenia?" Those respondents who answered yes were asked, "How did you come to know this information?" Respondents were assigned a value of one and categorized as current information consumers for mental health/alcoholism if they indicated that they had heard or read something about those conditions and if they were able to name the source of that information. All other respondents were assigned a value of zero and were classified as latent information consumers.

CHAPTER 6

No constructed variables were introduced in Chapter 6.

CHAPTER 7

Attentive Public for Biomedical Research

Building on previous work by Miller, (1983b, 1987a, 1995; Miller and Pardo, 2000; Miller *et al.,* 1997), measures of attentiveness to selected public policy areas were created from three batteries of questions: (1) interest in public policy issues; (2) perceived information about selected public policy issues; and (3) regular consumption of relevant magazines and newspapers. A respondent was classified as being attentive to biomedical research if he or she indicated that they were "very interested" in "issues about new medical discoveries," felt "very well informed" about "issues about new medical discoveries," and either read a newspaper on a daily basis or regularly read a news, health, or science magazine. Respondents who were "very interested" in issues about new medical discoveries, but who either did not feel that they were "very well informed" or did not regularly consume news about the topic, were classified as being a part of the interested public for biomedical research. All other individuals were classified as the residual public for biomedical research. In the structural equation models presented in Chapter 7, attentiveness to biomedical research was treated as a dichotomous variable, with the attentive public assigned a value of one, and all other respondents assigned a value of zero.

Attentive Public for Foreign Policy

Following the work of Almond (1950) and Rosenau (1974), respondents were classified as being attentive to foreign policy if they indicated that they were "very interested" in "international and foreign policy issues," felt "very well informed," about those issues, and either read a newspaper on a daily basis or regularly read a newsmagazine. Respondents who were "very interested" in international and foreign policy issues, but who either did not feel that they were "very well informed" or did not regularly consume news about the topic, were classified as being a member of the interested public for foreign policy. All other individuals were classified as the residual public for foreign policy.

Attentive Public for Economic Policy

Respondents were classified as being attentive to economic policy if they indicated that they were "very interested" in "economic issues and business conditions," felt "very well informed," about those issues, and either read a newspaper on a daily basis or regularly read a newsmagazine or business magazine. Respondents who were "very interested" in economic issues and business conditions, but who either did not feel that they were "very well informed" or did not regularly consume news about the topic, were classified as being a member of the interested public for economic policy. All other individuals were classified as the residual public for economic policy.

Attentive Public for Local Schools

Respondents were classified as being attentive to local schools if they indicated that they were "very interested" in "local school issues," and felt "very well informed," about those issues. Respondents who were "very interested" in local school issues, but did not feel that they were "very well informed" were classified as being a member of the interested public for local schools. All other individuals were classified as the residual public for local schools.

Attentive Public for Science and Technology Policy

Separate measures were created for attentiveness to science policy and attentiveness to technology policy, following the same procedures outlined above. A respondent was classified as being attentive to science policy if he or she indicated that they were "very interested" in "issues about new scientific discoveries," felt "very well informed," about those issues, and either read a newspaper on a daily basis or regularly read a newsmagazine or science magazine. Respondents who were "very interested" in issues about new scientific discoveries, but who either did not feel that they were "very well informed," or did not regularly consume news about the topic, were classified as being a member of the interested public for science policy. All other individuals were classified as the residual public for science policy.

A respondent was classified as being attentive to technology policy if he or she indicated that they were "very interested" in "issues about the use of new inventions and technologies," felt "very well informed," about those issues, and either read a newspaper on a daily basis or regularly read a newsmagazine or science magazine. Respondents who were "very interested" in issues about new inventions and technologies, but who either did not feel that they were "very well informed," or did not regularly consume news about the topic, were classified as being a member of the interested public for technology policy. All other individuals were classified as the residual public for technology policy.

A summary measure of attentiveness to science and technology policy was created by combining the two separate measures. Individuals classified as attentive to either science policy or technology policy were classified as being attentive to science and technology policy. Individuals who were a member of the interested public for at least one of the issues, but were not attentive to either issue, were classified as a member of the interested public for science and technology policy. All other individuals were classified as the residual public for science and technology policy. In the structural equation models presented in Chapter 7, attentiveness to science and technology policy was treated as a dichotomous variable, with the attentive public assigned a value of one, and all other individuals a value of zero.

Attentive Public for Environmental Issues

A respondent was classified as being attentive to environmental issues if he or she indicated that they were "very interested" in "issues about environmental pollution," felt "very well informed," about those issues, and either read a newspaper on a daily basis or regularly read a newsmagazine or science magazine. Respondents who were "very interested" in issues about environmental pollution, but who either did not feel that they were "very well informed," or did not regularly consume news about the topic, were classified as being a member of the interested public for environmental issues. All other individuals were classified as the residual public for environmental issues.

Attentive Public for Military and Defense Policy

A respondent was classified as being attentive to military and defense policy if he or she indicated that they were "very interested" in "issues about military and defense policy," felt "very well informed," about those issues, and either read a newspaper on a daily basis or regularly read a newsmagazine. Respondents who were "very interested" in issues about military and defense policy, but who either did not feel that they were "very well informed" about the topic, or who did not regularly consume news about the topic, were classified as being a member of the interested public for military and defense policy. All other individuals were classified as the residual public for military and defense policy.

Attentive Public for Nuclear Power Issues

A respondent was classified as being attentive to nuclear power issues if he or she indicated that they were "very interested" in "issues about nuclear energy to generate electricity," felt "very well informed," about those issues, and either read a newspaper on a daily basis or regularly read a newsmagazine or science magazine. Respondents who were "very interested" in issues about nuclear energy to generate electricity, but who either did not feel that they were "very well informed" about the topic or did not regularly consume information about the topic, were classified as being a member of the interested public for nuclear power issues. All other individuals were classified as the residual public for nuclear power issues.

Attentive Public for Space Exploration

A respondent was classified as being attentive to space exploration if he or she indicated that they were "very interested" in "issues about space exploration," felt "very well informed," about those issues, and either read a newspaper on a daily basis or regularly read a newsmagazine or science magazine. Respondents who were "very interested" in issues about space exploration, but who either did not feel that they were "very well informed" about the topic or did not regularly consume information about the topic, were classified as being a member of the interested public for space exploration. All other individuals were classified as the residual public for space exploration.

Attentive Public for Agriculture Policy

A respondent was classified as being attentive to agriculture policy if he or she indicated that they were "very interested" in "agriculture and farm issues," felt "very well informed," about those issues, and either read a newspaper on a daily basis or regularly read a newsmagazine. Respondents who were "very interested" in agriculture and farm issues, but who either did not feel that they were "very well informed" about the topic or did not regularly consume information about the topic, were classified as being a member of the interested public for agriculture policy. All other individuals were classified as the residual public for agriculture policy.

General Political Interest

Each respondent was asked: "Let me start by asking how interested you are in current news events. Would you say that you are very interested, moderately interested, or not at all interested in current news events?" A respondent was given four points if he or she said that they were "very interested" and two points if he or she said they were "moderately interested" in current news events. A respondent was given one additional point for being attentive to each of five issue areas—local schools, foreign policy, military and defense policy, economic and business conditions, and agricultural policy. A maximum of nine points is possible on the Index of General Political Interest. For use in the structural equation models, an ordinal measure of general political interest was created. Respondents with five or more points were classified as having a high level of general political interest, individuals with three or four points were classified as having a moderate level of general political interest, and respondents with two or fewer points were classified as having a low level of general political interest.

CHAPTER 8

Number of Newspapers Read per Year

Each respondent was asked, "Now let me change the topic slightly and ask you how you get information. First, how often do you read a newspaper: every day, a few times a week, once a week, or less than once a week?" The number of newspapers read per year was estimated on the basis of that question. Individuals who read a newspaper every day were estimated to read 360 newspapers each year. Respondents who read a newspaper a few times a week were estimated to read 100 newspapers a year, and those individuals who reported reading a newspaper once a week or less than once a week were estimated to read 12 newspapers a year.

Number of Newsmagazines Read per Year

An estimate of the number of newsmagazines read per year was created. Each respondent was asked to name up to five magazines that he or she reads on a regular basis (see the variable Newsmagazine Reading in Chapter 4 above). This number was then multiplied by 50 (as the most popular newsmagazines are published on a weekly basis), to produce the estimated number of newsmagazines read per year.

Number of Science Magazines Read per Year

An estimate of the number of science magazines read per year was created. Each respondent was asked to name up to five magazines that he or she reads on a regular basis (see the variable Science Magazine Reading in Chapter 4 above). This number was then multiplied by 11 (as the most popular science magazines are printed on a monthly basis), to produce the estimated number of science magazines read per year.

Number of Health Information Magazines Read per Year

An estimate of the number of health information magazines read per year was created. Each respondent was asked to name up to five magazines that he or she reads on a regular basis (see the variable Health Magazine Reading in Chapter 4 above). This number was then multiplied by 11 (as the most popular health magazines are printed on a monthly basis), to produce the estimated number of health magazines read per year.

Number of Hours of TV News Viewed per Year

Each respondent who indicated that he or she watched some television was asked, "About how many of those hours are news reports or news shows?" Responses of greater than 12 hours of news viewing per day were truncated to 12 hours in the computation of the average number of TV news hours viewed per day. The resulting number was multiplied by 350 to create an estimate of the number of hours of TV news viewed per year.

Number of Hours of Science Television Viewed per Year

A series of questions were included in the *Science and Engineering Indicators* studies to measure the public's science television viewing. Each respondent was asked, "Do you watch any television shows that focus primarily on science or nature?" Each respondent who replied affirmatively was then asked for the name of the show that he or she watched most often. After naming a show, the respondent was asked, "About how many times a month do you watch this show?" Responses greater than 50 times per month were truncated to 50. This cycle of questions was repeated three times, and the three estimates were added together to create an estimate of the number of science television shows viewed per month. This number was multiplied by 11 to produce an estimate of the number of hours of science television viewed per year.

Watched Some Episodes of Nova in Previous Year

All respondents who indicated that they watched any science television were asked, "Which science or nature show do you watch most often?" and were prompted for up to two additional shows. The verbatim responses were assigned numeric codes to represent different television shows, and a separate code was assigned for *Nova*. All respondents who named "*Nova*" as one of their three television shows were coded as having watched some episodes of *Nova*. All other individuals were coded as not watching *Nova*.

Watched Some Episodes of National Geographic TV

All respondents who indicated that they watched any science television were asked, "Which science or nature show do you watch most often?" and were prompted for up to two additional shows. The verbatim responses were assigned numeric codes to represent different television shows, and a separate code was assigned for *National Geographic TV*. All respondents who named "*National Geographic*" as one of their three television shows were coded as having watched some episodes of *National Geographic*. All other individuals were coded as not watching *National Geographic TV*.

Number of Hours of Radio News Listening per Year

All respondents who indicated that they listened to the radio were asked, "About how many of those hours are news reports or news shows?" Responses greater than 12 hours per day were truncated to 12 hours. The resulting number was multiplied by 350 to provide an estimate of the average number of hours of radio news listened to each year.

Access to a Computer

A number of questions were included in the *Science and Engineering Indicators* studies to measure the public's access to computers at work and home (see Chapter 4 variables). A measure of computer access was created from these questions containing the following three categories: (1) no access—the respondent did not use a computer at work and did not have a home computer, (2) access at home or work—the respondent had access to a computer in only one of the locations, or (3) access at home and work—the respondent used a computer at work and had a computer in their home.

Has an E-Mail Address

All respondents who reported being employed and using a computer at work were asked, "Do you have an e-mail address for use at work?" All respondents were asked if they had a home computer and, if so, did they have an e-mail address for that computer. The working of the questions was coordinated so that an individual who had previously reported that he or she had an e-mail address associated with their job were asked if they had a separate e-mail address for use with their home computer. All respondents with an e-mail address either at home or work were classified as having an e-mail address. All other respondents were classified as not having an e-mail address.

Estimated Number of Hours per Year On-line from Home

All respondents who reported that they subscribed to any network service at home were asked, "About how many hours a month do you use a dial-in or network service?" Responses of 60 or more hours were truncated to 60 hours. Respondents who did not subscribe to a network service were coded as spending zero hours per month on-line The resulting estimate of hours per month was multiplied by 11 to produce an estimate of the number of hours per year spent on-line from home.

Estimated Number of Hours per Year on the Web from Home and Work

Separate estimates of yearly home and work Web usage were created independently and then summed to estimate the number of hours of home and work Web use. All respondents who reported that they subscribed to an on-line service at home or who had Web television were asked, "Do you ever access the World Wide Web at home?" Those respondents who accessed the Web at home were asked, "During the last month, about how many hours have you spent on the Web at home?" Responses of 60 or more hours were truncated to 60. The resulting number was multiplied by 11 to provide an estimate of yearly home Web usage.

All respondents who reported being employed and using a computer at work were asked, "Do you have access to the World Wide Web through your work computer?" Those individuals responding affirmatively were asked, "During the last month, about how many hours have you spent on the Web at work?" Responses of 60 or more hours were truncated to 60, and the resulting number multiplied by 11 to provide an estimate of yearly work Web usage.

The measures of yearly home and work Web usage were summed to provide an estimate of the number of hours per year spent on the Web from home and work.

Looked for Science Information on the Web

The *Science and Engineering Indicators* studies included a series of questions to measure the public's use of the World Wide Web as a source of science information (see Chapter 4 variables). A respondent was categorized as having looked for science information on the World Wide Web if he or she named a scientific or technological topic in response to any of the four questions about information sought on the World Wide Web.

CHAPTER 9

Index of the Promise of Science and Technology

To assess a general attitude or schema toward science and technology, a set of attitude questions from the *Science and Engineering Indicators* studies were selected and subjected to a confirmatory factor analysis, using LISREL8. Four items loaded on a dimension that was characterized as reflecting the promise of science and technology. Using the technique described above (see Chapter 2), a factor score was computed for this dimension and then converted into a zero to 100 index. For analytic reasons, this Index of the Promise of Science and Technology was grouped into a five-category ordinal variable for use in the structural equation model analyses. The five categories were (1) zero through 20, (2) 21 through 40, (3) 41 through 60, (4) 61 through 80, and (5) 81 thru 100.

Index of Reservations about Science and Technology

In the confirmatory factor analysis described above, a second factor included four items that reflect reservations about the impact of science and technology. This second factor has a −.61 correlation with the promise of science and technology index described above, suggesting that they are strongly related negatively. The four items that loaded on this dimension were used to compute a factor score for reservations about science and technology, and the factor scores were converted to a zero to 100 scale using the same technique described above (see Chapter 2). For analytic reasons, this Index of Reservations about Science and Technology was grouped into a five-category ordinal variable for use in the structural equation model analyses. The five categories were (1) zero through 20, (2) 21 through 40, (3) 41 through 60, (4) 61 through 80, and (5) 81 thru 100.

Attitudes toward Support for Basic Scientific Research

In each of the *Science and Engineering Indicators* studies, each respondent was asked to indicate whether he or she strongly agreed, agreed, disagreed, or strongly disagreed with the statement: "Even if it brings no immediate benefits, scientific research which advances the frontiers of knowledge is necessary and should be supported by the federal government." A five-level ordinal measure was created from the responses to this question. Respondents who strongly agreed were assigned a value of five, those who agreed were assigned a value of four, those who were uncertain were assigned a value of three, those who disagreed were assigned a value of two, and those who strongly disagreed were assigned a value of one.

Attitudes toward Health Research Spending

The *Science and Engineering Indicators 2000* study included a set of questions that measured public attitudes toward spending for different areas. Two questions from this battery were used to create a typology representing three levels of support for government spending for health research. Each respondent was told, "We are faced with many problems in this country. I'm going to name some of these problems, and for each one, I'd like you to tell me if you think that the government is spending too little money on it, about the right amount, or too much." A list of areas was then read, including "Improving health care" and "Supporting scientific research." The responses to these two questions were combined to create the following typology: (1) high support for health research spending—responses that the government is spending too little for both of the areas; (2) moderate support for health research spending—responses that the government is spending too little on improving health care, but who are satisfied with the amount of spending on scientific research; (3) low support for health research spending—responses that the government is either spending "about the right amount" or "too much" on improving health care and conducting scientific research.

Attitude toward the Use of Animals in Biomedical Research

A summary measure of attitude toward the use of animals in biomedical research was created from two questions included in the *Science and Engineering Indicators 2000* study. Each respondent was asked if he or she strongly agreed, agreed, disagreed, or strongly disagreed with two statements: (1) "Scientists should be allowed to do research that causes pain and injury to animals like dogs and chimpanzees if it produces new information about human health problems and (2) "Scientists should be allowed to do research that causes pain and injury to animals like mice if it produces new information about human health problems." Respondents were given five points for strongly agreeing, four points for agreeing, three points for being uncertain, two points for disagreeing, and one point for strongly disagreeing to each of the two statements. The two numeric values were combined to create a variable that ranged from two (strongly disagreed with both statements) to ten (strongly agreed with both statements). A three-level ordinal measure was created for use in the structural equation model analyses, with a value of one assigned to respondents with four or fewer points, a value of two was assigned to respondents with five to seven points on the original index, and a value of three was assigned to respondents with eight to ten points on the combined measure.

CHAPTER 10

Awareness of Biotechnology

In the 1998 Biotechnology Study, each respondent was asked if they had heard of biotechnology prior to the interview, whether they had talked to anyone else about biotechnology in the previous year, and, if so, how frequently they talked to other adults about biotechnology. To provide a summary of prior experience, their responses were combined into a five-category ordinal variable: (1) respondent had not heard of biotechnology prior to the interview, (2) respondent had heard of biotechnology, but not spoken to anyone else about it, (3) respondent had heard of biotechnology and spoken to others about it rarely, (4) respondent had heard of biotechnology and spoken to others about it occasionally, and (5) respondent had heard of biotechnology and spoken to others about it frequently.

Attentive Public for Biotechnology

A measure of the attentive public for biotechnology was created from two questions in the 1998 Biotechnology Study. First, a dichotomous measure of interest in biotechnology was created based on responses to the following questions: "We've been discussing several issues to do with modern biotechnology. Some people think these issues are very important while others don't think so. On a scale from zero to ten, where zero is not at all important and ten is extremely important, how important are these issues for you personally?" Respondents who rated their interest in biotechnology as being seven or greater were assigned a value of one on interest in biotechnology; all other respondents were assigned a value of zero.

A dichotomous measure of informedness about biotechnology was created from the following question: "Now, using the same scale, how well informed would you say you are about biotechnology, if zero means you are not at all informed about biotechnology and ten means you are very well informed about biotechnology?" Respondents who rated their level of being informed about biotechnology as seven or greater were assigned a value of one on informedness about biotechnology; all other respondents were assigned a value of zero.

Respondents with a value of one on both interest and information about biotechnology, and who also either read a newspaper on a daily basis or regularly read a newsmagazine or science magazine, were classified as being a member of the attentive public for biotechnology and assigned an ordinal value of two. Respondents with a value of one for interest in biotechnology, but who did not qualify as a member of the attentive public were classified as being a member of the interested public for biotechnology and assigned an ordinal value of one. All other respondents were classified as being in the residual public for biotechnology and were assigned an ordinal value of zero. In the structural equation models presented in Chapter 10, a dichotomous measure of attentiveness was used, with the attentive public assigned a value of one, and all other individuals assigned a value of zero.

Index of the Promise of Biotechnology

Following the general procedures discussed above (see Chapter 9), a confirmatory factor analysis was conducted on eight attitudinal questions included in the 1998 Biotechnology Study. The eight questions were a part of a battery of items that asked each respondent to assess the likelihood of various consequences of biotechnology. Each respondent was told: "Now I am going to read you a list of things that might happen within the next 20 years as a result of modern biotechnology. For each one, please say whether you think it is likely or unlikely to happen within the next 20 years." Respondents were then read a list of possible events. For purposes of the analyses presented in this book, the responses were coded so that an answer of "likely" was assigned an ordinal value of three, "not sure" an ordinal value of two, and "unlikely" an ordinal value of one. The raw data was produced as a matrix of polychoric polyserial correlations along with an asymptotic covariance matrix using PRELIS2. The matrices necessary for the confirmatory factor analysis were then estimated using the Weighted Least Squares (WLS) method in LISREL8.

Four of the items loaded on one factor, labeled the promise of biotechnology. The four items, and their factor loadings (in parentheses), are: "Substantially reducing world hunger" (.72); "Getting more out of natural resources in third World countries" (.60); "Substantially reducing environmental pollution" (.54); and "Curing most genetic diseases" (.54). A factor score was created by multiplying the standardized response by its factor weight. This score was then converted to a zero to 100 metric by assigning a score of zero for the factor score reflecting the lowest level of agreement with the dimension and a score of 100 for the factor score reflecting the highest possible level of agreement with the dimension. An ordinal measure of the promise of biotechnology was created for use in the structural equation models presented in Chapter 10: (1) scores of 0 through 20, (2) scores from 21 through 40, (3) scores from 41 through 60, (4) scores from 61 through 80, and (5) scores from 81 through 100. An ordinal score of five on this measure reflects a high belief in the promise of biotechnology, while an ordinal score of one represents a low level of belief in the promise of biotechnology.

Index of Reservations about Biotechnology

Four of the original eight items used in the factor analysis that produced the Index of the Promise of Biotechnology loaded on a factor labeled reservations about biotechnology. The four items, and their factor loadings (in parentheses), are: "Replacing most existing food products with new varieties" (.74); "Producing designer babies" (.56); "Creating dangerous new diseases" (.48); and "Reducing the range of fruits and vegetables we can get" (.40). A factor score was created by multiplying the standardized response by its factor weight. This score was then converted to a zero to 100 metric by assigning a score of zero for the factor score reflecting the lowest level of agreement with the dimension and a score of 100 for the highest possible level of agreement with the dimension. An ordinal measure of the Index of Reservations about Biotechnology was created for use in the structural equation models presented in Chapter 10: (1) scores of 0 through 20, (2) scores from 21 through 40, (3) scores from 41 through 60, (4) scores from 61 through 80, and (5) scores from 81 through 100. An ordinal score of five on this ordinal measure reflects a high level of reservations about biotechnology, while an ordinal score of one represents a low level of reservations about biotechnology.

Index of Support for Biotechnology for Medical Purposes

Using the same techniques described above, a confirmatory factor analysis was conducted on four questions included in the 1998 Biotechnology Study using LISREL8. The four questions, and their factor scores, are: "All in all, using biotechnology to introduce human genes into bacteria to produce medicines and vaccines should be encouraged. Do you definitely agree, tend to agree, tend to disagree, or definitely disagree?" (.77); "Do you support or oppose the use of biotechnology to develop new medicines to treat human disease?" (.76); "All in all, using biotechnology to introduce human genes into animals to produce organs for human transplants should be encouraged. Do you definitely agree, tend to agree, tend to disagree, or definitely disagree?" (.63); and "All in all, using genetic testing to determine whether an unborn child has a genetic predisposition for a serious disease should be encouraged. Do you definitely agree, tend to agree, tend to disagree, or definitely disagree?" (.48). The three agree/disagree items were coded so that a response of "definitely agree" was assigned a value of five, "tend to agree," a value of four, "don't know" a value of three, "tend to disagree" a value of two, and "definitely disagree" a value of one. The question regarding support or opposition of biotechnology to develop new medicines was coded so that individuals who opposed were assigned a value of one, those who were unsure a value of two, and those who supported the application a value of three.

A factor score was created by multiplying the standardized response by its factor weight. This score was then converted to a zero to 100 metric by assigning a score of zero for the factor score reflecting the lowest level of agreement with the dimension and a score of 100 for the highest possible level of agreement with the dimension. An ordinal measure of the Index of Support for Biotechnology for Medical Purposes was created for use in the structural equation models presented in Chapter 10. Scores of 0 through 20 were assigned a value of 1, scores from 21 through 40 a value of 2, scores from 41 through 60 a score of 3, scores from 61 through 80 a score of 4, and scores from 81 through 100 a score of 5. A score of five on the ordinal measure reflects a high level of support for biotechnology for medical purposes, while a score of 1 represents a low level of support.

Index of Support for Biotechnology for Agricultural Purposes

A confirmatory factor analysis was conducted in LISREL8 on three questions included in the 1998 Biotechnology Study using the same techniques described for the Index of the Promise of Biotechnology to create a measure of the Index of Support for Biotechnology for Medical Purposes. The three questions, and their factor scores, are: "Now, please tell me whether you support or oppose the use of biotechnology in agriculture and food production?" (.69); "All in all, the use of modern biotechnology in the production of food and drinks should be encouraged. Do you definitely agree, tend to agree, tend to disagree, or definitely disagree?" (.72); "All in all, using biotechnology to insert genes from one plant into a crop plant should be encouraged. Do you definitely agree, tend to agree, tend to disagree, or definitely disagree?" (.89). The agree/disagree items were coded so that a response of "Definitely agree" was assigned a value of five, "tend to agree," a value of four, "don't know" a value of three, "tend to disagree" a value of two, and "definitely disagree" a value of one. The question regarding support or opposition of biotechnology in agriculture and food production was coded so that individuals who opposed were assigned a value of one, those who were unsure a value of two, and those who supported the application a value of three.

A factor score was created by multiplying the standardized response by its factor weight. This score was then converted to a zero to 100 metric by assigning a score of zero for the factor score reflecting the lowest level of agreement with the dimension and a score of 100 for the highest possible level of agreement with the dimension. An ordinal measure of the Index of Support for Biotechnology for Agricultural Purposes was created for use in the structural equation models presented in Chapter 10. Scores of 0 through 20 were assigned a value of 1, scores from 21 through 40 a value of 2, scores from 41 through 60 a score of 3, scores from 61 through 80 a score of 4, and scores from 81 through 100 a score of 5. A score of five on the ordinal measure reflects a high level of support for biotechnology for agricultural purposes, while a score of 1 represents a low level of support.

CHAPTER 11

No new constructed variables were introduced in Chapter 11.

CHAPTER 12

No new constructed variables were introduced in Chapter 12.

C

....

ANALYTIC PROCEDURES

....

Many analyses in this book use structural equation modeling techniques. This appendix provides a description of structural equation modeling for readers interested in learning more about these methods.

AN INTRODUCTION TO STRUCTURAL EQUATION MODELING

Research in the social and behavioral sciences is concerned with two broad problems: measurement and causal relationships (Jöreskog and Sörbom, 1993):

> *The first problem is concerned with the measurement properties—validity and reliability—of the measurement instruments. The second problem concerns the causal relationships among the variables and their relative explanatory power (p. 15).*

Structural equation models combine the two broad concerns of social science research: measurement and causal relationships. Discussions on measurement are conducted separately from other stages of research (Hayduk, 1987). Speaking of LISREL, the first structural equation modeling software package, Hayduk notes that:

> *LISREL integrates measurement concerns with structural equation modeling by incorporating both latent theoretical concepts and observed or mea-*

sured indicator variables into a single structural equation model. Furthermore, knowledge of the methodological adequacy of the data gathering process and the quality of particular questionnaire items (measurement instruments) can be directly incorporated into LISREL models by specifying (fixing) a specific proportion of the variance in an indictor to be error variance (pp. 87–88).

Structural equation models have two parts: measurement and structural equation models. Measurement is used to specify "how the latent variables or hypothetical constructs are measured in terms of the observed variables, and it describes the measurement properties (validity and reliability) of the observed variables" (Jöreskog and Sörbom, 1988, p. 2). Loehlin (1987) has described the measurement portion as a variant of confirmatory factor analysis. The structural equation model "specifies the causal relationships among the latent variables and describes the causal effects and the amount of unexplained variance" (Jöreskog and Sörbom, 1988, p. 2).

A structural equation model is a set of equations that provides an estimate for a set of relationships among independent variables and one or more dependent variables. Jöreskog and Sörbom (1988) define structural equation modeling as:

[It] estimates the unknown coefficients in a set of linear structural equations. Variables in the equation system may be either directly observed variables or unmeasured latent (theoretical) variables that are not observed but relate to observed variables. The model assumes that there is a "causal" structure among a set of latent variables, and that the observed variables are indicators or symptoms of the latent variables (p. 2).

This is similar to regression analysis which provides estimates of the relationship between a series of independent variables and a dependent variable. Three situations exist in which structural equation models should be used because regression parameters do not give relevant information: when observed variables contain measurement error, when the observed variables are interdependent, and when important explanatory variables have been omitted or not included in the model. These three situations occur frequently in social and behavioral science research.

Structural equation models are a theory-driven analytical technique. The analyst develops a hypothetical model specifying the anticipated relationships between a series of constructs based on theory. The theoretical model is tested with actual data. Statistical software packages are available for structural equation modeling, including LISREL, EQS, AMOS, CALIS, and M-PLUS. Each package provides goodness-of-fit measures to determine whether the model theorized by the analyst fits the data.

If the model does not fit the data, a variety of measures may be used to modify the model to better fit the data. However, Jöreskog and Sörbom (1993) caution:

> *If the model fits the data, it does not mean that it is the "correct" model or even the "best" model. In fact, there can be many equivalent models, all of which will fit the data equally well as judged by any goodness-of-fit measure. This holds not just for a particular data set but for any data set. The direction of causation and the causal ordering of the constructs cannot be determined by the data. To conclude that the fitted model is the "best", one must be able to exclude all models equivalent to it on a logical or a substantive basis (p. 114).*

Jöreskog and Sörbom (1993) distinguish among three different model testing scenarios in structural equation modeling: strictly confirmatory, alternative or competing models, and model generating. In strict confirmatory models, the researcher develops a model on the basis of theory, tests the model with empirical data, and accepts or rejects the model on the basis of the test. In alternative or competing models, the researcher develops and tests a series of models and selects the model that best fits the data. In the most common situation—model generating, the researcher develops an initial model based on theory and tests the model with empirical data. If the model does not fit the data, the analyst modifies the model and tests it again, using the same data. The goal of model generating "may be to find a model which not only fits the data well from a statistical point of view, but also has the property that every parameter of the model can be given a substantively meaningful interpretation" (Jöreskog and Sörbom, 1993, p. 115). In the analyses conducted for this book we followed the model generating process.

The path model presented in Figure C-1 was used to predict biomedical literacy in the United States. The model has two basic background, or exogenous, factors. Each respondent's gender and age were taken as being temporally and logically prior to the person's current level of biomedical literacy. This does not imply that gender or age causes differences in one's level of biomedical literacy, but that these variables are associated with biomedical literacy. The structural equation analysis identifies the intervening variables that account for, or explain, the bivariate correlations between background variables such as gender and age and outcome measures such as biomedical literacy.

Three intervening variables—the respondent's level of formal education, their exposure to college level science courses, and their reading of the news—were placed in the model between the background variables and biomedical literacy. Such intervening variables help explain the relationships

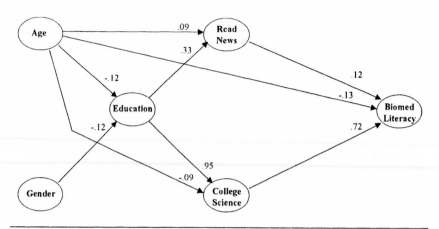

Figure C-1   A path model to predict biomedical literacy, 1999.

between background variables such as gender and age and outcome variables such as biomedical literacy.

The numbers above the arrows are the standardized beta coefficients for the paths. Standardized beta coefficients allow for comparisons of the relative effects of all of the factors in the model. All beta coefficients presented in this book are significant at the .05 level. Standardized beta coefficients range from -1.0 to $+1.0$ with values close to zero representing small paths, and values close to -1.0 or $+1.0$ representing large paths.

The arrow, on the left, from age to education indicates that age has an effect on the respondents' level of education. The number of the arrow, $-.12$, indicates the sign and size of the effect. The negative sign means that younger respondents tend to have higher levels of education than older respondents. No arrow between gender and college science courses means that once age and highest level of education are taken into account, there is no relationship between gender and college science courses.

The effects of background (or exogenous) variables and intervening variables on outcome factors such as biomedical literacy are important in structural equation models. The total effects of selected factors on various outcome variables are discussed in this book. Total effects are comprised of explained effects (sometimes called indirect effects) and residual effects (sometimes called direct effects). The total explained and residual effects of gender, age, education, reading the news, and college science courses on biomedical literacy are shown on Table C-1. Explained effects occur when intervening variables account for part, or all, of the relationship between background variables and outcome variables. Residual effects are represented by paths from any background or intervening variable to the outcome variable. Table C-1 explains the differences in these effects on biomedical literacy.

Table C-1   Explained, Residual, and Total Effects of Gender, Age, Education, College Science Courses, and Reading the News on Biomedical Literacy, 1999

| | Effects | | |
Variable	Explained (indirect)	Residual (direct)	Total
Gender (female is positive)	−.08	—	−.08
Age	−.12	−.13	−.28
Level of education	.72	—	.72
College science courses	—	.72	.72
Read news	—	.12	.12

No direct path leads from gender or education to biomedical literacy, indicating that gender and education have no significant residual, or direct, effect on biomedical literacy. An explained effect is obtained by analyzing other paths. There is a path of .33 from education to reading the news, and another path of .12 from reading the news to biomedical literacy. Similarly, there is a path of .95 from education to college science courses, and another path of .72 from college science courses to biomedical literacy. These paths indicate that reading the news and college science courses mediate, or explain, the relationship between a respondent's level of education and his level of biomedical literacy. When the path of .33 is multiplied by the path of .12 (education to reading the news to biomedical literacy) and added to the product of the paths of .95 and .72 (education to college science courses to biomedical literacy), a value of .72 is obtained, which is the value of the explained, or indirect, effect of education on biomedical literacy.

The explained, residual, and total effects of reading the news on biomedical literacy are provided in the last row of Table C-1. Because no intervening variables were included in this model between reading the news and biomedical literacy, reading the news can have no explained, or indirect, effects on biomedical literacy, and this null case is indicated by a dash.

SPECIFIC TECHNIQUES USED IN THIS BOOK

In structural equation modeling, latent constructs (such as the Promise of Science and Technology) can be measured by multiple indicators (each item from a questionnaire that might measure the Promise of Science and Technology) or by single indicators (a single Index of the Promise of Science and Technology). When multiple indicators are used, the analyst can allow the software program to calculate the reliability for each measure. All latent constructs that were included in the analyses presented in this book were measured by single indicators. Error variances were specified for each indicator based on their estimated relative reliability when compared to other indicators used in a model. The estimations of error variance used in the models ranged from a low of .01 for gender to a high of .30 for interest in health information.

Multiple measures were used to assess the fit of all of the models presented in this book. The Root Mean Square Error of Approximation (RMSEA) is a measure of discrepancy per degree of freedom. Values of .05 or less indicate a close fit. It is generally suggested that the 90 percent confidence interval for the RMSEA should be less than .08 (Jöreskog and Sörbom, 1993). Joreskog and Sorbom (1988) recommend using the χ^2 as a goodness-of-fit measure. Large χ^2 values indicate a bad fit, and small χ^2 values indicate a good fit. However, the χ^2 is extremely sensitive to large sample sizes. As a result, Joreskog and Sorbom (1988) recommend dividing the measure by the total degrees of freedom in cases of large sample size. Wheaton *et al.* (1977) recommend an χ^2 to a degree of freedom ratio of five or less, whereas Carmines and McIver (1981) suggest a more stringent ratio of two to three.

All of the structural equation models planned for this book used a large proportion of variables that were ordinal. When used to produce a simple covariance or correlation matrix, ordinal variables can result in distorted parameter estimates, incorrect χ^2 measures, and incorrect standard errors. A solution to this problem is to produce the raw data as a matrix of polychoric polyserial correlations, along with an asymptotic covariance matrix using PRESLIS2. These matrices can be estimated using the WLS method in LISREL (Jöreskog and Sörbom, 1993). At the time the analyses for this book were conducted, however, a problem had been found and announced concerning the accuracy of the asymptotic covariance matrix produced by the PRELIS software when both ordinal and interval measures were included in the same matrix. To avoid this problem and retain the use of the asymptotic covariance matrix in our computations, we followed the practice of using all dichotomous (nominal) or ordinal measures in our analyses. Interval level measures (such as the Index of the Promise of Biotechnology and the Index of Reservations about Biotechnology) were converted into ordinal variables (see Appendix B). We systematically compared the correlation matrices produced by this procedure against correlation matrices using mixtures of ordinal and interval measures of the same variables and found no significant differences between the two matrices.

ADDITIONAL INFORMATION ABOUT STRUCTURAL EQUATION MODELING

There are many excellent resources available for readers who want to obtain more detailed information about structural equation modeling. The journal *Structural Equation Modeling*, published four times a year by Lawrence Erlbaum Associates, provides numerous technical articles on structural equation modeling, as well as a review of current books in the field. The Structural Equation Modeling Discussion Network (SEMNET) is an open forum for ideas and questions about the methodology of structural equation modeling. Individuals can search the archives of SEMNET or join the list at http://bama.ua.edu/archives/semnet.html.

In addition to the above resources, there are many excellent books on structural equation modeling. For readers who want to do additional reading, we recommend the following books:

Bollen, K. A., and Long, J. S. (1993). *Testing Structural Equation Models.* Newbury Park, California: Sage.

Cudeck, R., du Toit, S., and Sörbom, D. (2001). *Structural Equation Modeling: Present and Future.* Chicago, Illinois: Scientific Software International.

Cuttance, P., and Ecob, R. (1987). *Structural Modeling by Example: Applications in Educational, Sociological, and Behavioral Research.* Cambridge: Cambridge University Press.

Hayduk, L. A. (1987). *Structural Equation Modeling with LISREL: Essentials and Advances.* Baltimore: The Johns Hopkins University Press.

Hayduk, L. A. (1996). *LISREL Issues, Debates, and Strategies.* Baltimore: The Johns Hopkins University Press.

Long, J. S. (1983). *Covariance Structure Models: An Introduction to LISREL.* Beverly Hills, California: Sage.

Schumacker, R. E., and Lomax, R. G. (1996). *A Beginner's Guide to Structural Equation Modeling.* Mahwah, New Jersey: Lawerence Erlbaum Associates.

REFERENCES

Aaronson, L. S., Mural, C. M., and Pfoutz, S. K. (1988). Seeking Information: Where do pregnant women look? *Health Education Quarterly, 15*(3), 335–345.

Akatsu, H., and Kuffner, J. (1998). Medicine and the Internet. *Western Journal of Medicine, 169,* 311–317.

Almond, G. A. (1950). *The American People and Foreign Policy.* New York: Harcourt, Brace and Company.

Anderson, N. H. (1971). *Integration theory and attitude change. Psychological Review, 78,* 171–206.

Atkin, C., and Arkin, E. (1990). Issues and initiatives in communicating health information to the public. In C. Atkin and L. Wallack (Eds.), *Mass Communication and Public Health Complexities and Conflicts.* Newsbury Park, California: Sage.

Atkin, C., and Wallack, L. (1990). *Mass Communication and Public Health: Complexities and Conflicts.* Newsbury Park, California: Sage.

Bailey, M. (1994, April 14–16). *Women and Support for the Animal Rights Movement, 1948– 1985.* Paper presented at the 1994 meeting of the Midwest Political Science Association, Chicago, Illinois.

Backer, T. E., Rogers, E. M., and Sopory, P. (1992). *Designing Health Communications Campaigns: What Works?* Thousand Oaks, California: Sage.

Baker, L. M., Wilson, F. L., and Kars, M. (1997). The readability of medical information on Info-Trac: Does it meet the needs of people with low literacy skills? *Reference & User Services Quarterly, 37,* 155–160.

Beaton, A. E., Martin, M. O., Mullis, I. V. S., Gonzalez, E. J., Smith, T. A., and Kelly, D. L. (1996a). *Science Achievement in the Middle School Years: IEA's Third International Mathematics and Science Study.* Boston: Center for the Study of Testing, Evaluation, and Educational Policy, Boston College.

Beaton, A. E., Mullis, I. V. S., Martin, M. O., Gonzalez, E. J., Kelly, D. L., and Smith, T. A. (1996b). *Mathematics Achievement in the Middle School Years: IEA's Third International Mathematics and Science Study.* Boston: Center for the Study of Testing, Evaluation, and Educational Policy, Boston College.

Beck, P. A., and Jennings, M. K. (1991). Family traditions, political periods, and the development of partisan orientations. *The Journal of Politics, 53,* 742–763.

Becker, H. K., Agopian, M. W., and Yeh, S. (1992). Impact evaluation of Drug Abuse Resistance Education (DARE). *Journal of Drug Education, 22,* 283–291.

Bimber, B. (1998). Toward an empirical map of political participation on the Internet. Paper presented at the 1998 Annual meeting of the American Political Science Association, Boston, September 3–6.

Bock, R. D., and Aitkin, M. (1981). Marginal maximum likelihood estimation of item parameters: Application of an EM algorithm. *Psychometrika, 46,* 443–459.

Bock, R. D., and Zimowski, F. M. (1997). Multiple-Group IRT. In W. J. van der Linden and R. K. Hableton (Eds.), *Handbook of Modern Item–Response Theory.* New York: Springer-Verlag.

Bowd, A. D., and Bowd, A. C. (1989). Attitudes toward the treatment of animals: A study of Christian groups in Australia. *Anthrozoos, 3*(1), 20–24.

Brockopp, D. Y., Hayko, D., Davenport, W., and Winscott, C. (1989). Personal control and the need for hope and information among adults diagnosed with cancer. *Cancer Nursing, 12,* 112–116.

Broida, J., Tingley, L., Kimball, R., and Miele, J. (1993). Personality differences between pro- and antivivisectionists. *Society and Animals, 1,* 129–144.

Buchanan, J. M., and Tullock, G. (1962). *The Calculus of Consent.* Ann Arbor: University of Michigan Press.

Bunn, M. D. (1993). Consumer perceptions of medical information sources: An application of multidimensional scaling. *Health Marketing Quarterly, 10*(3–4), 83–104.

Cangelosi, J. D., and Markham, F. S. (1994). A descriptive study of personal, institutional, and media sources of preventive health care information. *Health Marketing Quarterly, 12,* 23–36.

Carmines, E. G., and Stimson, J. A. (1981). Issue evolution, population replacement, and normal partisan change. *The American Political Science Review, 75,* 107–118.

Carmines, E. G., McIver, J. P., and Stimson, J. A. (1987). Unrealized partisanship: A theory of dealignment. *The Journal of Politics, 49,* 376–400.

Chi-Lum, B. (1999). Friend or foe? Consumers using the Internet for medical information. *Journal of Medical Practice Management, 14,* 196–198.

Coelho, P. C. (1998). The Internet: Increasing information, decreasing certainty. *Journal of the American Medical Association, 280,* 1454.

Connell, C. M., and Crawford, C. O. (1988). How people obtain their health information: A survey on two Pennsylvania counties. *Public Health Reports, 103,* 196–198.

Davey, G. C., Tallis, F., and Hodgson, S. (1993). The relationship between information-seeking and information-avoiding coping styles and the reporting of psychological and physical symptoms. *Journal of Psychosomatic Research, 37*(4), 333–334.

Davis, R. (1999). *The Web of Politics: The Internet's Impact on the American Political System.* New York: Oxford University Press.

Davis, J. A., and Smith, T. W. (Annual Series). *General Social Surveys, Cumulative Codebook.* Chicago: University of Chicago, National Opinion Research Center.

Deering, M. J. (1998). Health communication and health policy. In L. D. Jackson and B. K. Duffy (Eds.), *Health Communication Research: A Guide to Developments and Directions* (pp. 125–137). Westport, Connecticut: Greenwood Press.

Donohew, R. L., Nair, M., and Finn, S. (1984). Automacity, arousal, and information exposure. In R. N. Bostrom (Ed.), *Communication Yearbook 8* (pp. 267–284). Beverly Hills, California: Sage.

Donohue, G. A., Tichenor, P. J., and Olien, C. N. (1975). Mass media and the knowledge gap. *Communications Research, 2,* 3–23.

Donohue, G. A., Olien, C. N., and Tichenor, P. J. (1987). Media access and knowledge gaps. *Critical Studies in Mass Communications,* 87–92.

Downs, A. (1957). *An Economic Theory of Democracy.* New York: Harper and Row.

Friedman, S. M., Dunwoody, S., and Rogers, C. L. (1999). *Communicating Uncertainty: Media Coverage of New and Controversial Science.* Mahwah, New Jersey: Lawrence Erlbaum.

Gallagher, S. M. (1999). Rethinking access in an information age. *Ostomy Wound Management, 45,* 12–14,16.

Gallup, G. G. J., and Beckstead, J. W. (1988). Attitudes toward animal research. *American Psychologist, 43,* 474–476.

Galvin, S. L., and Herzog, H. A. (1992). The ethical judgment of animal research. *Ethics and Behavior, 2,* 263–286.

Hayduk, L. A. (1987). *Structural Equation Modeling with LISREL.* Baltimore: The Johns Hopkins University Press.

Heath, R. L., and Bryant, J. (2000). *Human Communication Theory and Research: Concepts, Contexts, and Challenges.* Mahwah, New Jersey: Lawrence Erlbaum.

Hennessy, B. C. (1972). A head note on the existence and study of political attitudes. In D. D. Nimmo and C. M. Bonjean (Eds.), *Political attitudes and public opinion.* New York: McKay.

Herzog, H. A., Betchart, N. S., and Pittman, R. B. (1991). Gender, sex role orientation, and attitudes toward animals. *Anthrozoos, 4,* 184–191.

Hibbard, J. H., and Pope, C. R. (1987). Women's roles, interest in health and health behavior. *Women and Health, 12,* 67–84.

Hickey, T., Rakowski, W., and Julius, M. (1988). Preventive health practices among older men and women. *Research on Aging, 10,* 315–328.

Hovland, C. I., and Weiss, W. (1951). The influence of source credibility on communication effectiveness. *Public Opinion Quarterly, 15,* 633–350.

Impicciatore, P., Pandolfini, C., Castella, N., and Bonati, M. (1997). Reliability of health information for the public on the world wide web: Systematic survey of advice on managing fever in children at home. *British Medical Journal, 314,* 1875–1880.

Jackson, L. D., and Duffy, B. K. (1998). *Health Communication Research: A Guide to Developments and Directions.* Westport, Connecticut: Greenwood Press.

Jacoby, W.G. (1994). Public attitudes toward government spending. *American Journal of Political Science, 38,* 336–361.

Jadad, A. R., and Gagliardi, A. (1998). Rating health information on the Internet: Navigating to knowledge or to Babel? *Journal of the American Medical Association, 279,* 611–614.

Jasper, J. M., and Nelkin, D. (1992). *Animal Rights Crusade.* New York: The Free Press.

Johnson, J. D., (1997). *Cancer-Related Information Seeking.* Cresskill, New Jersey: Hampton Press.

Johnson, J. D., and Meischke, H. (1994). Women's preferences for cancer-related information from specific types of mass media. *Health Care for Women International, 15,* 23–30.

Jöreskog, K., and Sörbom, D. (1988). *LISREL 7: A Guide to the Program and Applications.* Chicago, Illinois: SPSS Inc.

Jöreskog, K., and Sörbom, D. (1993). *Lisrel 8.* Chicago: Scientific Software International.

Katz, E. (1980). On conceptualizing media effects. In T. McCormack (Ed.), *Studies in Communications, Vol. I* (pp. 119–141). Greenwich, Connecticut: JAI Press.

Katz, E., and Lazarsfeld, P. F. (1955). *Personal Influence: The Part Played by People in the Flow of Mass Communications.* Glencoe: Free Press.

Kellert, S. R., and Berry, J. K. (1987). Attitudes, knowledge, and behaviors toward wildlife as affected by gender. *Wildlife Society Bulletin, 15,* 363–371.

Kim, J.-O., and Mueller, C. W. (1978). *Introduction to Factor Analysis: What It is and How to Do It.* Beverly Hills, California: Sage.

Kingdon, J. W. (1984). *Agendas, Alternatives, and Public Policies.* Boston: Little, Brown and Company.

Klapper, J. T. (1960). *The Effects of Mass Communication.* New York: Free Press.

Kreps, G. L., Bonaguro, E. W., and Query, J. L. (1998). The history and development of the field of health communication. In L. D. Jackson and B. K. Duffy (Eds.), *Health Communication Research: A Guide to Developments and Directions* (pp. 1–15). Westport, Connecticut: Greenwood Press.

Kreps, G. L., O'Hair, D., and Clowers, M. (1994). The influences of human communication on health outcomes. *The American Behavioral Scientist, 38,* 248.

Kreps, G. L., and Thornton, B. C. (1992). *Health Communication: Theory and Practice.* Prospect Heights, Illinois: Waveland Press.

Kubey, R., and Csikszentmihalyi, M. (1990). *Television and the Quality of Life: How Viewing Shapes Everyday Experience.* Hillsdale, New Jersey: Lawrence Erlbaum.

Lau, R. R., and Sears, D. O. (1986). *Political Cognition.* Hillsdale: Lawrence Erlbaum.

Lenz, E. R. (1984). Information seeking: A component of client decisions and health behavior. *Advances in Nursing Science, April,* 59–72.

Loehlin, J. C. (1987). *Latent Variable Models.* Hillsdale: Lawrence Erlbaum Associates.

Long, J. S. (1983). *Confirmatory Factor Analysis.* Beverly Hills, California: Sage.

Lynam, D. R., Milich, R., Zimmerman, R., Novak, S. P., Logan, T. K., Martin, C., Leukefeld, C., and Clayton, R. (1999). Project DARE: No effects at 10-year follow-up. *Journal of Consulting Clinical Psychology, 67,* 590–593.

Maibach, E., and Parrott, R. L. (1995). *Designing Health Messages: Approaches from Communication Theory and Public Health Practice.* Thousand Oaks, California: Sage.

Marwick, C. (2000). Ensuring ethical Internet information. *Journal of the American Medical Association, 283,* 1667.

McCallum, D. B., Hammond, S. L., and Covello, V. T. (1991). Communicating about environmental risks: How the public uses and perceives information sources. *Health Education Quarterly, 18,* 349–361.

McGinnies, E., and Ward, C. D. (1974). Persuadability as a function of source credibility and locus of control. *Journal of Personality, 42,* 360–371.

McQuail, D., and Windahl, S. (1993). *Communication Models for the Study of Mass Communication.* Second Edition. London: Longman.

Meissner, H. I., Potosky, A. L., and Convissor, R. (1992). How sources of health information relate to knowledge and use of cancer screening exams. *Journal of Community Health, 17,* 153–165.

Milburn, M. A. (1991). *Persuasion and Politics: The Social Psychology of Public Opinion.* Pacific Grove, California: Brooks/Cole.

Mileti, D. S., and Fitzpatrick, C. (1993). *The Great Earthquake Experiment: Risk Communication and Public Action.* Boulder: Westview Press.

Miller, J. D. (1983a). Scientific Literacy: A conceptual and empirical review. *Daedalus, 112*(2), 29–48.

Miller, J. D. (1983b). *The American People and Science Policy.* New York: Pergamon Press.

Miller, J. D. (1987a). Scientific literacy in the United States. In D. Evered and M. O'Connor (Eds.), *Communicating Science to the Public.* London: Wiley.

Miller, J. D. (1987b). The Challenger accident and public opinion: Attitudes toward the space programme in the USA. *Space Policy, 3,* 122–140.

Miller, J. D. (1989, January). *Scientific Literacy.* Paper presented at the 1989 annual meeting of the American Association for the Advancement of Science, San Francisco, California.

Miller, J. D. (1995). Scientific literacy for effective citizenship. In R. E. Yager (Ed.), *Science/Technology/Society as Reform in Science Education.* New York: State University of New York Press.

Miller, J. D. (1998). The measurement of civic scientific literacy. *Public Understanding of Science, 7,* 203–223.

Miller, J. D. (2001). *Public Perceptions of Biotechnology.* Cresskill, New Jersey: Hampton Press.

Miller, J. D., Kimmel, L., and Smith, T. (1999). *The causes and Treatment of Selected Diseases.* Final Report to the Office of Behavioral and Social Science (OBSSR) in the Office of the Director of NIH. Chicago, Illinois: Chicago Academy of Sciences.

Miller, J. D., and Pardo, R. (2000). Civic Scientific Literacy and Attitude to Science and Technology: A comparative analysis of the European Union, the United States, Japan, and Canada. In M. Dierkes and C. von Grote (Eds.), *Between Understanding and Trust: The Public, Science and Technology* (pp. 81–129). Amsterdam: Harwood Academic Publishers.

Miller, J. D., Pardo, R., and Niwa, F. (1997). *Public Perceptions of Science and Technology: A Comparative Study of the European Union, the United States, Japan and Canada.* Madrid: BBV Foundation Press.

Miller, J. D., and Pifer, L. K. (1995). *The Public Understanding of Biomedical Science in the United States.* Final Report to the Office of National Institutes of Health. Chicago, Illinois: Chicago Academy of Sciences.

Minsky, M. (1986). *The Society of Mind.* New York: Simon and Schuster.

Mullis, I. V. S., Martin, M. O., Beaton, A. E., Gonzalez, E. J., Kelly, D. L., and Smith, T. A. (1998). *Mathematics and Science Achievement in the Final Year of Secondary School.* Boston: Center for the Study of Testing, Evaluation, and Educational Policy, Boston College.

National Research Council (1996). *National Science Education Standards.* Washington, D.C.: National Academy Press.

National Science Board (NSB) (1981). *Science and Engineering Indicators—1980.* Washington, D.C.: U.S. Government Printing Office.

National Science Board (NSB) (1983). *Science and Engineering Indicators—1982.* Washington, D.C.: U.S. Government Printing Office.

National Science Board (NSB) (1985). *Science and Engineering Indicators—1985.* Washington, D.C.: U.S. Government Printing Office.

National Science Board (NSB) (1987). *Science and Engineering Indicators—1987.* Washington, D.C.: U.S. Government Printing Office.

National Science Board (NSB) (1989). *Science and Engineering Indicators—1989.* Washington, D.C.: U.S. Government Printing Office.

National Science Board (NSB) (1991). *Science and Engineering Indicators—1991.* Washington, D.C.: U.S. Government Printing Office.

National Science Board (NSB) (1993). *Science and Engineering Indicators—1993.* Washington, D.C.: U.S. Government Printing Office.

National Science Board (NSB) (1996). *Science and Engineering Indicators—1996.* Washington, D.C.: U.S. Government Printing Office.

National Science Board (NSB) (1998). *Science and Engineering Indicators—1998.* Washington, D.C.: U.S. Government Printing Office.

National Science Board (NSB) (2000). Science and Engineering Indicators—2000. Washington, D.C.: U.S. Government Printing Office.

Nibert, D. A. (1994). Animal rights and human social issues. *Society and Animals, 2*(2), 115–124.

Nicholson, J. (1999). NAA survey finds many online users read a daily newspaper. *Editor and Publisher* (132), 34–35.

Page, B. I., Shapiro, R. Y., and Dempsey, G. R. (1984). *Television News and Changes in Americans' Policy Preferences.* Paper presented at the Annual Meeting of the Midwest Political Science Association, Chicago, Illinois.

Parrott, R. L. (1995). Motivation to attend to health messages. In E. Mailbach & R. L. Parrott (Eds.), *Designing Health Messages: Approaches from Communication Theory and Public Health Process* (pp. 7–23). Thousand Oaks, California: Sage.

Paulos, J. A. (1988). *Innumeracy: Mathematical Illiteracy and Its Consequences* (First Edition ed.). New York: Hill and Wang.

Petrocik, J. R. (1987). Realignment: New party coalitions and the nationalization of the south. *The Journal of Politics, 49*, 347–375.

Pick, H. L., van den Broek, P., and Knill, D. C. (1992). *Cognition: Conceptual and Methodological Issues.* Washington: American Psychological Association.

Pifer, K. L. (1994). Adolescents and animal rights: Stable attitudes or ephemeral opinions. *Public Understanding of Science, 3*, 291–307.

Pifer, K. L. (1996). Exploring the gender gap in young adults' attitudes about animal research. *Society and Animals, 4*, 37–52.

Plous, S. (1991). An attitude survey of animal rights activists. *Psychological Science, 2*, 194–196.

Rakowski, W., Assaf, A. R., Lefebvre, R. C., Lasater, T. M., Niknian, M., and Carleton, R. A. (1990). Information-seeking about health in a community sample of adults: Correlates and associations with other health-related practices. *Health Education Quarterly, 17*, 379–393.

Ratzan (1993).

Rensberger, B. (1996). *Life Itself: Exploring the Realm of the Living Cell.* New York: Oxford University Press.

Robinson, J. P., and Levy, M. R. (1996). News media use and the informed public: A 1990s update. *Journal of Communications, 46*, 129–135.

Rogers, E. M. (1986). *Communication Technology: The New Media in Society.* New York: The Free Press.

Rosenau, J. (1961). *Public Opinion and Foreign Policy: An Operational Formulation.* New York: Random House.

Rosenau, J. (1963). *National Leadership and Foreign Policy: The Mobilization of Public Support.* Princeton: Princeton University Press.

Rosenau, J. (1974). *Citizenship between Elections.* New York: Free Press.

Rutherford, F. J., and Ahlgren, A. (1990). *Science for All Americans.* New York: Oxford University Press.

Salmon, C. T. (1989). *Information Campaigns: Balancing Social Values and Social Change.* Newbury Park, California: Sage.

Schank, R. (1977). *Scripts, Plans, Goals, and Understanding.* Hillsdale: Lawrence Erlbaum.

Schmidt, W. H., McKnight, C. C., Jakwerth, P. M., Cogan, L. S., Raizen, S. A., Houang, R. T., Valverde, G. A., Wiley, D. E., Wolfe, R. G., Bianchi, L. J., Yang, W.-L., Kang, S.-H., and Britton, E. D. (1998). *Facing the Consequences: Using TIMSS for a Closer Look at United States Mathematics and Science Education.* Dordrecht/Boston/London: Kluwer Academic Publishers.

Schramm, W., and Wade, S. (1967). *Knowledge and the Public Mind. A Preliminary Study of the Distribution and Sources of Science, Health, and Public Affairs Knowledge in the American Public. A report to the Office of Education (DHEW), Washington, D.C.* Stanford, CA: Stanford University Institute for Communication Research.

Schumacker, R. E., and Lomax, R. G. (1996). *A Beginner's Guide to Structural Equation Modeling.* Mahwah, New Jersey: Lawrence Erlbaum Associates.

Severin, W. J., and Tankard, J. W. (1992). *Communication Theories: Origins, Methods, and Uses in the Mass Media.* White Plains, New York: Longmans.

Silberg, W. M., Lundberg, G. D., and Musacchio, R. A. (1997). Assessing, controlling, and assuring the quality of medical information on the Internet. *Journal of the American Medical Association, 277*, 1244–1245.

Stanley, H. W. (1988). Southern partisan changes: Dealignment, realignment or both? *The Journal of Politics, 50*, 64–88.

Sternberg, R. J. (1988a). *The Nature of Creativity: Contemporary Psychological Perspectives.* Cambridge: Cambridge Univ. Press.

Sternberg, R. J. (1988b). *The Triarchic Mind: A New Theory of Human Intelligence.* New York, New York: Viking.

Sternberg, R. J. (1999). *The Nature of Cognition.* Cambridge, Massachusetts: MIT Press.

Sternberg, R. J., Forsythe, G. B., and Hedlund, J. (2000). *Practical Intelligence in Everyday Life.* Cambridge, UK: Cambridge Univ. Press.

Turk-Charles, S., Meyerowitz, B. E., and Gatz, M. (1997). Age differences in information-seeking among cancer patients. *International Journal of Aging and Human Development, 45,* 85–98.

U.S. Department of Commerce (1999). *Falling through the Net: Defining the Digital Divide.*

Wheaton, B., Muthén, B., Alwin, D., and Summers, G. (1977). Assessing reliability and stability in panel models. In D. R. Heise (Ed.), *Sociological Methodology 1977.* San Francisco: Jossey-Bass.

Worsley, A. (1989). Perceived reliability of sources of health information. *Health Education Research, 4,* 367–376.

Zimowski, F. M., Muraki, E., Mislevy, J. R., and Bock, R. D. (1996). *Bilog-MG: Multiple-Group IRT Analysis and Test Maintenance for Binary Items.* Chicago, Illinois: Scientific Software International.

SUBJECT INDEX

A

Acceptance rates
for biomedical communications to consumers, 163–164, 166–167, 168
for biomedical policy communications, 276–277, 281–282, 283
Adult literacy and numeracy, 296–297
Adult panel studies, 307–308
Adults with children at home
biomedical communication with, 129–133
biomedical literacy, 34–36
defining as audience for health information, 148
interest in health information, 54–55, 56–57, 61–62
media use patterns, 89, 90t, 91f
retention and recall of health information, 129–130, 132
science television viewing, 73
African-Americans, 13
attentiveness to biomedical research, 189, 190
biomedical literacy, 31, 32f, 33
health information sources used by, 125, 129, 136
informal adult education and, 62
interest in health information, 60–61, 62
retention and recall of health information, 110–111
Age, *see also* Older adults; Young adults
attentiveness to biomedical research and, 181, 184, 186, 187, 188–189

attentiveness to biotechnology and, 239
attitudes toward animal research and, 230, 232
biomedical literacy and, 31, 33, 37
computer and Internet use and, 81, 84
educational attainment and, 29–30
health newsletter subscription and, 81
interest in health information and, 55, 57–58, 60
newspaper reading and, 77
radio listening and, 75–76
rating of seriousness of specific diseases and, 63, 65t
reservations about science and technology and, 219
retention and recall of health information and, 104–105, 107
science television viewing and, 73
support for basic research spending and, 221–222
Agricultural biotechnology
attitudes toward, 250–256
implications for biomedical communications, 258
summary measure of acceptability, 251–252
AIDS, 63
Alcoholism
health information sources, 148
additional, 121, 122
primary, 118–121
used by men and women, 141–143

443

Printed in the United States
56001LVS00003B/10-36